Executive Function and Dysfunction

Identification, Assessment and Treatment

Executive Function and Dysfunction

Identification, Assessment and Treatment

Scott J. Hunter
Pritzker School of Medicine, University of Chicago, Chicago, IL, USA

Elizabeth P. Sparrow
Sparrow Neuropsychology, Raleigh, NC, USA

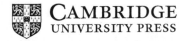

CAMBRIDGE UNIVERSITY PRESS
Cambridge, New York, Melbourne, Madrid, Cape Town,
Singapore, São Paulo, Delhi, Mexico City

Cambridge University Press
The Edinburgh Building, Cambridge CB2 8RU, UK

Published in the United States of America
by Cambridge University Press, New York

www.cambridge.org
Information on this title: www.cambridge.org/9780521889766

First published 2012

Printed and bound in the United Kingdom by the MPG Books Group

A catalog record for this publication is available from the British Library

Library of Congress Cataloging-in-Publication Data

Executive function and dysfunction : identification, assessment, and
treatment / [edited by] Scott J. Hunter, Elizabeth P. Sparrow.
    p.   cm.
Includes index.
ISBN 978-0-521-88976-6 (Hardback)
1. Clinical neuropsychology.   2. Developmental psychobiology.
3. Executive function.   I. Hunter, Scott J.   II. Sparrow, Elizabeth P.
QP360.E936 2012
616.8–dc23
                                                                 2012008940

ISBN 978-0-5218-8976-6 Hardback

Contents

Section III – Applications

Editor biographies

Scott J. Hunter obtained his PhD in Clinical and Developmental Psychology from the University of Illinois at Chicago, and completed a postdoctoral residency in Pediatric Neuropsychology and Developmental Disabilities at the University of Rochester. He is Associate Professor of Psychiatry and Behavioral Neuroscience, and Pediatrics, and Director of Neuropsychology at the University of Chicago. He serves on the editorial board of the journal *Behavioral Sciences* and is a reviewer for a number of additional peer-reviewed professional journals. Dr. Hunter's primary research concerns the identification of trajectories of attention and executive function development in youth with neurodevelopmental disorders and medical illness (epilepsy, cancer, neurofibromatosis, HIV/AIDS), and the impact of sociocultural and environmental risk factors (e.g., homelessness) on executive and regulatory development. He is co-editor, with Jacobus Donders, PhD, of *Pediatric Neuropsychological Intervention* (2007) and *Principles and Practice of Lifespan Developmental Neuropsychology* (2010), both published by Cambridge University Press.

Elizabeth P. Sparrow obtained her PhD in Clinical Psychology with a specialization in Neuropsychology from Washington University in St. Louis. She completed a postdoctoral residency in Pediatric Neuropsychology at Johns Hopkins School of Medicine/Kennedy Krieger Institute. She is Director of Sparrow Neuropsychology in Raleigh, NC and Neuropsychology Consultant for the North Carolina State University Psychoeducational Clinic. She serves on the editorial board of the *Journal of Attention Disorders* and is a guest reviewer for other peer-reviewed professional journals. Dr. Sparrow's research focuses on assessment and intervention for children, adolescents, and young adults who present with executive deficits. She is a co-author of the Conners' Adult ADHD Rating Scale and served as the clinical consultant for development of the Conners 3rd Edn, the Conners Comprehensive Behavior Rating Scales, and the Conners Early Childhood. Her first book, *The Essentials of Conners Behavior Assessments*, was published in 2010. She co-authored the *Guide to Assessment Scales in Attention-Deficit/Hyperactivity Disorder, 2nd Edn*. She has contributed chapters to several volumes, presented at numerous conferences, and co-authored publications in peer-reviewed journals. In her clinical work, she helps other professionals and parents better understand their children who have executive dysfunction.

Contributors

Laura Gutermuth Anthony, PhD
Division of Pediatric Neuropsychology,
Children's National Medical Center,
Department of Psychiatry & Behavioral
Sciences, George Washington University
Medical School, USA

Laura A. Barquero, MS
Department of Special Education, Peabody
College, Vanderbilt University, USA

Sabrina L. Benedict, BA
Department of Special Education,
Peabody College, Vanderbilt University,
USA

Laurie E. Cutting, PhD
Departments of Education & Human
Development, Radiology, and Pediatrics,
Vanderbilt University, Department of
Neurology, Johns Hopkins University
School of Medicine, USA

Jennifer P. Edidin, PhD
Department of Psychiatry & Behavioral
Neuroscience, University of Chicago, USA

Lev Gottlieb, MA
Division of Clinical Psychology,
Department of Psychiatry & Behavioral
Sciences, Feinberg School of Medicine,
Northwestern University, USA

Marsha Nortz Gragert, PhD
ABPP-Cn, Section of Psychology,
Department of Pediatrics,
Texas Children's Hospital,
Baylor College of Medicine, USA

Heather C. Harris, BS
Education and Brain Sciences Research
Laboratory, Vanderbilt University, USA

Emily J. Helder, PhD
Department of Psychology,
Calvin College, USA

Clayton D. Hinkle, MS
Institute of Psychology, Illinois Institute
of Technology, USA

Scott J. Hunter, PhD
Department of Psychiatry & Behavioral
Neuroscience, University of Chicago, USA

Lisa A. Jacobson, PhD
NCSP, Department of Neuropsychology,
Kennedy Krieger Institute, Department of
Psychiatry & Behavioral Sciences,
Johns Hopkins University School of
Medicine, USA

Kelly Janke, MA
Department of Psychology, University of
Wisconsin-Milwaukee, USA

Lisa S. Kahalley, PhD
Section of Psychology, Department of
Pediatrics, Texas Children's Hospital,
Baylor College of Medicine, USA

Niranjan S. Karnik, MD, PhD
Department of Psychiatry & Behavioral
Neuroscience, University of Chicago, USA

Jill Kelderman, PhD, ABPP
The Center for Pediatric Neuropsychology,
LLC, Palm Beach Gardens, FL, USA

Laura E. Kenealy, PhD
Division of Pediatric Neuropsychology,
Children's National Medical Center,
Departments of Pediatrics and Psychiatry &
Behavioral Sciences, George Washington
University Medical School, USA

Lauren Kenworthy, PhD
Division of Pediatric Neuropsychology,
Children's National Medical Center,
Departments of Pediatrics, Neurology, and
Psychiatry & Behavioral Sciences,
George Washington University Medical
School, USA

Bonnie Klein-Tasman, PhD
Department of Psychology,
University of Wisconsin-Milwaukee, USA

Megan Kramer, PhD
Department of Neuropsychology,
Kennedy Krieger Institute, Department of
Psychiatry & Behavioral Sciences,
Johns Hopkins University School of
Medicine, USA

Tory L. Larsen, BA
Division of Pediatric, Adolescent, and
Maternal HIV Infection Children's
Memorial Hospital Calvin College, USA

Esther R. Lindström, BA
Department of Special Education,
Peabody College, Vanderbilt University,
USA

Gianna Locascio, PsyD
Department of Neuropsychology,
Kennedy Krieger Institute, USA

E. Mark Mahone, PhD, ABPP
Department of Neuropsychology,
Kennedy Krieger Institute, Department
of Psychiatry & Behavioral Sciences,
Johns Hopkins University School of
Medicine, USA

Sharon Nichols, PhD
Neuroscience and Clinical Psychology
Programs, University of California
San Diego, USA

Iris Paltin, PhD
Division of Pediatric Neuropsychology,
Children's National Medical Center, USA

Cynthia Salorio, PhD
Departments of Pediatric Rehabilitation
and Neuropsychology, Kennedy Krieger
Institute, Departments of Physical
Medicine & Rehabilitation and Psychiatry
& Behavioral Sciences, Johns Hopkins
University School of Medicine, USA

Jillian M. Schuh, PhD
Section of Neuropsychology,
Department of Neurology,
Medical College of Wisconsin, USA

Beth Slomine, PhD, ABPP
Department of Neuropsychology,
Kennedy Krieger Institute,
Departments of Psychiatry & Behavioral
Sciences and Physical Medicine &
Rehabilitation, Johns Hopkins University
School of Medicine, USA

Elizabeth P. Sparrow, PhD
Sparrow Neuropsychology, PA,
Raleigh, NC, USA

Lindsay M. Wilson, MEd
Department of Special Education,
Peabody College, Vanderbilt University,
USA

Benjamin E. Yerys, PhD
Center for Autism Research,
Children's Hospital of Philadelphia,
USA

Frank A. Zelko, PhD
Department of Psychiatry and Behavioral
Sciences, Children's Memorial Hospital,
Feinberg School of Medicine,
Northwestern University, USA

Preface

Executive functioning (EF) is a complex construct with many facets, served by an intricate neurobiologic network that develops over the course of childhood, adolescence, and early adulthood. The behavioral manifestations of EF and executive dysfunction (EdF) go through periods of rapid growth during this same time. This book reviews the research literature on the development and neurobiology of EF. Conceptual assessment issues are discussed, with a focus on key elements of identifying EF/EdF in specific clinical conditions such as Disruptive Behavior Disorders (DBD), autism spectrum disorders (ASDs), learning disorders (LD), mood and anxiety disorders, seizure disorders, and human immunodeficiency virus (HIV), among others, including test performance, neuro-imaging, and clinical presentation. Several chapters are devoted to practical aspects of EdF, including research-based treatment strategies, educational implications, forensic cautions, and intervention resources.

The text is divided into three sections. Section I provides a foundation by reviewing models of EF, neuropsychological and neurobiological development, and key assessment considerations. Section II presents critical information on how EF deficits present in pediatric neurodevelopmental and acquired disorders. The book closes with a section addressing applications of the research, including remediation and educational implications of EF deficits, cautions for forensic neuropsychologists, and reflections on the volume as a whole.

This book is essential reading for medical, psychological, and educational professionals who work with children and adolescents in clinical and educational settings.

Acknowledgments

I would like to first acknowledge the trainees and colleagues who have collaborated with me, over the past 13 years, in an exploration of the ideas being presented in this volume, as part of the Pediatric Clinical Neurosciences Seminar at the University of Chicago. It is through this yearly course that I have been challenged to think deeply and critically about executive functioning, and to consider the trajectories of its development. I also thank my partner Richard Renfro, fellow child psychologist and behind-the-scenes supporter, for listening to and encouraging my efforts with this book. Finally, I deeply thank Elizabeth Sparrow, for agreeing to take the journey of writing and editing this book with me.

I dedicate this book to my patients and their families, for their trust and continued encouragement to better understand executive functioning and its variabilities.

Scott J. Hunter, PhD, 2012

I would like to thank and acknowledge my mentors. Each of them taught me to recognize and appreciate executive functioning in educational, clinical, and research settings, and to consider executive deficits whether tutoring, assessing, or conducting therapy. Thanks also to the children, adolescents, and young adults (and their families) with whom I have worked – your stories and successes have driven me to continue in this field. My valued colleagues and friends have provided much needed support to complete this volume. I very much appreciate the students and trainees who ask excellent questions, inspiring me to find better ways to explain these concepts. Finally, thank you to Scott Hunter for inviting me to share in this project.

I dedicate this volume to my family, who encouraged me to pursue this endeavor, especially my 91-year-old grandmother whose executive functions are still phenomenal.

Elizabeth P. Sparrow, PhD, 2012

Introduction

Elizabeth P. Sparrow and Scott J. Hunter

Executive functioning (EF) is a cognitive capacity that is difficult to define succinctly. Most explanations of EF reflect some degree of self-regulation as applied to cognition, emotion, behavior, adaptive functioning, and even moral reasoning and choice. In line with this, multiple models have been proposed to account for and explain the range of capacities and acts that represent EF, although the predominant models are adult-centric, and as a result, less applicable to thinking about EF developmentally. It is difficult to ignore the fact that nearly every neuropsychological evaluation in the clinical setting reveals and then attempts to address some aspect of executive dysfunction (EdF). EF deficits have a significant impact in multiple domains of a person's life and the lives of others around them, including parents, teachers, siblings, and peers. The pervasive and at times quite impairing nature of EdF calls for attention and emphasis from researchers and clinicians alike.

With this volume, the reader will find that we promote a model that emphasizes the plurality of executive *functions*, as opposed to a model that views EF as a singular (albeit still dynamic) cognitive capacity. Clinical and empirical data provide examples of dissociability within EF, at both the level of neural organization and skill demonstration. We also find that EF is best represented as a spectrum, such that too much or too little of a particular EF skill can represent EdF. For example, poorly controlled emotion and behavior are EF deficits in the Disruptive Behavior Disorders (Chapter 5), and overly controlled emotion and behavior are EF deficits in the Anxiety Disorders (Chapter 10). Even when none of the EF skills assessed show a significant deficit, the cumulative effect of multiple EF deficits can result in severe impairment (i.e., the whole is greater than the sum of the parts).[1] We address this directly in Chapters 2 and 4, in particular.

With this volume, we argue that it is important to examine the differences that exist for children and adolescents in EF and EdF, specifically between the occasional lapses into executive weakness that all people experience and "true EdF" that is persistent, pervasive, and severely impairing. We emphasize that it is important to recognize the range of factors that impact and moderate EF, including stable factors such as age, gender, ethnicity, personality, and genes, and more variable factors like self-care (fatigue, pain, stress, mood, and exercise), socioeconomic status, abuse, neglect, trauma, and social rejection. Each of these factors serves to influence how EF skills develop, vary in their presentation, and remain vulnerable, both environmentally and neurobiologically. These factors are discussed at multiple points in this volume, with particular emphasis found in the chapters comprising Section II, as well as Chapters 4, 19, and 20.

Executive Function and Dysfunction, ed. Scott J. Hunter and Elizabeth P. Sparrow. Published by Cambridge University Press. © Cambridge University Press 2012.

When EdF is present, it often impacts functioning widely, and hampers adjustment across academic, vocational/occupational, social and interpersonal, emotional and intrapersonal, behavioral, and adaptive functioning (see Chapters 4, 18, and 20 in particular). This also creates a recurring cycle between what EdF impacts and what impacts EdF; however, intervention has the potential to change this cycle. As a result, we place a significant emphasis across this volume on recognition and intervention for EdF.

The primary purpose of this volume is to provide a comprehensive summary of what is known about EF and EdF in childhood and adolescence, examine what these data mean in a practical sense, and consider future directions for clinical and research work. Throughout this volume, our perspective is developmental, with a focus on issues usually first seen in children and adolescents. As a result, EdF in conditions that usually show onset in adulthood, such as schizophrenia,[2,3,4,5,6] the personality disorders,[7,8] and the dementias,[9,10,11,12,13,14,15] are not covered in this volume. There are numerous review articles and texts available that address EF in the adult population, including the classic references by Stuss and Benson[16] and Lezak.[17] Books addressing EdF in pediatric populations tend to present very applied materials (i.e., worksheets for use in treatment) or very academic and theoretical perspectives, but have not integrated research and practice. This volume will fill the gap in the literature for EF in pediatric populations, as a guide for researchers and clinicians who work with children and adolescents on a daily basis.

This volume is organized into three sections. The first section provides an overview of the foundations for understanding EF and EdF. Chapter 1 reviews the historical context of EF and summarizes various efforts to define and model this complex concept. The development of EF, from infancy through young adulthood, is examined in Chapter 2. It is critical to have an understanding of this progression as individual differences[18] are superimposed on the "typical" leaps and plateaus in EF development. Chapter 3 reviews what is known about the neurobiology of EF, specifically its developmental neuroanatomical, and neurochemical correlates. Current research in this area argues against simplistic assignment of EF to the frontal lobes,[16] instead revealing the beautiful complexity of the executive networks that involve cortical, subcortical, and cerebellar areas, among others. Ironically, we are once again reaching what early scientists postulated in the 1800s, that " ... the frontal lobes are the seat of coordination and fusion of the incoming and outgoing products of the several sensory and motor areas of the cortex."[19] Chapter 4 concludes the first section with a discussion of key assessment principles and a consideration of areas to address when examining EF and EdF.

The chapters in Section II represent current advances in pediatric neuropsychology and EF by presenting examples of a variety of pediatric clinical conditions that are associated with EdF. Section II is composed of 12 chapters describing EF and EdF in a number of conditions that begin in childhood or adolescence, either acquired neurodevelopmentally or through insult to the developing brain. Each of these chapters has a similar structure to help the reader find material, including discussion of the clinical manifestations, neuroimaging data, neuropsychological findings, and future directions for research pertinent to each disorder or condition. This section includes a range of neurodevelopmental and acquired disorders involving EdF, not only the "usual suspects" such as Attention-Deficit/Hyperactivity Disorder (ADHD) and the autism spectrum disorders (ASDs), but also less frequently discussed examples, like the pediatric movement disorders, neurodevelopmental conditions secondary to trauma and insult, the seizure disorders, human immunodeficiency virus (HIV), and the sequelae of the childhood cancers. It was our goal with this section to address the range of potential conditions seen in clinical practice, as well as to provide guidance for those less common disorders that may occasionally be referred.

The chapters in Section III represent applications of this information. Chapter 17 reviews empirically supported interventions for EdF. Chapter 18 extends this with a consideration of educational implications, including research on school-based programs to improve EdF. Cautions and caveats regarding the consideration of EF and EdF in the forensic neuropsychology and child psychiatry setting are offered in Chapter 19. This volume concludes with Chapter 20, sharing reflections on key messages and goals for research and practice.

The reader is encouraged to mark the Appendices for easy reference while reading. Appendix I lists abbreviations used throughout the volume. Appendix II provides information about tests mentioned in the volume, including names, abbreviations, and quick references to learn more about each test. Unless specified otherwise, "child" is used in this volume to refer to children and adolescents.

The contributors to this volume were carefully considered and selected to represent a range of neurodevelopment professionals who work with EdF on a daily basis. The authors represent a mix of researchers, assessors, and interventionists, across both clinical and academic settings. With their contributions, these authors are not simply summarizing what others have written, but also extending the available research literature with clinical observations, new interpretations, and guidance for the future. We hope that this volume will provide practitioners and clinical consultants with a better understanding of both EF and EdF, and provide researchers and developers of intervention programs with an impetus for continued progress in the area. By examining the foundations, manifestations, and implications of EF and EdF, we hope to convincingly demonstrate the importance of addressing these issues for the many children and adolescents who present clinically for assessment and intervention, in order to support their effective transition to productive adulthood. We also hope to challenge our colleagues and professional peers towards a broader, more dynamic view of both EF and EdF, and how they unfold and alter across development, in anticipation of more effectively coaching and guiding the families who seek our consultation.

We anticipate that this volume will be of interest to psychologists (including neuropsychologists, school psychologists, developmental psychologists, and child clinical psychologists), pediatricians, pediatric neurologists, psychiatrists, rehabilitation physicians and pediatric physiatrists, and advanced trainees in these disciplines. Additionally, it may serve as a valuable resource for educators and even parents, to support their understanding of the children with whom they live and work on a daily basis.

References

1. Suchy Y. Executive functioning: Overview, assessment, and research issues for non-neuropsychologists. *Ann Behav Med* 2009; 37(2): 106–16.

2. Moritz S, Birkner C, Kloss M, *et al.* Executive functioning in obsessive-compulsive disorder, unipolar depression, and schizophrenia. *Arch Clin Neuropsychol* 2002; 17: 477–83.

3. Savla GN, Twamley EW, Delis DC, *et al.* Dimensions of executive functioning in schizophrenia and their relationship with processing speed. *Schizophr Bull* 2010; 16. [Epub ahead of print]

4. Klemm S, Schmidt B, Knappe S, Blanz B. Impaired working speed and executive functions as frontal lobe dysfunctions in young first-degree relatives of schizophrenic patients. *Eur Child Adolesc Psychiatry* 2006; 15(7): 400–8.

5. Raffard S, Bayard S, Gely-Nargeot MC, *et al.* Insight and executive functioning in schizophrenia: a multidimensional approach. *Psychiatry Res* 2009; **167**(3): 239–50.

6. Keshavan MS, Kulkarni S, Bhojraj T, *et al.* Premorbid cognitive deficits in young relatives of schizophrenia patients. *Front Hum Neurosci* 2010; **3**: 62.

7. Morgan AB, Lilienfeld SO. A meta-analytic review of the relation between antisocial behavior and neuropsychological measures of executive function. *Clin Psychol Rev* 2000; **20**: 113–56.

8. LeGris J, van Reekum R. The neuropsychological correlates of borderline personality disorder and suicidal behaviour. *Can J Psychiatry* 2006; **51**: 131–42.

9. Salmon DP, Bondi MW. Neuropsychological assessment of dementia. *Annu Rev Psychol* 2009; **60**: 257–82.

10. Stopford CL, Thompson JC, Neary D, *et al.* Working memory, attention, and executive function in Alzheimer's disease and frontotemporal dementia. *Cortex* 2010; **21**. [Epub ahead of print]

11. Allain P, Havet-Thomassin V, Verny C, *et al.* Evidence for deficits on different components of theory of mind in Huntington's disease. *Neuropsychology* 2011; **25**(6): 741–51.

12. Seelaar H, Rohrer JD, Pijnenburg YA, *et al.* Clinical, genetic and pathological heterogeneity of frontotemporal dementia: a review. *J Neurol Neurosurg Psychiatry* 2011; **82**(5): 476–86.

13. Johns EK, Phillips NA, Belleville S, *et al.* Executive functions in frontotemporal dementia and Lewy body dementia. *Neuropsychology* 2009; **23**(6): 765–77.

14. Woods SP, Tröster AI. Prodromal frontal/executive dysfunction predicts incident dementia in Parkinson's disease. *J Int Neuropsychol Soc* 2003; **9**(1): 17–24.

15. Oosterman JM, de Goede M, Wester AJ, *et al.* Perspective taking in Korsakoff's syndrome: the role of executive functioning and task complexity. *Acta Neuropsychiatrica* 2011; **23**: 302–8.

16. Stuss DT, Benson DF. *The Frontal Lobes*. New York: Raven Press, 1986.

17. Lezak MD. *Neuropsychological Assessment, Second edition*. New York: Oxford University Press, 1983.

18. Hughes C. Changes and challenges in 20 years of research into the development of executive functions. *Infant Child Developm* 2011; **20**(3): 251–71.

19. Bianchi L. The functions of the frontal lobes. *Brain* 1895; **18**: 497–530.

Models of executive functioning

Chapter 1

Scott J. Hunter and Elizabeth P. Sparrow

Scientists have approached executive functioning (EF) from a variety of perspectives, including neuroanatomical, neurochemical, evolutionary, syndrome-based, and statistical. Many have attempted to concisely define EF and executive dysfunction (EdF) by listing functions or underlying operations,[1,2] while others have focused on its neuroanatomical or neurophysiological correlates.[3] There is some degree of overlap among these descriptions, but no consensus. Perhaps the confusion regarding exactly what constitutes EF reflects the ways in which it has been examined historically. Early studies were *adult-based*, examining behaviors produced by brains that had already developed. These studies, while informative about adults with acquired EdF, did not take into account issues of development, such as how an insult impacts EF in a still-developing brain or how neurodevelopmental disorders impact brain and function. Early work in the field primarily examined the effects of insults to the *frontal lobes*, which led to a circular argument that "damage to the frontal lobes causes EdF, therefore EF must be regulated by the frontal lobes." This was later refined and modified with attribution of EF to the prefrontal cortex (PFC), but the assumption of one-to-one correspondence between function and structure, with limited consideration of the rich network we now know is involved in EF, remained the dominant model. Yet this model failed to account for evidence of intact functioning after removal of the frontal lobe,[4] EdF experienced after damage to other brain areas,[5] or evidence of EdF in the absence of a known neurologic insult (as is the case with some of the neurodevelopmental disorders).

Another key assumption in early work regarding EF was that there is a *homogenous* executive construct. This oversimplification led to a substantial degree of inflexibility in planning, executing, and interpreting studies. As Salthouse has observed, the *diversity of variables* used in assessing EF reveals a lack of agreement regarding the construct; different researchers use different tasks as the primary EF variable, and even standard EF batteries have very little overlap in tests used.[2] The lack of a "gold standard" significantly limits evaluation of EF measures beyond face and predictive validity. Efforts to examine construct validity generally find that performance on tests hypothesized to measure EF is moderately correlated with many other constructs, not just EF (i.e., low discriminant validity).[2]

Without a unifying plan or concept, investigations of EF and EdF have gone in a number of directions. Some researchers and clinicians continue to emphasize the simplistic explanation they learned early in their training, that EF is most related to the frontal lobes, and that it is primarily seen after brain injury or in Attention-Deficit/Hyperactivity Disorder (ADHD). Lack of agreement regarding what processes are part of EF contributes

Executive Function and Dysfunction, ed. Scott J. Hunter and Elizabeth P. Sparrow. Published by Cambridge University Press. © Cambridge University Press 2012.

to the confusion, as different definitions and classifications complicate comparisons of research findings. For example, opinions regarding whether working memory (WM) is part of EF impact interpretation of high correlations between EF measures and intelligence quotient (IQ) test results that are primarily moderated by the Working Memory Index (cf. data reported by Arffa).[6] This confusion regarding the EF construct limits cohesion in the field, and thus limits progress.

In this chapter, we present a historical context within which to understand current models of EF and EdF. We conclude with suggestions for reaching an improved, integrated model of EF that accounts for changes in neural networks and skills across child and adolescent development.

Evolutionary context

For many years, an assumption has been that EF is a singular, phylogenetically higher-order cognitive skill that identifies us as human and differentiates us both behaviorally and dynamically from other mammalian species. Bernstein and Waber, among others, have reminded us that this fallacious concept ignores the reality that problem solving is an inherent aspect of mammalian development.[7] Although it was initially believed that the size of the PFC was a critical difference between humans and other species, comparative analyses indicate that the frontal lobe to total brain volume ratio is consistent across primates, including humans.[8-10] It appears that white matter volume is a differentiating factor, with humans having more white matter than other primates.[11] However, it is difficult to know whether this represents basic species differences, or whether modern human brains reflect high levels of stimulation that cause greater interconnectivity.[12] Ultimately, it remains important to remember that, as highlighted by Bernstein and Waber:[7]

> "the frontal lobes are neither new in evolutionary terms nor special to humans: they have been part of the neural apparatus of the mammalian line for 176 million years. The goal-oriented behavior that these neural systems support is not only common to all mammals, but also critical to their survival and to the evolutionary success of the whole mammalian enterprise . . . [The EF-directed] control processes are – indeed, must be – inextricably embedded in the total package of biological systems that all animals need to obtain food, reproductive partners, and other critical resources" (p. 40).

Historical context

The concepts referred to as EF today have been considered for centuries. The Bible seems to mention EF in verses written in approximately 900 B.C., "A man without self-control is like a city broken into and left without walls."[13] In 1835, deNobele described impairment after damage to the frontal lobes,[14] although the more famous case is that of Phineas Gage, who was described by Harlow in 1848.[15-18] The importance of these cases was realized retrospectively, after prominent neuropsychologists began to draw attention to this concept.

In 1964, Teuber published a paper entitled, "The Riddle of the Frontal Lobes".[19] Much of his commentary could be reiterated today, nearly 50 years later. He wrote,

> "Man's frontal lobes have always presented problems that seemed to exceed those encountered in studying other regions of his brain . . . these assorted aspects of frontal lobe dysfunction, in infrahuman species, are dissociable, since any one of these symptoms can be shown to occur

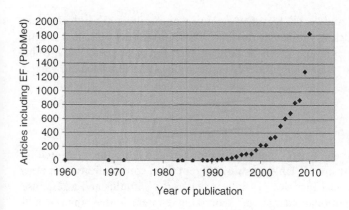

Fig. 1.1. Number of articles indexed in PubMed that included EF or EdF (search terms ="executive function "OR" executive dysfunction" OR "executive functions" OR "executive dysfunction" OR "dysexecutive "OR" executive deficit "OR" executive deficits")

without the others ... Despite the conspicuous efforts and ingenuity that went into behavioral analysis of these frontal lobe symptoms, their interpretation, in terms of some basic alterations in carnivore or simian behavior, remains elusive ... During the first third of this century, there developed a substantial majority opinion which ascribed to the frontal lobes all the highest conceivable functions – from "abstract behavior," foresight, and intellectual synthesis, to capacity for ethical behavior, control of affect, awareness of self, and recent memory. In the early forties and through the fifties of the century, the pendulum swung in the other direction – toward a denial of any especial importance of human prefrontal structures" (p. 25).

A next landmark in the consideration of EF is "the frontal lobe syndrome" described by Luria in 1969.[20,21] This term was coined at a time when EF deficits were believed to occur in conjunction with insults to the frontal lobes. Although Luria[22] did not explicitly refer to EF in writing, he did attribute deficits in the ability to solve complex problems to the frontal lobes as the locus for the "complex process of formation and execution of a programme" (p. 219).

The first intentional use of "executive" in the published literature was noted in Baddeley and Hitch's model of the "central executive," which is discussed later in this chapter.[23] This concept gradually gained popularity, including Schaie's description of the "executive stage of adult cognitive development" that he postulated emerged in the 30s and 40s.[24] Shallice[25] used the phrase "executive functions and their disorders" in a 1982 publication applying the Norman and Shallice supervisory attentional system concept to explain performance of patients with brain lesions (p. 199). Although the first edition of Lezak's well-referenced volume[26] did not include a section about EF, she addressed many of the components we now consider as such. In the second edition,[27] she included a chapter entitled "Executive Functions and Motor Performance," describing the problems inherent in assessing EF.

Although the earliest publications about EdF in clinical populations focused on brain injury, the late 1980s showed an emerging interest in the EF concept as it was exhibited in other clinical conditions including schizophrenia,[28] ADHD,[29] and phenylketonuria (PKU).[30] This slow trickle of research quickly became a torrent, with the 1990s showing an explosion of articles regarding EF in various conditions. The number of articles per year focusing on and addressing this concept has only increased (see Fig. 1.1).

In the following sections, a handful of influential models will be examined, including evolution of language, the central executive, the Supervisory Attentional System, Theory of

Mind, self-regulation, "hot" and "cold" EF, the Cognitive Complexity and Control theory, and structural equation modeling with latent variables. These models are presented roughly in the order of publication, although it can be difficult even for theorists to know whose idea came first. Each of these models has influenced other models and impacted our current views of EF and EdF.

Evolution of language

Bronowski, a physicist, mathematician, linguist, philosopher, and educator, presented his theory in 1967 to explain why human language was different from communication in other species.[31] Elements of his model included (1) a delay between a stimulus and a response, (2) separation of affect/emotional charge, or processing content rather than simply responding to affective charge, or self-regulation of emotion, (3) prolongation of reference, or the capacity to recall the past to inform future decisions while keeping in mind the present situation (much like what we now call WM), (4) internalization of language, referring to private self-reflection and self-exploration allowing consideration of options before responding, and (5) reconstitution, analyzing parts of a situation and synthesizing them to construct a new response. He summarized these steps as allowing humans to disengage from their current context and influence their environment by understanding it, and connected the ability to delay response to development of the frontal lobes.[32] Although Bronowski's model focused on language, it showed consideration of what would come to be called EF in a few years. This model was a primary influence for Barkley's[33] model of executive functions in ADHD (see below).

Working memory (central executive)

In 1974, Baddeley and Hitch published a chapter describing their three-part model of WM[23] that was developed in response to concerns about the existing model that a short-term store held information until it could be entered into long-term memory (LTM). Their tripartite model was controlled by a system of limited attentional capacity, the "central executive," which was subserved by two storage or "slave" systems, the phonological loop and visuospatial sketchpad. Baddeley and Hitch were not the first to use the term "working memory," but they were the first to include specific mention of an executive component.[34] This model of a unitary attentional executive within a WM system was challenged by findings of intact immediate memory in patients with severely impaired LTM, findings that surpassed the capacity of finite slave systems. The original central executive was not believed to have any integrational capacity, which meant the model could not explain facilitation of short-term memory (STM) by LTM (as occurs in chunking) nor did it allow for crosstalk between the visuospatial and auditory slave systems. After the proposal of a dual-process control by Norman and Shallice[35] (see below), Baddeley added the "episodic buffer" to his model, a finite system controlled by the central executive that holds information long enough to be integrated.[36] Baddeley ties the central executive in this model to a distributed neural network, writing "[t]he central executive is likely to engage multiple brain regions in a functionally coherent network, including dorsolateral prefrontal cortex" (p. 836).[34] The central executive model has been criticized for creating a homunculus within the brain.[37]

Attentional control (supervisory attentional system)

The information processing model of attentional control was presented by Norman and Shallice in 1980.[35] Rather than a single executive, Norman and Shallice proposed two control processes: (1) routine habits, or pre-existing "schemas," that control a specific overlearned action or skill, and (2) an intentional "supervisory attentional system" (SAS) that comes online when a situation is non-routine. This grew out of the information processing movement related to artificial intelligence solutions to problem solving. Even in routine situations, "contention scheduling" selected a certain number of schemas to activate, inhibiting the others until environmental demands changed. The SAS serves to bias contention scheduling such that different schemas are activated.

In a subsequent paper, Shallice referenced Luria's work with frontal lobe lesions, stating that the study of executive functions and their disorders was a good area for interaction of cognitive psychology and neuropsychology.[25] He then evaluated what his model could predict about "high-level cognitive impairment" (p. 202). Shallice hypothesized that an inoperative SAS would leave a person reliant on the contention scheduling system; this would produce predictable behaviors that were slow to change (i.e., perseveration). In the presence of strong environmental triggers that activated schemas, the person would have difficulty inhibiting (i.e., distractibility), and in the absence of strong environmental triggers he would likely do nothing at all (i.e., apathy). He drew strong parallels between these predictions and observations of animals and humans with frontal lobe lesions. Like the central executive model, the SAS has been criticized for creating a homunculus within the brain.[37]

Theory of mind

The concept "theory of mind" was first described by Hebb in a 1958 lecture.[38] The term appeared again in 1978 when Premack and Woodruff[39] discussed its relevance to understanding chimpanzees, defining theory of mind as the ability to attribute mental states not only to self, but also to others (e.g., "I *think* John likes you," or, "I *guess* she will be happy with this gift."). They postulated that this ability allowed chimpanzees to make inferences about what others believe to be the case and thus make predictions about their probable actions. They concluded with a discussion of preliminary data from human children showing that they did not show evidence of inferred mental states until about 4 years old.

Alan Leslie presented on theory of mind in autism at a 1983 conference,[40] later publishing a paper with Uta Frith and her doctoral student, Simon Baron-Cohen, on the subject.[41] They described a model of "metarepresentational development . . . being able to conceive of mental states: that is, knowing that other people know, want, feel, or believe things" (p. 38), saying that the ability to form second-order representations was a prerequisite for existence of this theory of mind which subserves social skills.

Frith and colleagues examined theory of mind with a variety of clever manipulations dealing with beliefs and false beliefs. In the well-known "Sally and Anne scenario" (an example of a "false-belief" task), Sally puts a marble in a basket and then leaves the room. Anne hides Sally's marble in her box. Sally returns, and the experimenter asks, "Where will Sally look for her marble?" If theory of mind is present, the child will recognize that Sally expects the marble to be where she left it, and he says she will look in the basket. In the absence of theory of mind, the child does not discriminate between his knowledge and Sally's knowledge, and he says Sally will look in the box. There were four questions asked: Naming (names for each girl in the story), Belief (where does Sally believe the marble is), Reality (where is the marble really), and Memory (where was the marble in the beginning). All members of the clinical samples (children with autism and children with Down Syndrome) and normal control groups replied accurately to the Naming, Reality, and Memory questions. The Belief question was answered accurately by 85% of the normal control group, 86% of the Down Syndrome group, and 20% of the autism group ($p < 0.001$); the children with autism pointed to the current marble location when asked where Sally would look for the marble. In other words, the children with autism did not demonstrate a theory of mind.

Over 1500 articles about theory of mind have been published since that time, many examining the construct in autism. Theory of mind has been explored in typical development[42–44] as well as in clinical groups beyond autism, including disruptive behaviors,[45,46] Fetal Alcohol Spectrum Disorders (FASD),[47] traumatic brain injury (TBI),[48] bipolar disorder,[49] and schizophrenia.[50] Although there are differing views regarding whether theory of mind has EF components, whether EF is a prerequisite for theory of mind, whether theory of mind is a prerequisite for EF, or whether theory of mind is actually an example of an EF skill, results from a number of analyses show a close relationship between theory of mind and EF,[45,46,51–56] with a meta-analysis finding a strong effect size of 1.08 for the relationship.[57]

Self-regulation in ADHD

In 1997, Barkley proposed a formal model of executive dysfunction in ADHD.[33] His model reflected a core deficit in "behavioral inhibition" that influenced four specified EF skills (WM, internalized speech, self-regulation of affect/motivation/arousal, and reconstitution); all five of these components impacted the motor control systems.[33] Barkley[58] proposed that "behavioral inhibition sets the occasion for the executive functions to occur" (p. 193). He[58] described behavioral activation as playing a support role, writing, "I would not consider arousal or activation to be executive functions in themselves" (p. 194). He criticized past descriptions of the central executive, saying they produce another black box or homunculus within the brain. Barkley[58] proposed instead that the central executive might actually be "time, or the individual's sense of the future," (p. 202) in that review of the past and future-directed goals represent self-regulation relative to time.

The influence of Bronowski's[31] model on Barkley's[33,58] work is clear, as the new model expanded Bronowski's five elements beyond language, adding an explicit component of the motor control system. The element of time can be linked to Fuster's premise that "cross-temporal contingencies," as subserved by temporal organization, temporal integration, attention, "executive working memory," and preparatory set, are critical for the timely organization of behavior and language.[59,60] Barkley also acknowledges the influence of Douglas' early work on self-regulation as an underlying deficit in ADHD,[61] Goldman-Rakic's WM model,[62] and Damasio's somatic marker hypothesis.[63]

Barkley's model is considered by some critics to be incomplete, and in need of broader validation than just with a sample of individuals with ADHD. As well, it is likely that this model serves to capture some but not all of the processes underlying what we conceptualize as EF. However, it does facilitate and foster an empirical approach to examining how EF interacts with and is guided by broader cognitive capacities.

"Hot" and "Cold" EF

In 1962, Abelson[64] used the terms "hot cognition" to refer to "cognition dealing with affect-laden objects" and "cold cognition" to describe cognition associated with problem solving (p. 277); these terms were used incidentally during his introduction of computer simulation of human attitudes and interpersonal perceptions. During a presentation in 1979, social psychologist Zajonc[65] described his thoughts about the relationships between thought and affect, invoking the terms "hot" and "cold" cognition (giving credit to Abelson for these terms). These terms were applied to a theory of delayed gratification by Mischel and colleagues.[66,67] They described a "cool," cognitive, "knowing" system, and a "hot," emotional, "going" system, further elaborating that the cool system, associated with contemplation and strategy, was the basis for self-regulation and self-control, whereas the hot system, impulsive and passionate, was the basis for emotionality. They posited that the balance between these two systems explained willpower, and was regulated by development and stress.

Shortly after this, an article about prefrontal cortex function referred to "hot" stimuli (i.e., more likely to lead to reflexive and possibly inappropriate reactions) in relation to the inhibitory function of the orbital PFC and "cold" stimuli (i.e., less likely to invoke a strong response) in relation to the dorsal regions of the PFC.[68] Zelazo and colleagues expanded this application of the hot and cool terms to EF in typical and atypical development.[37] They observed that most of the EF literature focused on relatively cool EF which is activated by abstract, decontextualized problems, neglecting hot EF such as social and emotional dyscontrol. Rather than a dichotomy, Zelazo and colleagues view tasks and functioning as relative levels of hot and cool EF. They posit that EF tasks differ in "motivational significance," with hot EF tasks involving motivationally and emotionally salient stimuli, decisions, and outcomes, in other words, everyday decision making,[69] and suggest that an emotionally salient problem might be best solved through cool EF.[70]

While this approach has broadened and refined the description of EF, it has continued to emphasize a cortico-centered interpretation, with a strong focus on frontal systems at the expense of broader neural networks. This distinction continues to resonate with Luria's earlier hypotheses concerning the functional units of the brain, particularly the role of the arousal-motivational (limbic and reticular activating system) aspects of problem solving.[71]

Cognitive complexity and control theory

Zelazo and colleagues are also associated with the Cognitive Complexity and Control theory (CCC theory),[72] first described in 1997 and revised in 2003 (CCC-r theory),[73] which posits that one must have reflective awareness of one's knowledge to use that knowledge to guide behavior in the presence of interference. The CCC theory is based on two different systems, a lower-level, unconscious, automatic, response-based system and a higher-level, conscious, representational system. Child development leads to growth in the representational system which in turn increases the complexity of explicit rule systems, which then increase a child's reflexive awareness of rules. In other words, EF gains occur because children can formulate, hold in WM, and use more complex hierarchies of rules as they develop.[74] The CCC-r theory expands on the original theory by adding inhibition of rules (in addition to activation of rules) and the role of conscious reflection on rules (also called the Levels of Consciousness model).[73,75] Three major transitions in children's development include: (1) shift from explicit representation of a goal to explicit representation of a rule around 2 years old, (2) shift to explicit representation of a relation between two rules around 3 years old, and (3) shift to explicit representation of a higher-order rule that integrates two incompatible pairs of rules.[72] The four rule types in CCC theory are ranked by complexity, moving from *single stimulus-reward associations*, to *condition-action rules* (i.e., if-then contingencies), then *univalent rule pairs* (i.e., each stimulus has one response), and the most complex, *bivalent rule pairs* (i.e., each stimulus has two possible responses, with the correct response context-dependent); higher-order rule generation involves combinations among these four rule types.[74] Additional work has attempted to link each rule type to areas of the PFC.[76] The CCC theory has been criticized on several counts, including arbitrary decisions about task complexity[77] and examples of adults failing to use higher order rule generation.[78]

Structural equation modeling with latent variables

Friedman and Miyake began publishing on executive functions from the cognitive psychology perspective in 2000, with several papers addressing verbal and spatial WM,[79] dual-task methodology and the central executive,[80] and assessment of EF.[81,82] They expressed concern about using traditional statistical procedures like correlations and factor analysis, noting inherent problems with EF tasks such as task impurity (i.e., an EF test does not measure solely EF), low internal and test-retest reliability, and lack of construct validation, and proposed the use of a new procedure, latent variable analysis.[82] These latent variables (i.e., shared constructs underlying the various EF tasks) are hypothetically purer than manifest variables (i.e., individual test results), allowing a clearer examination of how EF skills may be interrelated. This is theorized to reduce complications from task impurity and construct validity issues.

Friedman and Miyake chose to examine relationships among shifting, updating/monitoring WM, and inhibition of prepotent response in their first latent variable analysis, with the goal of evaluating whether they were unitary or separable (and if separable, to identify their relative contributions to scores on the selected tasks).[82] Their investigation of these relationships with college students supported that these three EF skills were indeed separable, but moderately correlated (suggesting a unitary underlying factor), and that they contributed differentially to performance on EF tasks. They posited that the underlying factor might be inhibition (harkening back to an earlier model proposed by Bronowski). Friedman and Miyake cautioned that they had selected these three EF skills as a starting place, but that this model was by no means representative of EF as a whole. Their continued work with structural equation modeling and latent variable analysis in combination with researchers from other fields has contributed significantly to our understanding of EF, the heritability of EF, the relationships among EF skills, and various EF skills involved in standard EF tasks.

Summary and future directions

Despite endeavors to describe, define, and model EF, there is still no gold standard for understanding this construct. There is consensus that EF is a complex and critical component of successful human life, subserved by an intricate network of neural resources. Behavioral changes after brain injury, described as early as the 1800s, continue to be part of our definition for EdF. Although the early descriptions were closely linked to frontal lobe impairment, there is clear evidence that EdF can be observed subsequent to other types of neural insult, including subcortical and cerebellar damage. Elements of early models continue to be recognized as EF, including inhibition, WM, self-regulation, integration of past with present and anticipated future consequences in decision-making, internalized thought processes, segregation of complex problems into smaller components, and manipulation and integration of small components to create a response. Structural equation modeling with latent variables has begun to clarify some of the relationships among the EF skills and other psychological constructs, and offers a quantitative way to evaluate various hierarchical models of EF from operational, neuroanatomical, and even neurochemical perspectives. Awareness of EdF as part of neurodevelopmental conditions has increased, and there is growing recognition of the complicated interactions between development and EF.

Much remains to be learned about gene-environment interactions and how these influence the ongoing development of EF across childhood and adolescence. Studies are using behavioral and neuroimaging methodologies to examine how individuals come to show significant differences in EF development. Differences in how genes guide the development of specific neural circuits controlling expression of EF across development remain elusive in both typical development and neurodevelopmental disorders. Sociocultural and biopsychosocial factors also appear to contribute to the development of EF, such as the impact of homelessness and chronic stress on childhood development (see Chapters 19 and 20). What is increasingly becoming clear is that no existing model, neuropsychological test, or neuroimaging approach is adequate to describe this complex domain of capability. Although our ability to identify and target potential risks is improving, our understanding of the impact of EdF is still developing. As this knowledge increases, our ability to measure and intervene will continue to improve, enhancing our models and approaches to EF.

References

1. Jurado MB, Rosselli M. The elusive nature of executive functions: a review of our current understanding. *Neuropsychol Rev* 2007; **17**(3): 213–33.

2. Salthouse TA. Relations between cognitive abilities and measures of executive functioning. *Neuropsychology* 2005; **19**(4): 532–45.

3. Stuss DT, Benson DL. *The Frontal Lobes*. New York: Raven Press, 1986.

4. Hebb DO. Intelligence in man after large removals of cerebral tissue: report of four left frontal lobe cases. *J Gen Psychol* 1939; **21**: 73–87.

5. Tranel D, Hyman BT. Neuropsychological correlates of bilateral amygdala damage. *Arch Neurol* 1990; **47**(3): 349–55.

6. Arffa S. The relationship of intelligence to executive function and non-executive function measures in a sample of average, above average, and gifted youth. *Arch Clin Neuropsychol* 2007; **22**(8): 969–78.

7. Bernstein JH, Waber DP. Executive capacities from a developmental perspective. In Meltzer L. ed. *Executive Function in Education: From Theory to Practice*. New York: Guilford Press; 2007, 39–54.

8. Jerison HJ. Evolution of prefrontal cortex. In: Krasnegor NA, Lyon GR, Goldman-Rakic PS, editors. *Development of the Prefrontal Cortex*. Baltimore, MD: Brookes; 1997, 9–26.

9. Semendeferi K, Damasio H, Frank R, Van Hoesen GW. Evolution of the frontal lobes: a volumetric analysis based on three-dimensional reconstructions of magnetic resonance scans of human and ape brains. *J Hum Evol* 1997; **32**(4): 375–88.

10. Semendeferi K, Lu A, Schenker N, Damasio H. Humans and great apes share a large frontal cortex. *Nat Neurosci* 2002; **5**(3): 272–6.

11. Schoenemann PT, Sheehan MJ, Glotzer LD. Prefrontal white matter volume is disproportionately larger in humans than in other primates. *Nat Neurosci* 2005; **8**: 242–52.

12. Ardila A. On the evolutionary origins of executive functions. *Brain Cogn* 2008; **68**(1): 92–9.

13. The Holy Bible. *Revised Standard Version.* Grand Rapids, MI: Zondervan Bible Publishers, 1971; Proverbs **25**: 28.

14. Lyketsos CG, Rosenblatt A, Rabins P. Forgotten frontal lobe syndrome or 'executive dysfunction syndrome'. *Psychosomatics* 2004; **45**: 247–55.

15. Harlow, JM. Passage of an iron bar through the head. *Boston Med Surg J* 1848; **39**: 389–93.

16. Macmillan M. *An Odd Kind of Fame: Stories of Phineas Gage.* Cambridge, MA, US: The MIT Press; 2000.

17. Macmillan M, Lena ML. Rehabilitating Phineas Gage. *Neuropsychol Rehabil* 2010; **20**(5): 641–58.

18. Ratiu P, Talos IF, Haker S, Lieberman D, Everett P. The tale of Phineas Gage, digitally remastered. *J Neurotrauma* 2004; **21**(5): 637–43.

19. Teuber HL. The riddle of frontal lobe function in man. 1964. *Neuropsychol Rev* 2009; **19**(1): 25–46.

20. Luria AR. Frontal lobe syndromes. In: Vinken PJ, Bruyn GW, eds. *Handbook of Clinical Neurology.* Vol **2**. Amsterdam: North Holland; 1969, 725–57.

21. Meyer A. The frontal lobe syndrome, the aphasias and related conditions. A contribution to the history of cortical localization. *Brain* 1974; **97**(3): 565–600.

22. Luria AR. *The Working Brain.* Middlesex, England: Penguin Books; 1973.

23. Baddeley A, Hitch G. Working memory. In Bower GH, ed. *Recent Advances in Learning and Motivation.* Vol. 8. New York: Academic; 1974.

24. Schaie KW. Toward a stage theory of adult cognitive development. *Int J Aging Hum Dev* 1977–1978; **8**(2): 129–38.

25. Shallice T. Specific impairments of planning. *Phil Trans Roy Soc Lond B Biol Sci* 1982; **298**(1089): 199–209.

26. Lezak MD. *Neuropsychological Assessment.* New York: Oxford University Press; 1976.

27. Lezak MD. *Neuropsychological Assessment.* 2nd edn. New York: Oxford University Press; 1983.

28. Morice R. Beyond language – speculations on the prefrontal cortex and schizophrenia. *Aust N Z J Psychiatry* 1986; **20**(1): 7–10.

29. Hamlett KW, Pellegrini DS, Conners CK. An investigation of executive processes in the problem-solving of attention deficit disorder-hyperactive children. *J Pediatr Psychol* 1987; **12**(2): 227–40.

30. Welsh MC, Pennington BF, Ozonoff S, Rouse B, McCabe ER. Neuropsychology of early-treated phenylketonuria: specific executive function deficits. *Child Dev* 1990; **61**(6): 1697–713.

31. Bronowski J. Human and animal languages. In Bronowski J, ed. *A Sense of the Future.* Cambridge, MA: MIT Press, 1977; 104–31.

32. Bronowski J, Bellugi U. Language, name, and concept. *Science.* 1970; **168**(3932): 669–73.

33. Barkley RA. Behavioral inhibition, sustained attention, and executive functions: constructing a unifying theory of ADHD. *Psychol Bull* 1997; **121**(1): 65–94.

34. Baddeley A. Working memory: looking back and looking forward. *Nat Rev Neurosci* 2003; **4**(10): 829–39.

35. Norman DA, Shallice T. Attention to action: willed and automatic control of behavior. Center for Human Information Processing. In Davidson RJ, Schwarts GE, Shapiro D, eds. *Consciousness and Self-regulation.* Vol. 4. New York: Plenum Press; 1986, 1–18.

36. Baddeley AD. The episodic buffer: a new component of working memory? *Trends Cogn Sci* 2000; **4**: 417–23.

37. Zelazo PD, Müller U. Executive function in typical and atypical development. In Goswami, U. ed. *Blackwell Handbook of Childhood Cognitive Development.* Malden: Blackwell Publishing; 2002, 445–69.

38. Hebb DO. Intelligence, brain function and the theory of mind. *Brain* 1959; **82**: 260–75.

39. Premack D, Woodruff G. Does the chimpanzee have a theory of mind? *Behav Brain Sci* 1978; **1**: 515–26.

40. Leslie AM. Pretense and representation: The origins of theory of mind. *Psychol Rev* 1987; **94**: 412–26.

41. Baron-Cohen S, Leslie AM, Frith U. Does the autistic child have a "theory of mind"? *Cognition* 1985; **21**(1): 37–46.

42. Dumontheil I, Apperly IA, Blakemore SJ. Online usage of theory of mind continues to develop in late adolescence. *Dev Sci* 2010; **13**(2): 331–8.

43. Walker RF, Murachver T. Representation and theory of mind development. *Dev Psychol* 2012; **48**(2): 509–20.

44. Grant MG, Mills CM. Children's explanations of the intentions underlying others' behaviour. *Br J Dev Psychol* 2011; **29**: 504–23.

45. Hughes C, Dunn J, White A. Trick or treat? Uneven understanding of mind and emotion and executive dysfunction in "hard-to-manage" preschoolers. *J Child Psychol Psychiatry* 1998; **39**(7): 981–94.

46. Fahie, CM, Symons, DK. Executive functioning and theory of mind in children clinically referred for attention and behavior problems. *J Appl Devel Psychol* 2003; **24**(1): 51–73.

47. Rasmussen C, Wyper K, Talwar V. The relation between theory of mind and executive functions in children with fetal alcohol spectrum disorders. *Can J Clin Pharmacol* 2009; **16**(2): e370–80.

48. Walz NC, Yeates KO, Taylor HG, Stancin T, Wade SL. Theory of mind skills 1 year after traumatic brain injury in 6- to 8-year-old children. *J Neuropsychol* 2010; **4**: 181–95.

49. Schenkel LS, Marlow-O'Connor M, Moss M, Sweeney JA, Pavuluri MN. Theory of mind and social inference in children and adolescents with bipolar disorder. *Psychol Med* 2008; **38**(6): 791–800.

50. Stretton J, Thompson PJ. Frontal lobe function in temporal lobe epilepsy. *Epilepsy Res* 2012; **98**: 1–13.

51. Bishop DV. Annotation: autism, executive functions and theory of mind: a neuropsychological perspective. *J Child Psychol Psychiatry* 1993; **34**(3): 279–93.

52. Frye, Douglas. Development of intention: The relation of executive function to theory of mind. In: Zelazo PD, Astington JW, Olson DR, eds. *Developing Theories of Intention: Social Understanding and Self-control*. Mahwah, NJ: Lawrence Erlbaum Associates Publishers; 1999, 119–32.

53. Carlson SM, Moses LJ, Claxton LJ. Individual differences in executive functioning and theory of mind: an investigation of inhibitory control and planning ability. *J Exp Child Psychol* 2004; **87**(4): 299–319.

54. Pellicano E. Individual differences in executive function and central coherence predict developmental changes in theory of mind in autism. *Dev Psychol* 2010; **46**(2): 530–44.

55. Pellicano E. Links between theory of mind and executive function in young children with autism: clues to developmental primacy. *Dev Psychol* 2007; **43**(4): 974–90.

56. Müller U, Liebermann-Finestone DP, Carpendale JI, Hammond SI, Bibok MB. Knowing minds, controlling actions: the developmental relations between theory of mind and executive function from 2 to 4years of age. *J Exp Child Psychol* 2011; **111**(2): 331–48.

57. Perner J, Lang B. Development of theory of mind and executive control. *Trends Cogn Sci* 1999; **3**(9): 337–44.

58. Barkley RA. *ADHD and the Nature of Self-control*. New York, NY: The Guilford Press; 1997.

59. Fuster JM. The prefrontal cortex, mediator of cross-temporal contingencies. *Hum Neurobiol* 1985; **4**(3): 169–79.

60. Fuster JM. The prefrontal cortex – an update: time is of the essence. *Neuron* 2001; **30**(2): 319–33.

61. Douglas, VI. Higher mental processes in hyperactive children: Implication for training. In Knight R. Bakker D. eds. *Treatment of Hyperactive and Learning Disordered Children*. Baltimore, MD: University Park Press; 1980, 65–92.

62. Goldman-Rakic PS. Architecture of the prefrontal cortex and the central executive. In Grafman J, Holyoak KJ, Boller F, eds, *Annals of the New York Academy of Sciences*; 1995; 769, 71–83.

63. Damasio AR. *Descartes' Error: Emotion, Reason and the Human Brain.* New York, NY: Putnam; 1994.

64. Abelson RP. Computer simulation of "hot cognition" In Tomkins SS, Mesick S, eds. *Computer Simulation of Personality.* New York: Wiley; 1963, 277–302.

65. Zajonc, RB. Feeling and thinking: preferences need no inferences. *Am Psychol* 1980; **35**(2): 151–75.

66. Metcalfe J, Mischel W. A hot/cool-system analysis of delay of gratification: dynamics of willpower. *Psychol Rev* 1999; **106**(1): 3–19.

67. Mischel W, Aydak O, Berman, MG, *et al.* Willpower over the life span: Decomposing self-regulation. *Soc Cogn Affect Neurosci* 2011; **6**: 252–6.

68. Miller EK, Cohen JD. An integrative theory of prefrontal cortex function. *Ann Rev Neurosci* 2001; **24**: 167–202.

69. Prencipe A, Kesek A, Cohen J, Lamm C, Lewis MD, Zelazo PD. Development of hot and cool executive function during the transition to adolescence. *J Exp Child Psychol* 2010; **108**(3): 621–37.

70. Kerr A, Zelazo PD. Development of "hot" executive function: the children's gambling task. *Brain Cogn* 2004; **55**(1): 148–57.

71. Luria AR. *Higher Cortical Functions in Man.* New York, NY: Basic Books; 1962.

72. Zelazo, PD, Frye D. Cognitive complexity and control: a theory of the development of deliberate reasoning and intentional action. In Stamenov M, ed. *Language Structure, Discourse, and the Access to Consciousness.* Amsterdam, Holland: John Benjamins; 1997, 113–53.

73. Zelazo PD, Müller U, Frye D, Marcovitch S. The development of executive function in early childhood: VI. The development of executive function: cognitive complexity and control. *Monogr Soc for Res Child Dev* 2003; **68**(3): 93–119.

74. Zelazo PD, Müller U. Executive function in typical and atypical development. In Goswami, U, editor. *The Wiley-Blackwell Handbook of Childhood Cognitive Development,* 2nd ed. New York, NY: Wiley-Blackwell; 2011, 574–603

75. Zelazo PD. Language, levels of consciousness, and the development of intentional action. In Zelazo PD, Astington JW, Olson DR, editors. *Developing Theories of Intention: Social Understanding and Self-control.* Mahwah, NJ: Lawrence Erlbaum Associates Publishers; 1999, 95–117.

76. Bunge SA, Zelazo, PD. A brain-based account of the development of rule use in childhood. *Curr Dir Psychol Sci* 2006; **15**(3): 118–21.

77. Perner J. About + belief + counterfactual. Children's reasoning and the mind. In Mitchell P, Riggs KJ, eds. *Children's Reasoning and the Mind.* Hove, England: Psychology Press/Taylor & Francis; 2000, 367–401.

78. Kirkham NZ, Cruess L, Diamond, A. Helping children apply their knowledge to their behavior on a dimension-switching task. *Dev Sci* 2003; **6**(5): 449–76.

79. Friedman NP, Miyake A. Differential roles for visuospatial and verbal working memory in situation model construction. *J Exp Psychol Gen* 2000; **129**(1): 61–83.

80. Hegarty M, Shah P, Miyake A. Constraints on using the dual-task methodology to specify the degree of central executive involvement in cognitive tasks. *Mem Cogn* 2000; **28**(3): 376–85.

81. Miyake A, Emerson MJ, Friedman NP. Assessment of executive functions in clinical settings: problems and recommendations. *Sem Speech Lang* 2000; **21**(2): 169–83.

82. Miyake A, Friedman NP, Emerson MJ, Witzki AH, Howerter A, Wager TD. The unity and diversity of executive functions and their contributions to complex "Frontal Lobe" tasks: a latent variable analysis. *Cogn Psychol* 2000; **41**(1): 49–100.

The developmental neuropsychology of executive functions

Scott J. Hunter, Jennifer P. Edidin, and Clayton D. Hinkle

The predominant view regarding EF among clinical and research neuropsychologists has historically been one of modularity. As a result, EF skills have been most commonly equated with frontally-focused neural systems that are presumed to drive and regulate their performance. Consequently, it is a still popular belief within the field of neuropsychology that EF skills are best characterized as a set of control capabilities that only fully emerge as an individual achieves adult maturity.[1-2] This belief holds despite the exponential growth of developmental neuropsychology and the empirical literature addressing developmental evidence of EF. Although the research has shown that it is risky to extrapolate from adult models of brain function to patterns of neural development and consequent behavior in children,[3-5] there remains a tendency to do so, particularly with regard to EF.

A corollary belief is that effective EF is achieved by late adolescence or early adulthood when neural systems directed by the frontal lobes are reaching their final period of myelination and adult patterning.[6-8] While this belief is increasingly understood as developmentally erroneous, given that some EF skills reach adult levels of performance at younger ages, it serves as a reminder that much in neuropsychology remains adult "privileged" in theories and models.[4,9] This impacts how we can guide "real" thinking about EF skills and their expression at varying points in development.

The accumulation of evidence indicates that, while there is a lengthy developmental trajectory for EF in humans, aspects of executive capability and its behavioral representations can be observed beginning in late infancy.[4,10-15] However, the development of EF is not necessarily linear, but rather a process that occurs in "spurts" (p. 75).[3-4] As such, our current thinking about what it means to "be executive" is one of metaphor, with varied representations across time and age. As Bernstein and Waber[4] have suggested, "it may be useful to think of executive capacities as a resource and not a set of functions that can themselves be meaningfully and reliably parsed" (p. 50). Furthermore, to become executive can be considered developmentally as an unfolding transaction between increasingly differentiated neural networks and the behavioral interactions that take place in response to environmental, social, and learning demands.[4]

It is the aim of this chapter to discuss the emergence, consolidation, and refinement of EF across infancy, childhood, adolescence, and early adulthood. By examining this developmental path, we present an informed model of the functions of emerging EF that engage with and influence increasing cognitive and regulatory responses, helping the reader to

Executive Function and Dysfunction, ed. Scott J. Hunter and Elizabeth P. Sparrow. Published by Cambridge University Press. © Cambridge University Press 2012.

consider relationships between neuropsychological development as discussed in this chapter and neural development as discussed in Chapter 3.

In the following pages of this chapter, we will aim to define what it means to be executive when development is taken into account. While clearly acknowledging that there is a developmental trajectory for the frontal lobes that parallels the emergence of self-directed and flexible problem solving, we also attempt to define what is meant when we discuss EF skills at differing age levels. As will be discussed in Chapter 3, various components of the executive neural system come online to support and direct increasing levels of self-control, as newer elements of EF emerge across time. This chapter provides a broader understanding of what it means to be executive, including how this appears in typical variations in EF skill development across time and with emerging psychopathology and developmental disability. By better understanding the variabilities that underline EF, we anticipate an opportunity to better outline potential mechanisms for intervention and accommodation.

A developmental neuropsychological framework for thinking about EF

In their chapter addressing EF development and appropriate models for outlining its trajectories, Bernstein and Waber[4] specifically remind us that EF and their coordination through the frontal lobes are not a unique capacity to humans, and are in fact seen across all mammalian species (see Chapter 1). EF skills are not unique to humans and their enhanced information processing needs, but are instead an integral part of mammalian brain development that has emerged across time to facilitate higher-order problem solving and goal-oriented behavior.[16] As such, we must consider the development of EF from an evolutionary standpoint, recognizing that our nervous system is "biologically wired" for adaptation, flexibility, and control. A core enterprise of the developing neural systems is an unfolding of the capacities and regulatory efforts that are needed for humans to become effective learners and successfully adaptive organisms. The vertical and horizontal developmental processes that underscore brain development lead to communications and controls that become more automatic and efficient with age and experience.[17] This guides our understanding of what it means to become executive across childhood and adolescence, as a representation of the resourcefulness and adaptability we possess that emerge over time. We become quite adept at engaging and utilizing cognitive controls in tandem with their ongoing maturation. But the system is prepared to provide effective, albeit less mature or adaptive supports from an early point in development, in line with emerging needs.[11]

Setting the frame: a review of essential building blocks of the executive network

As discussed above, the cognitive capacities that emerge across time to become executive capability are initially broad in scope; with refinement, they become intrinsic to many different aspects of information processing and behavior. They span the emergence of such foundational skills as orientation and attention, to the later appearing, highly complex aspects of problem solving, such as strategy identification and implementation. When considering EF from a developmental perspective, it becomes important to consider that the capacity to become executive is built upon multiple emergent cognitive skills; appreciating what it means to become executive requires understanding how each component capability builds across time (See Table 2.1). It is the goal of this section to frame the discussion of emergent EF, through a review of the skills that support its growth and elicitation.

Attention

The attentional system is a principal, supportive component of the emerging executive system. It is particularly active, from birth, as a means for directing engagement with the environment and subserving learning for the developing organism.[10,18–21] Over the course of infancy and into toddlerhood, the child becomes increasingly adept at directing engagement, taking in information from the environment, and establishing a foundation of schema and representations about the here and now that support and guide subsequent learning and adaptation to environmental demands and challenges.[22] As such, attention and attentional control interact neurodevelopmentally with the establishment of memory processes,[23] establishing the cognitive structures that are required for executive and behavioral control. As a result, emerging attentional and resulting goal directed behaviors in infancy and toddlerhood appear in tandem across time, and serve as early representatives of developing EF skills.[3,12,20,24]

The infant, through increasing awareness of the events and experiences taking place around her, also comes to recognize that she has an increasing influence on the information she encodes from the environment. This fosters, through direct and indirect interactions with objects and persons, a cognitive and behavioral dialogue. Motor, sensory, and emerging cognitive capacities interact to form representations between the infant and her environment, facilitating a set of experiences that form her immediate context. The infant gains increased control of her engagement with the environment; this is initially a passive response of directed engagement, then a process of exploration secondary to the hard-wired preference for novelty. It then becomes an active process, of seeking increased attachment and interaction. As people, events, and experiences become more familiar, the infant can more effectively detach herself attentionally from those events and experiences that she finds familiar, over-stimulating, and/or uncomfortable, and seeks, through behavioral and vocal responses, a specific form of support or nurturance.[25] Through mechanisms such as directed attention, purposeful reaching, and exploration, the young child begins to understand that she has a causal effect on the environment; this awareness coincides with what can be called early problem-solving skill, where action is engaged upon to reach goals and desires.

Behavioral and affective regulation

Self-regulation improves over the course of infancy, toddlerhood, and the elementary school years. Although directive parenting initially guides this developing capacity, the infant and then child herself develops expectations and reactions that guide how behavior plays out.[20,26–29] Through "hands-on" experience, observation, and imitation, the child becomes increasingly aware that her actions cause reactions. Using active recall of such experiences, the child makes behavioral choices. Strategy begins to play a larger role in her behavior, so that by late toddlerhood, examples of purposeful and even "stealth" behaviors are observed (e.g., hiding games, early denials of responsibility).[30–31] These efforts to guide outcome are clearly examples of emerging EF skills – problem solving, monitoring, strategy identification and implementation, and even rudimentary flexibility (e.g., finding another

Table 2.1. *Development of executive functions*

Executive function	Developmental period in which EF emerges	Studies
Attention Joint	Infancy/toddlerhood	• Carpenter M, Nagell K, Tomasello M. Social cognition, joint attention, and communicative competence from 9 to 15 months of age. *Monogr Soc Res Child Dev* 1998; **63**(4): 1–143. • Hoehl S, Reid V, Mooney J, Striano T. What are you looking at? Infants' neural processing of an adult's object-directed eye gaze. *Developmental Sci* 2008; **11**(1): 10–16. • Hood BM, Willen JD, Driver J. Adult's eyes trigger shifts of visual attention in human infants. *Psychol Sci* 1998; **9**(2): 131–4.
Regulation and control	Infancy/toddlerhood	• Harman C, Rothbart MK, Posner MI. Distress and attention interactions in early infancy. *Motiv Emot* 1997; **21**(1): 27–43. • Sheese BE, Rothbart MK, Posner MI, White LK, Fraundorf SH. Executive attention and self-regulation in infancy. *Infant Behav Dev* 2008; **31**(3): 501–10.
Sustained	Infancy/toddlerhood	• Richards JE, Casey BJ. Heart rate variability during attention phases in young infants. *Psychophysiology* 1991; **28**(1): 43–53. • Courage ML, Reynolds GD, Richards JE. Infants' attention to patterned stimuli: developmental change from 3 to 12 months of age. *Child Dev* 2006; **77**(3): 680–95.
Impulse Control and Self Regulation Behavioral and affective regulation	Infancy/toddlerhood	• Wentworth N, Haith MM, Karrer R. Behavioral and cortical measures of infants' visual expectations. *Infancy* 2001; **2**(2): 175–95. • Bernier A, Carlson SM, Whipple N. From external regulation to self-regulation: early parenting precursors of your children's executive functioning. *Child Dev* 2010; **8**(1): 326–39. • Diener ML, Mangelsdorf SC, MCHale JL, Frosch CA. Infants' behavioral strategies for emotion regulation with fathers and mothers: Associations with emotional expressions and attachment quality. *Infancy* 2002; **3**(2): 153–74. • Diener ML, Mangelsdorf SC. Behavioral strategies for emotion regulation in toddlers: associations with maternal involvement and emotional expressions. *Infant Behav Dev* 1999; **22**(4): 569–83. • Roque L, Verissimo M. Emotional context, maternal behavior and emotion regulation. *Infant Behav Dev* 2011; **34**(4): 617–26.

Table 2.1. (cont.)

Executive function	Developmental period in which EF emerges	Studies
Inhibition	Infancy/ toddlerhood	• Calkins SD, Fox NA, Marshall TR. Behavioral and physiological antecedents of inhibited and uninhibited behavior. *Child Dev* 1996; **67**(2): 523–40. • Bernier A, Carlson SM, Whipple N. From external regulation to self-regulation: early parenting precursors of your children's executive functioning. *Child Dev* 2010; **81**(1): 326–39. • Morasch KC, Bell MA. The role of inhibitory control in behavioral and physiological expressions of toddler executive function. *J Exp Child Psychol* 2011; **108**(3): 593–606.
Self-monitoring	Infancy/ toddlerhood	• Moore C, Mealiea J, Garon N, Povinelli DJ. The development of body self-awareness. *Infancy* 2007; **11**(2): 157–74. • Rochat P. Self-perception and action in infancy. *Exp Brain Res* 1998; **123**: 102–9. • Elsner B, Ascersleben G. Do I get what you get? Learning about the effects of self-performed observed actions in infancy. *Conscious Cog* 2003; **12**(4): 732–51.
Working memory	Infancy/ toddlerhood	• Diamond A. Evidence of robust recognition memory early in life even when assessed by reaching. *J Exp Psychol* 1995; **59**(3): 419–56. • Bell MA, Adams SE. Comparable performance on looking and reaching versions of the A-not-B task at 8 months of age. *Infant Behav Dev* 1999; **22**(2): 221–35. • Hoehl S, Reid V, Mooney J, Striano T. What are you looking at? Infants' neural processing of an adult's object-directed eye gaze. *Dev Sci* 2008; **11**(1): 10–16. • Gilmore RO, Johnson MH. Working memory in infancy: six-month-olds' performance on two versions of the oculomotor delayed response task. *J Exp Child Psychol* 1995; **59**(3): 397–418.
Cognitive Flexibility Two-dimensional	Early childhood	• Smidts DP, Jacobs R, Anderson V. The Object Classification Task for Children (OCTC): a measure of concept generation and mental flexibility in early childhood. *Dev Neuropsychol* 2004; **26**(1): 385–401. • Jacques S, Zelazo P. The Flexible Item Selection Task (FIST): a measure of executive function in preschoolers. *Dev Neuropsychol* 2001; **20**(3): 573–91. • Bennet J, Muller U. The development of flexibility and abstraction in preschool children. *Merrill Palmer Quart* 2010; **56**(4): 455–73.

Table 2.1. (*cont.*)

Executive function	Developmental period in which EF emerges	Studies
Three-dimensional	Middle childhood	• Anderson V, Anderson P, Northam E, Jacobs R, Catroppa C. Development of executive functions through late childhood and adolescence in an Australian sample. *Dev Neuropsychol* 2010; **20**(1): 385–406. • Crone EA, Ridderinkof KR, Worm M, Somsen RJM, van der Molen MW. Switching between spatial stimulus-response mappings: a developmental study of cognitive flexibility. *Dev Sci* 2004; **7**(4): 443–55.
Planning and Organization Planning	Early childhood	• Espy KA, Kaufman PM, Glisky ML, McDiarmid MD. New procedures to assess executive functions in preschool children. *Clin Neuropsychol* 2001; **15**(1): 46–58. • Luciana M, Nelson CA. Assessment of neuropsychological function through use of the Cambridge Neuropsychological Testing Automated Battery: Performance in 4- to 12-year-old children. *Dev Neuropsychol* 2002; **22**(3): 595–624. • Kaller CP, Rahm B, Spreer J, Mader I, Unterrainer JM. Thinking around the corner: the development of planning abilities. *Brain Cogn* 2008; **67**(3): 360–70.
Organization	Middle childhood	• Anderson P, Anderson V, Garth J. Assessment and development of organizational ability: the Rey Complex Figure organizational strategy score (RCF-OSS). *Clin Neuropsychol* 2001; **15**(1): 81–94. • Anderson VA, Anderson P, Northam E, Jacobs R, Catroppa A. Development of executive functions through late childhood and adolescence in an Australian sample. *Dev Neuropsychol* 2001; **20**(1): 385–406.
Problem Solving and Decision Making Affective decision making	Early childhood	• Kerr A, Zelazo, PD. Development of "hot" executive function: The children's gambling task. *Brain Cogni* 2004; **55**(1): 148–57. • Garon N, Moore C. Complex decision-making in early childhood. *Brain Cogni* 2004; **55**(1): 158–70.
Problem solving	Infancy/toddlerhood	• Chen Z, Siegler RS. Across the great divide: Bridging the gap between understanding toddlers' and older children's thinking. *Monogr Soc Res Child* 2000; **65**(2): 1–108. • Berger SE, Adolph KE, Kavookijan AE. Bridging the gap: Solving spatial means-ends relations in a locomotor task. *Child Dev* 2010; **81**(5): 1367–75. • Goubet N, Rochat O, Maire-Leblond C, Poss S. Learning from others in 9–18-month-old infants. *Infant Child Dev* 2006; **15**(2): 161–77.

Table 2.1. (cont.)

Executive function	Developmental period in which EF emerges	Studies
Metacognition	Early childhood	• Whitebread D, Coltman P, Pasternak DP, et al. The development of two observational tools for assessing metacognition and self-regulated learning in young children. *Metacogn Learn* 2009; **4**(1): 63–85. • Robson S. Self-regulation and metacognition in young children's self-initiated play and reflective dialogue. *Int J Early Years Educ* 2010; **18**(3): 227–41.
Affective decision making	Early adulthood	• Crone EA, van der Molen MW. Developmental changes in real life decision making: performance on a gambling task previously shown to depend on the ventromedial prefrontal cortex. *Dev Neuropsychol* 2004; **25**(3): 251–79. • Cauffman E, Steinberg L. (Im)maturity of judgment in adolescence: Why adolescents may be less culpable than adults. *Behav Sci Law* 2000; **18**(6): 741–60.
Information Processing	Early childhood	• Espy KA. The Shape School: assessing executive function in preschool children. *Dev Neuropsychol* 1997; **13**(4): 495–9. • Riva D, Nichelli F, Devoti M. Developmental aspects of verbal fluency and confrontation naming in children. *Brain Lang* 2000; **71**(2): 267–84.

way to obtain a cookie after being told "no"). As she comes to better understand the relationship between her actions and the responses of others around her, the young child increasingly shows creativity in both her choices and actions taken; this too may serve as a further representation of EF skill.

Working memory

The capacity to keep information online and to use that information effectively is a skill that emerges across infancy and early childhood. Although difficult to assess in preverbal young infants, research by Diamond[32] has demonstrated that by early toddlerhood, children are able to keep a representation of setting and place in mind, and can act on this information in the moment. This example of WM has been associated with the initial emergence of dorsolateral prefrontal cortex (DLPFC) control. What is less often discussed, however, is how subcortical memory networks work with developing frontal pathways to facilitate WM, including engaging with, encoding, and using information in the moment.[23,28] These types of neural connections underlie the development of WM and its corollary skill, inhibitory control, facilitating an increased set of problem-solving skills[33] (see also Chapter 3). As the individual matures, these systems work more effectively and flexibly, supporting increased automaticity in the child's environmental interactions and increasing control over choice and behavioral action.[15,17] The engagement of memory provides the foundation for many key EF skills to develop; attention to information being processed and stored in WM becomes self-directed and sustained impulse control emerges and improves. Orientation and engagement occur in response to the child's efforts to guide and shape experience. Learning becomes more automatic and less effortful, subserved by an increased set of goals and desires.

Executive functions in infancy and toddlerhood

There is overwhelming evidence that EF can be observed as early as infancy, and certainly during the preschool years. These earliest stages appear in the form of increasing attention and emerging self-regulation. Studies of attention and engagement, and the processing of novel information by infants and toddlers, conducted over the past 30 years, have substantially broadened our understanding of how and when EF skills emerge.[23,34] Work in the domain of developmental cognitive neuroscience has contributed significantly to the understanding that, although immature, the neural systems that emerge to direct and manage cognitive development are evident and engaged from infancy forward. We now understand that structural maturation of the frontal and subcortical circuits within the brain, given their complex and vast connections with the broader information processing and association regions, coordinates the trajectory of EF skills. Although the PFC experiences a protracted period of development, reflecting ongoing myelination and dendritic branching,[35] it nonetheless is active from infancy forward, monitoring and guiding multiple aspects of cognitive and behavior regulatory skill.

The majority of studies have converged to suggest that, where developmentally appropriate approaches to measurement are taken,[12,24,36-37] emerging EF skills are reliably and validly observed in children as young as 3 years of age. However, because the frontal lobes are active and engaged at birth, albeit in an immature, but still coordinated communication network with cerebellar, subcortical, and broader cortical circuits, it has also been suggested that developing capacities for regulating attention towards and away from objects and experiences, and the increasing demonstration of goal-directed motor behaviors may serve as indicators of executive controls in developing infants and young toddlers.[20,25,29,34] It is, however, important to recognize the term EF is seldom used in tandem with describing these behaviors, likely given that these capacities, specifically attention, exist as primary skills on their own; and they are genetically mediated developmentally, given their immaturity.[38] Nonetheless, it is important when understanding how regulation and control develop that we begin to appreciate the dependency EF skill development has on these early cognitive skills.

During the first 2 years of life, the infant moves from a situation of substantial dependence, with little actual behavioral control at all, to becoming an individual with an increasing capacity to appreciate and then direct increasing levels of engagement and interaction with the environment. Cortical development and its increasing coordination, given synaptic overproduction, pruning and sculpting based on experience, and myelination of emerging white matter tracts[39-40] contributes to the infant's ability to better take in and represent sensory experiences, and through coordination with increasing hippocampal development, remember and associate these experiences as knowledge stores. Genetic and environmental transactions contribute to the underlying neural patterning that unfolds, across the regions of the brain. This, in turn, supports increased capacities for taking in, through orientation, engagement, and sustained attention; and memorizing, through familiarity and an increased capacity to disengage with what is already experienced, and to engage with novel sources of stimulation.[10,14,18,21] Infants around 9 months of age, for example, struggle to inhibit previously learned responses, whereas most infants can effectively inhibit a prepotent response and shift to a new response set by their first birthday.[41] Recognition memory and eventually representational memory both reflect the infant's capacity for assimilating and accommodating experiences.[32,42] Marcovitch and Zelazo[43] reported findings from several studies that indicate an age-related improvement in WM, beginning in infancy and continuing throughout the lifespan, as evidenced by performance on delayed response tasks. Essentially, this pattern suggests that improved WM skill may occur as a consequence of PFC development. These capacities to represent the world and direct efforts at further learning serve as the foundation skills for becoming goal-directed and ultimately executive.

It is equally important to recognize that these skills emerge through a dynamic interaction the individual has with the environment. Attachment and subsequent engagement with the primary caretaker fosters the infant's security, which in turn allows for increased opportunity to venture out and take on more individual exploratory control.[44] As emotion regulation begins to come online, so too does an increasing capacity for exerting an impact on the environment, in order to gain greater independence and take in broader knowledge. The underlying control circuits, which include coordinated communications between the cerebellum, subcortex, developing PFC, association areas, and processing regions of the brain, foster and support the developing capacities for memory, categorization, and motor and emotional engagement.[45] The infant seeks to take in and make sense of what is around her, and to attempt to better engage with the opportunities the environment presents. This facilitates stronger associations between information sources; and with the increasing laying down of myelin, is more rapidly taken in and understood.[46–48]

Another element that supports increasing skill at early problem solving and association is the emergence of language. As the older infant begins to engage with sounds, and is supported in efforts to form words through interactions with others in the environment, she begins to recognize that greater control can be exacted. Over the course of toddlerhood, the child observes that words direct and guide not only self-initiated action, but also those of others.[47] This further serves to provide an awareness of internal and external controls that are possible, and is over time more effectively utilized in order to drive and respond to environmental contingencies. Language has been described by Barkley[49] (by way of Bronowski; see Chapter 1) as one of the preeminent cognitive capacities that direct later executive capabilities; specifically, language, as it becomes internalized, guides inhibitory controls and assists in the synthesis of higher order executive capacities such as WM, self-monitoring, and strategy identification and implementation.[10,50] Consequently, it is believed that early language skills promote the ongoing recognition by the child that cause and effect are intertwined, and that actions can lead to desired, or even undesired consequences.

Over time, the infancy and toddler period provide the foothold for developing self-control mechanisms, ones that will be required to facilitate greater success at social engagement and learning across time.[51] Through increasing directed responses to the environment, the infant comes to recognize that she has a capacity for dictating and altering how and when information is presented. As intentional behaviors, like reaching, come more fully into play, with the expanding capacity for limb movement and eventually, walking, the infant comes to understand more directly that having a purpose and following through on action can lead to the obtainment of an object that is desired. Through interactions with others, specifically the primary objects of attachment (mother, father, siblings), the youngster begins to understand that there are both appropriate and inappropriate responses. Language development facilitates how information is absorbed, processed, practiced internally, and responded to environmentally. Through the emerging skills that underlie self-control, mainly attention, engagement, gross and fine motor control, memory, and expressive and receptive language, the toddler moves toward greater self-sufficiency and enters the learning environment as an actor.[52,53]

Executive functions in the early school years

The preschool years leading into kindergarten are a period of substantial and rapid change in the developing brain and an important phase in the development of EF skills, particularly self-control and self-concept. In line with the concurrent processes of neural proliferation and more active pruning, which reflects and determines increasing efficiencies in basic information processing, and coupled with increasing myelination of the frontal and prefrontal systems, the preschool age child begins to show fairly dramatic increases in EF skills. These include growing capacity for inhibitory control, increased engagement and sustained attention, developing WM, and motor persistence.[54-55] By 3 years of age, most children can inhibit "instinctive" behaviors reasonably well, and significant improvements in response speed and verbal fluency become evident.[41,56-57] Basic planning skills and the ability to switch rapidly between two simple response sets are exhibited by children between 3 and 4 years of age.[41,57] Simultaneously, a wider range of behaviors and actions are demonstrated by the youngster, across multiple cognitive and regulatory domains. Concurrent with this is recognition of rules and an increased reliance on them as behavioral guides, as well as growing efforts at thwarting such rules in a display of independence. The emergence of these increased capacities for behavior regulation and cognitive efficiency serve to prepare the preschooler for increased demands in the domains of socialization and learning.

The increased display of authority and even defiance is a common experience for parents of toddlers; this signals the emergence of self-control. Three- and 4-year-old preschoolers frequently say "no" as a response to requests and edicts adults present to them. This reflects several aspects of increasing EF skills in relation to growing independence; notably a sense of one's self as an authority, awareness that other's wishes and goals may be out of synch with one's own desires, and finally, an expression, using increased skill with language, at directing a situation and its outcome.[58] Although most preschoolers are easily thwarted from these efforts to exert control, these efforts do represent their desire to guide and direct others in order to meet their own wants and needs.[58] To reach the point where "no" becomes an option, the preschooler must first recognize that she has agency and an impact on the immediate environment; this is a culmination of much of what has been emerging across the first 2 years of life, and is now at a crucial point for being sculpted into individual action.

The preschooler is also at an important point where she realizes the potential for shared purpose around such demands as behavior and emotion regulation. Recollection of previous responses to requests and desires motivates improved efforts at gaining increased independence or support. These memories are then expressed more directly as requests and demands through the use of language; purpose dictates action or the choice of inaction in response to a request. Contingencies are understood and internalized more readily, and challenged more directly. Negotiating emerges as a particular strategy in older preschoolers, as they begin to understand that the adults around them seek reasons for their decisions and actions.[58]

Coupled with increased awareness of other's intentions, the preschooler also begins to more directly engage in practice, through play, of the rules and regulations that guide behavior. Direction and intention become dominant aspects of skill during the preschool period. Preschool age is a time where children begin to show an active awareness of time in the short and long term, hold information more readily in mind, and use that information to guide choice and action. Yet there remains an immaturity to the system, a propensity for short-term versus delayed gratification, that underscores the continued vulnerability to disinhibition and the lack of fully engaged internal controls that characterize this period developmentally.[59] Temper tantrums, inattention across time, frustration and irritability when tired, and varied interests all serve as reminders that the system of regulation is still quite immature, and in need of external scaffolding and support.[59-60]

It is also during the preschool period that biologically determined tendencies associated with temperament continue to influence and direct the expression of emerging cognitive skills.[61-62] This is particularly seen with the executive capabilities. As has been shown by research by Mary Rothbart and her associates, as well as in studies by Jerome Kagan, Nathan Fox, and others, core features of temperament interact with emerging cognitive skills, and guide and influence their engagement[61]. Attention, in particular, has been shown to be particularly sensitive to features of temperament; inhibited infants and toddlers show delayed acquisition of attentional control, and as these youngsters approach preschool age, reticence and anxiety emerge as strong influences on self-direction and interaction.[63-64] Kagan's work looking at the development of shyness, in particular, has fostered a stronger understanding of the relationship between behavioral inhibition and a delay in self-expression, independence, and social collaboration.[65-66] Consequently, it has become quite important to consider how executive development interacts with temperament, both identifying contributors to risk and resilience from the preschool period forward and guiding efforts at intervention.

Lastly, it is important to reiterate that the prevalent task for the preschool period is preparation for more active learning. In order for children to move towards acquiring the skills that foster reading, written expression, and mathematical problem solving, they must be able to direct effort towards demands placed on them, and to collaborate on day-to-day problem solving.[67] This requires increased aspects of self-control, engagement with the environment, and motivation.[68-69] Separately, it becomes important for the preschooler to inhibit self-directed goals, in order to work collaboratively with others, both socially and in the learning environment.[70] The environment for the preschooler changes from one of primarily self-direction, albeit with parental monitoring and influence, to one that is more directly managed by others; to accommodate to this change, the child is required to stop and reconsider an idea or option before moving forward. This is a critical example of EF in this developmental period; absence of this "stop and think" skill can be an early indication of continuing EdF. As such, it is not surprising that one of the more prevalent periods for diagnosis of a potential executive concern is at the transition point between preschool/ kindergarten age and first through third grade, when demands for self-direction and control increase dramatically.

Executive functions in the middle childhood years

Middle childhood is one of the principal periods during which EF skills are required to support successful learning and development of academic skills.[15,24] As children move through the first three grades, they are supported as they learn to identify what is important and integrate new information with existing knowledge. From the fourth grade forward, however, an increased expectation is placed on the learner to more skillfully and strategically manage integrated academic demands.[71-72] Significant demands are placed on WM, inhibition, self-monitoring, and intentionality, in order to facilitate independent problem solving and efficiency. For the typically developing middle school child, demands are met with variable engagement of EF skills, while learning success proceeds in a forward line, indicating a growing capacity for independence. In fact, there is considerable evidence to suggest that many types of inhibitory control, for example, are fully developed between 10 and 12 years of age.[54,73] Similar gains in processing speed, verbal fluency, multi-dimensional switching, and planning and organizational skills typically occur during middle childhood.[54,41,74]

Middle childhood also proves to be a period that demands increased attention across time, with expectations for vigilance and sustained motivation put forth. Successful learning comes to require increased behavioral regulation.[69] By age 6, children demonstrate marked improvements on impulse control tasks, and by age 9, most children can self-monitor and regulate their own actions reasonably well.[41,56,75] Children who effectively manage these increased demands for attention and regulation often show strong capacities for inhibition, delayed gratification, persistence, and verbal self-talk to guide demands for control. Emotional regulation, particularly regulation of frustration, anxiety, and irritability, underscores the increasing capacity for meeting increased daily demands and challenges. In contrast, difficulties with attentional and behavioral control, such as are commonly seen with ADHD and the disruptive behavior disorders (DBD), highlight a likely disruption in unfolding EF skills; inefficiency, inattention and distractibility, and poor self-control emerge as the predominant pattern of symptoms as increased challenge occurs.[75-77]

The improved capacity for self-regulation is necessary to meet additional demands that emerge during the middle childhood period, particularly in the realm of social affiliations. Youngsters at this age begin to more strongly affiliate with same aged peers, and collaborative opportunities, across play and learning, frequently take place. This social affiliation serves to likely increase opportunities, neurologically and neurobehaviorally, for strengthening and extending the aspects of executive control to a wider sphere of engagement and influence. In particular, shared efforts at problem solving involve the school-age child in situations where ideas and goals can be elaborated and then modified, given the opportunity to take in and consider other's viewpoints. Demands for collaboration and compromise serve to challenge self-oriented efforts and provide the child with a broadened set of expectations and contingencies to master. Weaknesses in social comprehension and in-the-moment problem solving can serve to challenge efforts at social engagement. And it is not uncommon to observe that the child who is unable to take another's perspective, or who struggles to step back and consider the broader options being presented during a group activity is frequently a child with an executive deficit, that impacts multiple domains of socialization and academic functioning.[78]

Executive functions in adolescence

Adolescence is a principal period for the engagement of metacognition, the capacity to know what is required, evaluate options, and make a strategic choice to meet that current demand. Continued development in the executive neural network may help explain why adolescence is characterized by inconsistencies in engagement of higher-order skills.[79–81] Frontal functioning continues to slowly come on line during this time,[79] particularly in the DLPFC and orbitofrontal cortex (OFC) regions. There is also a significant decrease in grey matter and increase in white matter that takes place across the cortex during adolescence.[79–80] Coupled with this period of substantial brain structural change is a substantial alteration in context; specifically, social awareness and expectations, and hormonal and physical changes combine to alter the impact and salience of self and the environment.[82] As such, adolescents show variability in their awareness, decision-making, and capacity for problem solving that is highly influenced by cognitive abilities and their emotional, social, and physical situations.[38] Consequently, it has been theorized by some[83] that EF development in adolescence "may be modulated by affective or social context" (p. 827). Luna and Sweeney[84] have described adolescence as a period of "transition to efficient brain collaboration," to reflect the aggregation of imaging and behavioral data that suggest that, as the brain becomes more adult like in its functioning, over the course of this period, its executive networks consolidate and refine in their interaction. Behavior becomes more synchronized and engaged, and the influences on behavior and emotion become better controlled.

Efforts at independence and capacities for managing multidimensional learning and behavioral demands improve significantly during adolescence. This is a reflection of increased attentional control, improved flexibility and increased processing speed, greater capacity for inhibition, and improvements in WM, strategic planning, and problem solving, which are likely linked to ongoing pruning and myelination in the frontal cortex that occurs throughout adolescence.[54,85] Although their respective developmental trajectories differ, Anderson[3,41] suggests that the capacities for information processing, cognitive flexibility and goal setting are largely mature by age 12. Other researchers, however, point out that many components of EF, including set shifting, WM updating, inhibition, and planning continue to improve considerably throughout adolescence and into early adulthood.[3,41,67,86] A brief regression of planning skills occurs between 12 and 13 years of age, during which time a preference for conceptual strategies gives way to a more cautious, piecemeal approach; this pattern resolves rather quickly, however, and a return to refined strategy and improved decision making is typically observed.[41,87] Some research has linked this phenomenon to the proliferation of synapses that occurs at the onset of puberty.[85] Emotion regulation becomes well enhanced with these executive improvements; affective decision making becomes less a reflection of reactivity to the environment and its demands, and is moreso, a guided and directed effort toward self-control and the enactment of socially appropriate rules.[81,88]

Deficits in development of executive controls across adolescence help us understand current and emerging vulnerabilities to psychopathology. The capacity to think through before acting, to contain one's response in order to assess its appropriateness, and to determine the most effective choice of action given a desired outcome are frequently observed to be variable skills in adolescents; nonetheless, in the typically developing teenager, these skills become more and more effective in their demonstration across time.[88] In youth who are showing EdF, the knowledge that a particular response is optimal does not serve to lead to the most effective choice or outcome. In fact, as adolescents become more self-conscious with the start of pubertal maturation, they get involved in risky and sometimes reckless behavior and they become increasingly sensitive to the opinions and evaluations of others.[81,83] This creates a challenging set of experiences with peers and adults. Distinguishing between what is developmentally appropriate and what might reflect an underlying EdF remains an active area of research in executive development.

Executive functions in early adulthood

The timing of mature adulthood has become less and less certain as we have become more knowledgeable about EF skill development and, in particular, the protracted period under which frontal systems unfold. Although the task of the young adult is to become more independent and capable of effective decision making, research has shown that there continues to be a slow, but certain trajectory of development in this capacity that takes place into the third decade of life.[38,89] The ongoing balance between myelination of the orbitofrontal region of the PFC, and the maturation of association and regulatory regions, specifically white matter tracts, reflects the continued structural refinement in the brain that underserves increased EF skills.[80,89] It is, in fact, during the 20s that individuals show their EF skill peak; WM, strategy development, flexibility, goal setting, and efficiency with problem solving all reach their maximum level as adulthood is entered.[90–92] This supports the growing capacity for individuation and life planning that is demanded of young adults at this point in time.

It is during early adulthood when the accumulated impact of developmental disability in the form of EdF can come to have its most significant effect. Difficulties with meeting the challenges associated with college level learning, choosing a career, and setting a path towards meeting life goals commonly occur. A young adult with significant EdF often struggles to meet adult-level expectations in line with typically developing peers, and as a result, shows increased vulnerability to mood, behavior, and substance-use disorders.[81] As well, independent efforts at support can be varied in their success for these individuals, particularly when they have not been ongoing to this point. While change and improved capability is definitely possible, it is often a challenge for the young adult to identify and then implement, independently, solutions and strategies for managing EdF. As such, it is best if one can build on efforts that have been lifelong whenever possible. This can facilitate both faster change and less stressful routes to improvement in capability. Unfortunately, this is not always possible.

What is definitive when considering early adulthood and executive development is the greater association with frontal functioning that can be made. With the coming fully online of the frontal systems, much of what is considered executive is now particularly managed and directed through these mature circuits. Nonetheless, broader networks remain at play; newer and novel learning experiences remain broad in their elicitation of executive programming, while familiar demands are met with greater efficiency and ease, given the more directly automatic responses that are engaged to manage them. This is ultimately the best reflection of what it means to be an adult; to be able to meet familiar and frequent demands in a highly flexible, automatic manner, with ongoing self-monitoring taking place just outside of awareness. This facilitates such skills as higher order reading comprehension, written communication, and even driving; it is the executive system in the background that is monitoring and engaging the appropriate cognitive processes that underserve these problem solving tasks.

Summary and future directions

The development of EF skills begins soon after birth, as the infant begins to interact with her environment, and continues into adulthood. Improvements in cognitive capacities like attention, behavioral regulation, and WM during the first two years of life enable the child to direct her engagement with the environment such that they provide the foundation for increased learning and growing skill at problem solving. The primary caregiver, the acquisition of language, and improved self-control together facilitate interaction with the environment during infancy and toddlerhood.

The focus of the early childhood years is to prepare for learning that is more active; it is supported by improvements in inhibition, WM, verbal fluency, and planning abilities. Throughout the school years, academic demands increase and EF continue to evolve in order to support ongoing needs for managing complexity, increasing learning efficiency, and enhancing academic skill. The structural changes taking place across the brain reflect increased maturation and support improved fluency in both behavioral and regulatory skills. As myelination and increased synaptic pruning continue into adolescence, there is improved synchrony among neural networks. These anatomical changes, coupled with other physiological changes, and new environmental experiences and demands, give rise to the variability in problem solving and decision making abilities characteristic of this developmental period.

Although the brain continues to change throughout life, it is during young adulthood that the PFC reaches maturity and capacity, such that EF skills peak during this time. Young adults can meet demands flexibly and automatically; they make decisions, problem solve, plan, and strategize both efficiently and effectively. This collaboration between behavior, experience, and brain maturation reflect improved EF.

Alterations in this developmental trajectory can have pervasive and long lasting consequences. Whereas EdF during childhood is typically evidenced by difficulty meeting academic demands, during adolescence, EdF may be associated with poor decision making and engagement in high-risk behaviors, some of which are associated with other physical and psychological sequelae. During young adulthood, EdF may affect an individual's ability to meet adult-level expectations, such as maintaining a job and paying bills. Individuals who have difficulty achieving developmentally appropriate EF skills are vulnerable to a range of psychopathology, including mood, learning, and disruptive behavior disorders, which may further exacerbate problems in functioning.

Research to date has brought us quite far in understanding how EF skills emerge and mature across time; and yet, we remain still at the forefront in terms of our knowledge. Ongoing studies are required to continue to move us forward in how we make sense of the increasing capacity brain maturation brings to EF, as well as how to recognize EdF and intervene appropriately. Several avenues of continued emphasis are identified. First, neuropsychology remains adult "privileged" with regard to models and theories. This conflicts with our growing understanding of brain development and the resulting models of what it means, broadly and specifically, to be executive. Second, developmental neuropsychological research, which is informed by our increased understanding of early brain systems and their engagement, and that takes a longitudinal, lifespan perspective may better inform us about how neural development during childhood and adolescence, and its consequent effects on behavioral and emotional function influence and guide adult capacity. In line with this, studies that continue to clarify and support our understanding of the processes that define the development of EF through childhood and adolescence are still needed, particularly given that many studies overtime continue to present with conflicting results. Third, as we come to appreciate the lack of sensitivity and reliability of measures that serve as downward extensions of those created for adults, the production of developmentally appropriate, psychometrically sound measures of emerging EF is strongly warranted. And lastly, as will be discussed in the chapters that follow, the literature would also benefit greatly from research that examines a broader host of environmental effects (e.g., socio-economic status, birth status, nutrition, and environmental stress) on the developing brain and EF. This would not only provide insight about environmental and sociological pressures that alter typical development, but also may highlight periods where developmentally informed interventions may be effective.

References

1. Lezak M. *Neuropsychological Assessment*, 3rd edn. New York: Oxford University Press; 1995.

2. Fuster JM. Frontal lobe and cognitive development. *J Neurocytol* 2002; **31**(3–5): 373–85.

3. Anderson PJ. Towards a developmental model of executive function. In Anderson V, Jacobs R, Anderson P, eds. *Executive Functions and the Frontal Lobes: A Lifespan Perspective*. Philadelphia, PA: Taylor & Francis; 2008, 3–21.

4. Bernstein JH, Waber DP. Executive capacities from a developmental perspective. In Meltzer L, ed. *Executive Function in Education: From Theory to Practice*. New York, NY: Guilford Press; 2007, 39–54.

5. Pennington BF. *Diagnosing Learning Disorders, Second Edition: A Neuropsychological Framework*. New York, NY: Guilford Press; 2009.

6. Fuster JM. *The Prefrontal Cortex: Anatomy, Physiology and Neuropsychology of the Frontal Lobe*, 2nd edn. New York: Raven Press; 1989.

7. Shallice T. *From Neuropsychology to Mental Structure*. New York: Cambridge University Press; 1990.

8. Stuss DT, Benson DF. *The Frontal Lobes*. New York: Raven Press; 1986.

9. Anderson V, Jacobs R, Anderson PJ. *Executive Functions and the Frontal Lobes: A Lifespan Perspective*. New York, NY: Taylor & Francis; 2008.

10. Carpenter M, Nagell K, Tomasello M. Social cognition, joint attention, and communicative competence from 9 to 15 months of age. *Monogr Soc Res Child Dev* 1998; **63**(4): 1–143.

11. Diamond A, Barnett WS, Thomas J, Munro S. Preschool program improves cognitive control. *Science* 2007; **318**(5855): 1387–8.

12. Espy KA. Using developmental, cognitive, and neuroscience approaches to understand executive control in young children. *Dev Neuropsychol* 2004; **26**(1): 379–84.

13. Hoehl S, Reid V, Mooney J, Striano T. What are you looking at? Infants' neural processing of an adult's object-directed eye gaze. *Developmental Sci* 2008; **11**(1): 10–16.

14. Hood BM, Willen JD, Driver J. Adult's Eyes Trigger Shifts of Visual Attention in human infants. *Psychol Sci* 2011; **9**(2): 131–4.

15. Mahone EM, Slomine BS. Managing dysexecutive disorders. In Hunter S, Donders J, eds. *Pediatric Neuropsychological Intervention*. Cambridge, UK: Cambridge University Press; 2007, 287–313.

16. Jerison HJ. Evolution of prefrontal cortex. In: Krasnegor NA, Lyon GR, Goldman-Rakic, eds. *Development of the Prefrontal Cortex*. Baltimore, MD: Brookes; 1997, 9–26.

17. Williamson J. A lifespan review of developmental neuroanatomy. In Donders J, Hunter, SJ, eds. *Principles and Practice of Lifespan Developmental Neuropsychology*. Cambridge, UK: Cambridge University Press; 2010, 3–16.

18. Courage ML, Reynolds GD, Richards JE. Infants' attention of patterned stimuli: Developmental change from 3 to 12 months of age. *Child Dev* 2006; 77(3): 680–95.

19. Harman C, Rothbart MK, Posner MI. Distress and attention interactions in early infancy. *Motiv Emotion* 1997; 21(1): 27–43.

20. Posner MI, Rothbart MK. *Educating the Human Brain*. Washington, DC: American Psychological Association; 2007.

21. Richards JE, Casey BJ. Heart rate variability during attention phases in young infants. *Psychophysiology* 1991; 28(1): 43–53.

22. Espy KA, Kaufmann PM, McDiarmid MD. Executive functioning in preschool children: performance on A-Not-B and other delayed response tasks. *Brain Cognition* 1999; 41(2): 178–99.

23. Nelson CA, de Haan M, Thomas KM. *Neuroscience of Cognitive Development: The Role of Experience and The Developing Brain*. Hoboken, NJ: John Wiley & Sons, Inc; 2006.

24. Anderson V, Anderson PJ, Jacobs R, Smith MS. Development and assessment of executive function: From preschool to adolescence. In Anderson V, Jacobs R, Anderson P, eds. *Executive Functions and the Frontal Lobes: A Lifespan Perspective*. Philadelphia, PA: Taylor & Francis; 2008, 123–54.

25. Sheese BE, Rothbart MK, Posner MI, White LK, Fraundorf SH. Executive attention and self-regulation in infancy. *Infant Behav Dev* 2008; 31(3): 501–10.

26. Bernier A, Carlson SM, Whipple N. From external regulation to self-regulation: early parenting precursors to young children's executive functioning. *Child Dev* 2010; 81(1): 326–39.

27. Diener ML, Mangelsdorf SC, Mchale JL, Frosch CA. Infants' behavioral strategies for emotion regulation with fathers and mothers: associations with emotional expressions and attachment quality. *Infancy* 2002; 3(2): 153–74.

28. Nelson CA, Zeanah CH, Fox NA, Marshall PJ, Smyke AT, Guthrie D. Cognitive recovery in socially deprived young children: The Bucharest Early Intervention Project. *Science* 2007; 21:318(5858): 1937–40.

29. Wentworth N, Haith MM, Karrer R. Behavioral and cortical measures of infants' visual expectations. *Infancy* 2001; 2(2): 175–95.

30. Calkins SD. The emergence of self-regulation: biological and behavioral control mechanisms supporting toddler competencies. In Brownell CA, Kopp CB, eds. *Socioemotional Development in the Toddler Years: Transitions and Transformations*. New York, NY: Guilford Press, 1–45.

31. Sethi A, Mischel W, Aber JL, Shoda Y, Rodriguez ML. The role of strategic attention deployment in development of self-regulation: predicting preschoolers' delay of gratification from mother-toddler interactions. *Dev Psychol* 2000; 36(6): 767–77.

32. Diamond, A. Evidence of robust recognition memory early in life even when assessed by reaching behavior. *J Exp Child Psychol* 1995; 59(3): 419–56.

33. Best JR, Miller PH, Jones LL. Executive functions after age 5: Changes and correlates. *Dev Rev* 2010; 29(3): 180–200.

34. Nelson CA, Luciana M. *Handbook of Developmental Cognitive Neuroscience*, 2nd edn. Cambridge, MA: The MIT Press; 2008.

35. Casey BJ, Giedd JN, Thomas KM. Structural and functional brain development and its relation to cognitive development. *Bio Psychol* 2000; 54(1–3): 241–57.

36. Diamond, A. Normal development of prefrontal cortex from birth to young adulthood: Cognitive functions, anatomy, and biochemistry. In Stuss DT, Knight RT, eds. *Principles of Frontal Lobe Function.* London, UK: Oxford University Press; 2002, 466–503.

37. Welsh M, Pennington B, Groisser D. A normative-developmental study of executive function: a window on prefrontal function in children. *Dev Neuropsychol* 1991; 7: 131–49.

38. De Luca CR, Leventer RJ. Developmental trajectories of executive functions across the lifespan. In Anderson V, Jacobs R, Anderson P, eds. *Executive Functions and the Frontal Lobes: A Lifespan Perspective.* Philadelphia, PA: Taylor & Francis; 2008, 23–56.

39. Huttenlocher PR. Synaptic density in human frontal cortex – developmental changes and effects of aging. *Brain Res* 1979; **163**(2): 195–205.

40. Huttenlocher PR, Dabholkar AS. Regional differences in synaptogenesis in human cerebral cortex. *J Comp Neurol* 1997; **387**(2): 167–78.

41. Anderson P. Assessment and development of executive function (EF) during childhood. *Child Neuropsychol* 2002; **8**(2): 71–82.

42. Gilmore RO, Johnson MH. Working memory in infancy: six-month-olds' performance on two versions of the oculomotor delayed response task. *J Exp Child Psychol* 1995; **59**(3): 397–418.

43. Marcovitch S, Zelazo PD. A hierarchical competing systems model of the emergence and early development of executive function: *Dev Sci* 2009; **12**(1): 1–18.

44. Schieche M, Spangler G. Individual differences in biobehavioral organization during problem-solving in toddlers: the influence of maternal behavior, infant–mother attachment, and behavioral inhibition on the attachment–exploration balance. *Dev Psychobiol* 2005; **46**(4): 293–306.

45. Richmond J, Nelson CA. Accounting for change in declarative memory: A cognitive neuroscience perspective. *Dev Rev* 2007; **27**(3): 349–73.

46. Deoni SCL, Mercure E, Blasi A, *et al.* Mapping infant brain myelination with magnetic resonance imaging. *J Neurosci* 2011; **31**(2): 784–91.

47. Herschkowitz N. Neurological bases of behavioral development in infancy. *Brain Dev* 2000; **22**(7): 411–16.

48. Picton TW, Taylor MJ. Electrophysiological evaluation of human brain development. *Dev Neuropsychol* 2007; **31**(3): 249–78.

49. Barkley RA. Genetics of childhood disorders: XVII. ADHD, Part 1: The executive functions and ADHD. *J Am Acad Child Psychol* 2000; **39**(8): 1064–8.

50. Vaughn BE, Kopp CB, Krakow JB. The emergence and consolidation of self-control from eighteen to thirty months of age: Normative trends and individual differences. *Child Dev* 1984; **55**(3): 990–1004.

51. Kochanska G, Murray KT, Harlan ET. Effortful control in early childhood: Continuity and change, antecedents, and implications for social development. *Dev Psychol* 2000; **36**(2): 220–32.

52. Lindsey EW, Cremeens PR, Colwell MJ, Caldera YM. The structure of parent-child dyadic synchrony in toddlerhood and children's communication competence and self-control. *Soc Dev* 2009; **18**(2): 375–96.

53. Olson SL, Bates JE, Sandy JM, Schilling EM. Early developmental precursors of impulsive and inattentive behavior: From infancy to middle childhood. *J Child Psychol* 2002; **43**(4): 435–47.

54. Brocki KC, Bohlin G. Executive functions in children aged 6 to 13: A dimensional and developmental study. *Dev Neuropsychol* 2004; **26**(2): 571–93.

55. Kochanska G, Murray K, Jacques TY, Koenig AL, Vandegeest KA. Inhibitory control in young children and its role in emerging internalization. *Child Dev* 1996; **67**(2): 490–507.

56. Diamond A, Taylor C. Development of an aspect of executive control: development of

the abilities to remember what I said and to "do as I say, not as I do." *Dev Psychobiol* 1996; **29**(4): 315–34.

57. Espy KA. The Shape School: Assessing executive function in preschool children. *Dev Neuropsychol* 1997; **13**(4): 495–9.

58. Kuczynski L, Kochanska G. Development of children's noncompliance strategies from toddlerhood to age 5. *Dev Psychol* 1990; **26**(3): 398–408.

59. Cole PM, Tan PZ, Hall SE, *et al.* Developmental changes in anger expression and attention focus: Learning to wait. *Dev Psychol* 2011; **47**(4): 1078–89.

60. Potegal M, Kosorok MR, Davidson RJ. Temper tantrums in young children: 2. Tantrum duration and temporal organization. *J Dev Behav Pediatr* 2003; **24**(3): 148–54.

61. Rothbart MK, Sheese BE, Rueda MR, Posner MI. Developing mechanisms of self-regulation in early life. *Emot Rev* 2011; **3**(2): 207–13.

62. Wolfe CD, Bell MA. Working memory and inhibitory control in early childhood: Contributions from physiology, temperament, and language. *Dev Psychobiol* 2004; **44**(1): 68–83.

63. Chang F, Burns BM. Attention in preschoolers: Associations with effortful control and motivation. *Child Dev* 2005; **76**(1): 247–63.

64. Rothbart MK, Ellis LK, Rueda MR, Posner MI. Developing mechanisms of temperamental effortful control. *J Pers* 2003; **71**(6): 1113–43.

65. Kagan J, Reznick JS, Snidman N. Biological bases of childhood shyness. *Science* 1988; **240**(4849): 167–71.

66. Kagan J, Reznick JS, Gibbons J. Inhibited and uninhibited types of children. *Child Dev* 1989; **60**(4): 838–45.

67. Brock LL, Rimm-Kaufman SE, Nathanson L, Grimm KJ. The contributions of "hot" and "cool" executive function to children's academic achievement, learning-related behaviors, and engagement in kindergarten. *Early Child Res Q* 2009; **24**(3): 337–49.

68. Senn TE, Espy KA, Kaufmann PM. Using path analysis to understand executive function organization in preschool children. *Dev Neuropsychol* 2004; **26**(1): 445–64.

69. Valiente C, Lemery-Chalfant K, Castro KS. Children's effortful control and academic competence mediation through school liking. *Science* 2007; **53**(1): 1–25.

70. Tarullo AR, Milner S, Gunnar MR. Inhibition and exuberance in preschool classrooms: Associations with peer social experiences and changes in cortisol across the preschool year. *Dev Psychol* 2011; **47**(5): 1374–88.

71. Denckla MB. Biological correlates of learning and attention: what is relevant to learning and attention-deficit hyperactivity Disorder? *J Dev Behav Pediatr* 1996; **17**(2): 114–19.

72. Denckla MB. Introduction: ADHD and modifiers of the syndrome: influences on educational outcomes. *Dev Disabil Rev* 2008; **14**(4): 259–60.

73. Brocki K, Fan J, Fossella J. Placing neuroanatomical models of executive function in a developmental context: Imaging and imaging-genetic strategies. In Pfaff DW, Kieffer, BL, eds. *Molecular and Biophysical Mechanisms of Arousal, Alertness, and Attention*. 2008. Boston, MA: Blackwell Publishing, 246–55.

74. Williams BR, Ponesse JS, Schacher RJ, Logan GD, Tannock R. Development of inhibitory control across the life span. *Dev Psychol* 1999; **35**(1): 205–13.

75. van der Meere J, Stemerdink N. The development of state regulation in normal children: An indirect comparison with children with ADHD. *Dev Neuropsychol* 1999; **16**(2): 213–25.

76. Berlin L, Bohlin G, Nyberg L, Janols L. How well do measures of inhibition and other executive functions discriminate between children with ADHD and controls? *Child Neuropsychol* 2004; **10**(1): 1–13.

77. Geurts HM, Verté S, Oosterlaan J, Roeyers H, Sergeant JA. ADHD subtypes: Do they differ in their executive functioning profile? *Arch Clin Neuropsych* 2005; **20**(4): 457–77.

78. Fahie CM, Symons DK. Executive functioning and theory of mind in children clinically referred for attention and behavior problems. *J Appl Dev Psychol* 2003. **24**(1): 51–73.

79. Sowell ER, Thompson PM, Leonard CM, Welcome SE, Kan E, Toga AW. Longitudinal mapping of cortical thickness and brain growth in normal children. *J Neurosci* 2004; **24**(38): 8223–31.

80. Giedd JN, Blumenthal J, Jeffries NO, *et al.* Brain development during childhood and adolescence: A longitudinal MRI study. *Nat Neurosci* 1999; **2**(1): 861–3.

81. Pharo H, Sim C, Graham M, Gross J, Hayne H. Risky business: Executive function, personality, and reckless behavior during adolescence and emerging adulthood. *Behav Neurosci* 2011; **125**(6): 970–8.

82. Steinberg L. Cognitive and affective development in adolescence. *Trends Cogn Sci* 2005; **9**(2): 69–74.

83. Crone EA. Executive functions in adolescence: Inferences from brain and behavior. *Developmental Sci* 2009; **12**(6): 825–30.

84. Luna B, Sweeney JA. The emergence of collaborative brain function: fMRI studies of the development of response inhibition. In Dahl RE, Spear LP, eds. *Adolescent Brain Development: Vulnerabilities and Opportunities*. New York, NY: New York Academy of Sciences; 2004, 296–309.

85. Blakemore S, Choudhury S. Development of the adolescent brain: Implications for executive function and social cognition. *J Child Psychol Psychiatry* 2006; **47**(3–4): 296–312.

86. Tamnes CK, Østby Y, Fjell AM, Westlye LT, Due-Tønnessen P, Walhovd KB. Brain maturation in adolescence and young adulthood: Regional age-related changes in cortical thickness and white matter volume and microstructure. *Cereb Cortex* 2010; **20**(3): 534–48.

87. Anderson P, Anderson V, Garth J. Assessment and development of organizational ability: The Rey Complex Figure Organizational Strategy Score (RCF-OSS). *Clin Neuropsychol* 2001; **15**(1): 81–94.

88. Smith DG, Xiao L, Bechara A. Decision making in children and adolescents: Impaired Iowa Gambling Task performance in early adolescence. *Dev Psychol* 2011: 1–8. doi: 10.1037/a0026342.

89. Sowell ER, Thompson PM, Tessner KD, Toga AW. Mapping continued brain growth and gray matter density reduction in dorsal frontal cortex: Inverse relationships during postadolescent brain maturation. *J Neurosci* 2001; **21**(22): 8819–29.

90. De Luca CR, Wood SJ, Anderson V, *et al.* Normative data from the Cantab. I: Development of executive function over the lifespan. *J Clin Exp Neuropsychol* 2003; **25**(2): 242–54.

91. Huizinga M, Dolan CV, van der Molen MW. Age-related change in executive function: Developmental trends and a latent variable analysis. *Neuropsychologia* 2006; **44**(11): 2017–36.

92. Salat DH, Tuch DS, Greve DN, *et al.* Age-related alterations in white matter microstructure measured by diffusion tensor imaging. *Neurobiol Aging* 2005; **26**(8): 1215–27.

The neurobiology of executive functions

Scott J. Hunter, Clayton D. Hinkle, and Jennifer P. Edidin

Executive functions are a set of interdependent, progressively acquired, higher-order cognitive skills that emerge in tandem with the expansion and integration of cerebellar, subcortical, corticocortical, and prefrontal neural networks across early childhood, through adolescence, and into early adulthood. Because the development of neural systems that support EF is so protracted, it is vulnerable across time to alterations in its unfolding trajectory, resulting in multiple possible routes to EdF. This chapter provides a summary of the underlying neuroanatomical and neurochemical substrates of EF development that support the behavioral and cognitive capacities discussed in Chapter 2. Although a primary emphasis of this chapter is typical EF development, discussion of abnormalities in and insults to the developing circuits that support EF are also considered.

Neurodevelopment

In contrast to models that describe the neural underpinnings of EF in adults, which emphasize modularity and take a reductionist approach to characterizing the "how and where" of executive capabilities, given their focus on the frontal lobes,[1] models of early brain development and its role in the establishment of EF are much less "tidy" and "bounded".[2–5] Instead, the boundaries of what constitutes EF in childhood and the description of specific structures supporting its elicitation are less distinct and are more broadly situated anatomically.[5] As a result, the classical emphasis on frontal cortical networks that characterizes adult neuropsychology is inadequate when thinking about EF developmentally. Instead, when considering the developmental neurobiology of EF, it is important to think about how the whole brain organizes and establishes its connections over time and across neural space, in order to best understand and make sense of the increasingly automatic and controlled responses that emerge neuropsychologically.[3,5,6]

Prenatal and early childhood periods

The early development of capacities seen as executive involves a broad set of neural structures that begin to emerge first across prenatal development, and then over the first years of life. Initial prenatal neural patterning, which is still quite incomplete at birth, establishes a foundation required for the neonate and later, the growing infant, to become an actor in and on the environment. As pregnancy progresses, the developing fetal brain grows significantly, in an initially "bottom-up" and then progressively more "top-down"

Executive Function and Dysfunction, ed. Scott J. Hunter and Elizabeth P. Sparrow. Published by Cambridge University Press. © Cambridge University Press 2012.

manner, with regard to the emerging networks being laid down and engaged. As Stiles has discussed, by midgestation, much of the formal process of neuronal production and glial proliferation has taken place; from that point forward, the brain is actively involved in the finer aspects of sculpting that subserve the emerging expression of capacity and capability.[7] With the active initiation of cortical network formation, the brain prepares to fully engage in information processing, through a series of "exuberant" and "eliminative" steps (p. 257) that facilitate engagement and consolidation of the systems that will guide sensation, perception, learning, and ultimately, effectiveness.[7] Importantly, however, this process of development is nonlinear and highly responsive to transactions taking place both within and outside of the individual.[8–10]

During the immediate postnatal period, neurogenesis continues, but slows and becomes more limited. This stage is most notable for the proliferation and migration of glial progenitors, which differentiate in response to injury or insult.[7,11] Following migration, these glial progenitors, particularly the oligodendrocyte progenitor cells, initiate the process of myelination, which is essential for axonal conduction. Additionally, oligodendrocytes are responsible for the production of trophic factors that maintain axonal integrity and neuronal survival.[11] Additionally, dendritic arborization and synaptogenesis accompany the increase in myelination taking place, in a hierarchical fashion, fostering increasing maturation of the communicative networks supporting central nervous system (CNS) elaboration.[12]

Early brain development is remarkable for an overproduction of neurons, glial cells, neural processes, and synapses.[7] A brief period of glial cell apoptosis occurs several days following differentiation, and a protracted period of neural pruning and sculpting begins that extends across childhood, adolescence, and into early adulthood. As pruning occurs, the number of synapses gradually decreases.[7,11] At their peak, the number of synapses in the early postnatal period is roughly twice the amount seen in the adult brain.[11,13] These processes ensure more precise neural connections, which in turn greatly increase the efficiency of communication across brain regions.

Over the first 2 to 3 years of life, brain development is marked by a period of substantial myelination. Changes in gross brain structure during this time are subtler than during early development.[7,11] Imaging research has highlighted considerably larger gray matter volumes in the cerebral cortex and subcortical nuclei in school-age children, compared with adults.[11,14,15] Over the course of early childhood, ongoing myelination and reductions in synaptic density in the cortex continue to characterize brain development, contributing to structural refinements and growing efficiency in communication across the developing neural networks. It is these ongoing refinements that support the emergence of increasingly efficient cognitive processing, and over time, that foster increased EF. As has come to be well understood, it is not only the integrity of the developing frontal lobes that serves to influence emerging EF, but also the functionality and communicative capacity of the whole brain itself.[10]

Childhood and pre-adolescence

Childhood is a period of continued myelination and refinement of the networks supporting unfolding EF, including synaptic pruning and the continued elaboration of neural linkages between frontal, limbic, and cingulate circuits.[7,11] As important white matter tracts are formed and distributed communication patterning takes place across the cortex, refinements in the subcortical-cerebellar and subcortical-frontal loops also occur.[6,16] Additionally, communication between the cortex and other cerebral structures becomes more efficient and coordinated. Each of these neural alterations supports an increased capacity for learning and action during this developmental period.

Neuroimaging, particularly diffusion tensor imaging (DTI) research, has been critical in assisting our understanding of the course of this expanding pattern of brain development in middle childhood. Children between the ages of 5 and 12 show robust development in key tracts, including the anterior cingulate cortex (ACC), corpus callosum, the inferior and superior longitudinal fasciculi, and the inferior fronto-occipital fasciculi, as measured by increases in fractional anisotropy (FA) of these fiber tracts.[7,11,15,17] These processes support improved neural communication that emerges to permit enhanced, complex information processing. Similarly, development of gray matter in the frontal lobes increases until around 10 to 12 years of age, further supporting opportunities for enhanced coordination and communication.[11,18]

As individuals approach adolescence, notable changes in gray matter volume occur, including a pattern of cortical thinning, first in the primary sensory-motor cortex and then in the secondary, multimodal, and supramodal cortical areas.[11,18] This pattern of cortical thinning is thought to be a result of a combination of two processes: (1) increased myelination, which coincides with reductions in some grey matter areas as regions of white matter expand, and (2) regressive tissue loss in some brain structures.[11] In a series of postmortem studies of children's brains, clear age-related structural changes within the PFC reflected this thinning process. Specifically, neuronal density in layer III of the PFC sharply declines between the ages of 2 and 7, at which point, synaptic density levels are around 10% above those of an average adult.[19] Similarly, Huttenlocher has shown a peak in synaptic density occurring around 3.5 years of age, which then gradually decreases through adolescence,[20] coinciding with thinning. Of note, recent research has shown an inverted U-shaped pattern of cortical maturation that illustrates an increase in cortical thickness during childhood, peaking around age 13, and is then followed by a steady decline as adolescents enter early adulthood.[21,22]

In line with this, Tamnes and colleagues found age-related improvements in performance on a WM updating task to be associated with developmentally appropriate cortical thinning in several areas, including the left inferior frontal gyrus and the superior medial parietal areas in the right hemisphere.[21] The relationship between increased myelination (both within the PFC and between the PFC and other subcortical regions) and the improved coordination across the ACC, limbic, and frontal regions provide support for the role of myelination and network refinement in developing EF.[23]

Adolescence

Adolescence is a critical period of PFC and broader neural development, during which the brain essentially rewires itself in an effort to direct and increase efficiency in neurocognitive functioning and behavior regulation. Between the ages of 11 and 13, the mechanisms of attentional control, information processing, cognitive flexibility, and goal-setting behavior approach maturity.[4] Studies have shown that WM improves as a child enters adolescence and moves into adulthood, as a result of improved processing speed efficiency and inhibitory control.[24,25] The left PFC, in conjunction with subcortical structures including the thalamus and putamen, has been implicated in performance on sustained attention tasks,[26] with strong leaps forward in capability during the adolescence period. Sowell and colleagues suggest that improvement in many aspects of cognitive functioning seen during this period, including reduced reaction time, may result from cortical changes (e.g., increased myelination, enhanced sculpting) that take place both in the PFC and more broadly across the brain.[27] They also suggest that improved accuracy on neurocognitive tasks can be attributed to the effects of synaptic pruning that continue during this period.[18]

Prencipe and colleagues have characterized adolescence as a period during which there is a marked transition from a rather diffuse pattern of functional activation within the PFC and broader EF-associated structures during EF tasks, to a more specialized, focal pattern of neural activation.[23] It appears that the collaborative process of neural myelination and synaptic pruning is responsible for more efficient processing of information and continued development of EF. The neural correlates of EF continue changing and improving in adolescence and into young adulthood.[23] In one study, a gambling task was administered to examine how patterns of functional activity across several brain areas differ in adolescents and young adults. Results indicated that, when making high-risk choices, young adults exhibited higher levels of activity in the OFC and dorsal ACC, both considered important regions in emotion regulation and response monitoring.[23] Prencipe and colleagues suggested that young adults are more likely than adolescents to carefully consider the risk associated with an activity before performing it. Young adults also demonstrated increased activation in the posterior medial PFC during a low-penalty task, relative to adolescents.[23] This series of studies illustrate important changes that emerge across adolescence, with regard to in how situations that involve high, low, or uncertain amounts of risk are processed and managed at the neural level.

Entering adulthood

As individuals approach adulthood, the fronto-parietal attention network becomes more fully integrated, and brain functions and processes associated with attention and EF generally become increasingly localized and modular.[27] In line with these findings, research suggests that EF development peaks in the third to fourth decade of life and begins to gradually decline as individuals enter late adulthood.[28] This decline in EF mirrors the gradual decrease of white matter volume in late adulthood.[11] Although the PFC is one of the last brain regions to develop, it is also typically the first area to degenerate in normal aging.[29]

Neuroanatomical underpinnings

The neural systems that underlie the development of EF begin to form in utero. As a child develops, these networks mature in a hierarchical fashion, reorganizing and strengthening connections between the frontal, subcortical, and cerebellar regions, and the processing and association regions distributed broadly across the cortex. This process contributes to the emergence and specialization of EF, and its alterations underlie the development of EdF. These connections enhance communication (1) vertically and horizontally, which allows for coordination among multiple regions of the brain, including the cerebellum, subcortical structures, and broader cortical areas, and (2) forward and backward to facilitate feedback. Thus, development and myelination of the white matter tracts that form the network among brain areas is critical in development of EF. As reviewed below, this executive network links a number of neuroanatomical regions implicated in EF (see Table 3.1).

Table 3.1. *Neurodevelopment of EF-linked structures*

Structure	Developmental timeframe	Executive functions	References
Cerebellum	Between ages of 5 and 24, hemispheric lobes follow inverted U-shaped developmental trajectory; vermis size does not change during this timeframe. Reaches peak size by age 11.3 (boys) and 15.6 (girls)	Emotional Processing Fluency Sequencing Inhibition Concept Formation/Cognitive Flexibility Motor Control	• Giedd JN, Stockman M, Weddle C, *et al.* Anatomic magnetic resonance imaging of the developing child and adolescent brain and effects of genetic variation. *Neuropsychol Rev* 2010; **20**(4): 349–61. • Ramnani N, Behrens TE, Johansen-Berg H, *et al.* The evolution of prefrontal inputs to the cortico-pontine system: diffusion imaging evidence from Macaque monkeys and humans. *Cereb Cortex* 2006; **16**(6): 811–18. • Riva D, Giorgi C. The cerebellum contributes to higher functions during development: evidence from a series of children treated for posterior fossa tumors. *Brain* 2000; **123**(5): 1051–61. • Steinlin M. Cerebellar disorders in childhood: cognitive problems. *Cerebellum* 2008; **7**(4): 607–10. • Timmann D, Daum I. Cerebellar contributions to cognitive functions: a progress report after two decades of research. *Cerebellum* 2007; **6**(3): 159–62.
Limbic system: anterior cingulate cortex	4 months: spindle cells can first be discerned. Cortical thickness peaks around 10.5 years of age; increased myelination, pruning, and dendritic branching contribute to	Attentional Control Emotional Processing and Regulation Inhibition	• Allman JM, Hakeem A, Erwin JM, Nimchinsky E, Hof P. The anterior cingulate cortex: the evolution of an interface between emotion and cognition. *Ann NY Acad Sci* 2001; **935**: 107–17.

Table 3.1. (cont.)

Structure	Developmental timeframe	Executive functions	References
	development through second decade of life Late adulthood: atrophic changes in white matter linked to decline in EF	Self-Monitoring Working Memory	• Eshel N, Nelson EE, Blair J, Pine DS, Ernst M. Neural substrates of choice selection in adults and adolescents: development of the ventrolateral prefrontal and anterior cingulate cortices. *Neuropsychologia* 2007; **45**(6): 1270–9. • Shaw P, Kabani NJ, Lerch JP, *et al.* Neurodevelopmental trajectories of the human cerebral cortex. *J Neurosci* 2008; **28**(14): 3586–94.
Prefrontal cortex	6 weeks: neuroblasts for frontal regions develop Birth to 10–12 years: gray matter development; peaks at 9.5 years in girls and 10.5 years in boys Adolescence – adulthood: dramatic increase in local gray matter density loss; net brain volume increase linked to increased myelination	Inhibition Organization Goal-Directed Behavior Working Memory Information Processing Cognitive Flexibility Attention	• Giedd JN, Stockman M, Weddle C, *et al.* Anatomic magnetic resonance imaging of the developing child and adolescent brain and effects of genetic variation. *Neuropsychol Rev* 2010; **20**(4): 349–61. • Sowell ER, Trauner DA, Garnst A, Jernigan TL. Development of cortical and subcortical brain structures in childhood and adolescence: a structural MRI study. *Dev Med Child Neurol* 2002; **44**(1): 4–16.
Orbitofrontal prefrontal cortex	Inverted-U shape developmental trajectory, peaking at 10.5 years in girls and 14.0 years in boys	Behavioral Inhibition Decision Making Affective	• Giedd JN, Stockman M, Weddle C, *et al.* Anatomic magnetic resonance imaging of the developing child and adolescent brain and effects of

Region	Functions	Development	References
	Regulation Motivation Working Memory Cognitive Inhibition Reversal Learning		genetic variation. *Neuropsychol Rev* 2010; **20**(4): 349–61.
Dorsolateral prefrontal cortex	Set Shifting Planning Response Selection Decision Making Judgment Working Memory Impulse Control	Development of DLPFC is protracted over several years of postnatal life Increases in white matter volume and the gray matter "peak" preceding cortical thinning occurs latest in high association areas like the DLPFC; onset of puberty thought to be "lower limit" of maturity in the DLPFC Adolescence – adulthood: some gray matter loss, but relatively small compared to earlier years; DLPFC growth during this time linked to cortical thinning	• Alexander GE, Goldman PS. Functional development of the dorsolateral prefrontal cortex: an analysis utilizing reversible cryogenic depression. *Brain Res* 1978; **143**(2): 233–49. • Giedd JN, Stockman M, Weddle C, *et al.* Anatomic magnetic resonance imaging of the developing child and adolescent brain and effects of genetic variation. *Neuropsychol Rev* 2010; **20**(4): 349–61. • Sowell ER, Trauner DA, Garnst A, Jernigan TL. Development of cortical and subcortical brain structures in childhood and adolescence: a structural MRI study. *Dev Med Child Neurol* 2002; **44**(1): 4–16.
Ventral medial prefrontal cortex	Emotional Processing Initiation Decision Making	Development occurs over the first three decades of life, Shift from VmPFC to DmPFC over time for emotional processing	• Hooper CJ, Luciana M, Conklin HM, Yarger RS. Adolescents' performance on the Iowa Gambling Task: implications for the development of decision making and ventromedical prefrontal cortex. *Dev Psychol* 2004; **40**(6): 1148–58.

Table 3.1. (cont.)

Structure	Developmental timeframe	Executive functions	References
			• Decety J, Michalska KJ. Neurodevelopmental changes in the circuits underlying empathy and sympathy from childhood to adulthood. *Dev Sci* 2010; **13**(6): 886–99. • Moriguchi Y, Ohnishi T, Mori T, Matsuda H, Komaki G. Changes of brain activity in the neural substrates for theory of mind during childhood and adolescence. *Psychiatry Clin Neurosci* 2007; **61**(4): 355–63.
Subcortical structures	2–3 years: considerable gray matter growth Considerably higher gray matter volumes in school-age children compared to adults	Sustained Attention	• Courchesne E, Chisum HJ, Townsend J, et al. Normal brain development and aging: quantitative analysis at in vivo MR imaging in healthy volunteers. *Radiology* 2000; **216**(3): 672–82. • Sowell ER, Trauner DA, Garnst A, Jernigan TL. Development of cortical and subcortical brain structures in childhood and adolescence: a structural MRI study. *Dev Med Child Neurol* 2002; **44**(1): 4–16. • Stiles J, Jernigan TL. The basics of brain development. *Neuropsychol Rev* 2010; **20**(4): 327–48.
Basal ganglia	4–12 years: increasing coordination of basal ganglia and other brain systems linked to marked improvements in inhibitory control during this time;	Inhibition Sustained Attention	• Lenroot RK, Giedd JN. Brain development in children and adolescents: insights from anatomical

Region	Development	Function	Reference
	caudate nucleus follows an inverted U-shaped developmental trajectory, peaking at 7.5 years in girls and 10.0 years in boys	Coordination of Complex Movement	magnetic resonance imaging. *Neurosci Biobehav Rev* 2006; **30**: 718–29.
Temporal lobe	Gray matter development: peaks at 10.0 years in girls and 11.0 years in boys	Inhibition	• Giedd JN, Stockman M, Weddle C, et al. Anatomic magnetic resonance imaging of the developing child and adolescent brain and effects of genetic variation. *Neuropsychol Rev* 2010; **20**(4): 349–61.
Amygdala	Significant volume increase during adolescence noted in males; indicative of a relatively high number of androgen receptors in the amygdala	Emotional Processing	• Giedd JN, Stockman M, Weddle C, et al. Anatomic magnetic resonance imaging of the developing child and adolescent brain and effects of genetic variation. *Neuropsychol Rev* 2010; **20**(4): 349–61.
Parietal lobe	Gray matter development: peaks at 7.5 years in girls and 9 years in boys. Postadolescent years: stabilization of regressive gray matter density changes; increased myelination linked to parietal lobe growth during this time	Cognitive Flexibility Goal-Directed Behavior Working Memory	• Giedd JN, Stockman M, Weddle C, et al. Anatomic magnetic resonance imaging of the developing child and adolescent brain and effects of genetic variation. *Neuropsychol Rev* 2010; **20**(4): 349–61. • Sowell ER, Trauner DA, Garnst A, Jernigan TL. Development of cortical and subcortical brain structures in childhood and adolescence: a structural MRI study. *Dev Med Child Neurol* 2002; **44**(1): 4–16.
Other Broad cortical network	Embryonic day 42: neuron production in humans begins Embryonic day 108: cortical neurogenesis is largely complete		• Stiles J, Jernigan TL. The basics of brain development. *Neuropsychol Rev* 2010; **20**(4): 327–48.

Table 3.1. (cont.)

Structure	Developmental timeframe	Executive functions	References
	Midgestation – late prenatal period: neurons migrate to different brain regions; make connections with other neurons to establish rudimentary neural networks Immediate postnatal: proliferation/ migration of glial progenitors Early childhood: synaptogenesis; glial cell apoptosis; neural pruning 2–3 years: increased myelination; gray matter growth 4–6 years: brain size increases four-fold; reaches 90% of adult size Late childhood – early adolescence: gray matter begins to decline		
Corpus callosum, inferior and superior longitudinal fasciculi, inferior fronto-occipital fasciculi	5–12 years: robust fiber tract development (all structures) Size increase during adolescence (corpus callosum); some evidence to suggest robust increases in mid sagittal CC area between ages 4–20		• Giedd JN, Stockman M, Weddle C, *et al. Anatomic magnetic resonance imaging of the developing child and adolescent brain and effects of genetic variation. Neuropsychol Rev* 2010; **20**(4): 349–61.

The executive network

The neural systems supporting EF are complex and widely distributed, integrating the PFC with the brainstem, cerebellum, pons, and wider cortex, as well as the networks within the limbic system and routing through subcortical structures.[4,10,16] Despite the intricacy of this network, damage to any one of the developing neural systems can potentially lead to cognitive, behavioral, and regulatory deficits.[4,16] For instance, the frontal lobes are very well connected to the rest of the brain via white matter tracts such as the corpus callosum. Consequently, a disruption in these connections can essentially take the frontal lobes offline. In much the same way, EdF cannot be tied to disruptions within the PFC alone,[4] given the likelihood that insult at any point within the neural network can lead to broader executive disruption.

Coordinated communication between the cerebellum, subcortical structures, PFC, and association and processing regions of the brain supports development of memory, categorization, motor skill, and emotional engagement.[30] As such, developmentally, EF is not solely linked to one specific brain region, but is instead distributed widely; with maturation, EF is associated with more clearly domain specific networks, although not exclusively. In children, cognitive functions are much less localized; rather, they are highly dependent on the coordinated efforts of a broader, whole brain network.[31]

Lesion, electrophysiological, and imaging studies in humans and other primates have elucidated the interplay between the PFC and white matter tracts in directing inhibitory control. Tsujimoto has suggested that, since white matter is comprised mainly of myelinated axons,[22] increases in white matter volume within the PFC are responsible for much of the associated improvement observed in aspects of cognitive functioning developmentally. In examining cortical activation in the context of neuropsychological tasks, imaging technologies including magnetic resonance imaging (MRI), functional magnetic resonance imaging (fMRI), electroencephalography (EEG), DTI, and near-infrared spectroscopy have all increasingly served as sensitive measures critical to better understanding the impact of both the broader and more specific brain regions on EF.[22,26,30,32] Through such methods, structural development, and activity that occurs within select regions of the brain, has been reliably observed in tandem with emergent aspects of functional and behavior change associated with EF. This contrasts with the reliance on "frontal lobe tasks" used in earlier studies examining the neural correlates of EF, including the WCST, the Tower of London, random generation tasks, and verbal fluency tasks.[33] When performances on such tasks are linked with neuroimaging technologies, studies find a pattern of broad cortical and subcortical activation, across both youth and adults, although this pattern of activation becomes increasingly specific with increased age.[10] Studies have indicated that the employment of several brain regions is important in the successful elicitation of multiple discrete EF skills.[5,34] As a result, recent research has expanded our understanding of just how complex and overlapping the EF systems truly are.

Overall, EF is a multidimensional construct that includes a number of cognitive processes, emotional responses, and behavioral actions,[4] and involves, with maturation, an increasingly centralized but still broadly distributed network of neural structures directing their performance. While factor analytic studies have yielded several models of EF, it is generally accepted that these specific "domains are interrelated and interdependent" (4, p. 73). Mounting evidence suggests that "the presence of frontal lesions does not necessarily involve executive dysfunction," and "executive processes are not exclusively based upon a network of prefrontal regions" (34, p. 210). Although the frontal lobes are key components of the neural network supporting development of EF, other principal structures include the ACC, parietal lobes, temporal lobes, cerebellum, and subcortical structures. The preponderance of research has examined the PFC and sub-regions in adults, as reflected in the information summarized below; this should not be taken to mean that the PFC is more important than these other network components however. As Diamond has reiterated, although the PFC may serve as a coordinating structure for EF, it is the broader neural network that establishes and sustains the development and display of EF across time.[35]

The prefrontal cortex

Although we now recognize that EF involves a broadly distributed network, the important role of the PFC in the development of EF is well documented and has received the most significant research to date. As such, it is an important structure to attend to when considering EF across development.[10,35] The PFC is located anterior to the premotor cortex and, in humans, accounts for approximately one quarter to one-third of the cortex.[36] The neural connections between the PFC, motor and sensory cortices, and subcortical structures of the brain are responsible for attention regulation, inhibiting and engaging thoughts and actions, and organizing goal-directed behavior.[37] As the individual matures, the broad set of neural signals responsible for learning and behavior become increasingly integrated and coordinated through these PFC-associated circuits. This streamlining of higher-order skill, which ultimately drives many behavioral outcomes, occurs in tandem with several neuro-developmental processes in the maturing brain. Specifically, the refining of the cortical network underlying EF coincides with broader refinements in both synaptogenesis and myelination, contributing to the increased coordination of executive related communication and behavioral regulation.

Early in life, subcortically directed neural processing primarily accounts for the infant's ability to engage with and understand sensory input, more fully engage with the environment, and consolidate and recall such experiences over time. These experiences bolster associations between information sources, which are more fully integrated and better understood with the continued myelination of the maturing brain. As the connections between the subcortical structures and the PFC grow, increased control over attention and memory emerges. Across infancy and into toddlerhood, multiple growth spurts are associated with increases in attentional control and WM capacity. Subsequent brain growth spurts occur between 6–8, 10–12, and 14–16 years of age,[16,38] eliciting further refinement in the coordination and communication between the PFC and broader regulatory and executive networks.

During the first years of life, PFC growth and the concurrent development of facilitating linkages with broader cortical networks are associated with increases in representation and memory.[35] As a child moves towards middle childhood, improvements occur in PFC-associated networks and their communication. Between the ages of 7 and 9 years, PFC development is tied to rapid improvements in information processing and cognitive flexibility.[4,16] These enhancements in the frontal system and its associated networks promote communication required for the increasing analysis and integration of complex information and effective and efficient decision making.[4] The PFC is especially engaged in processes of inhibition and subsequent strategy development and monitoring.[34,35]

Given the increasingly central role of the PFC in the successful development of executive skill over time, insult to this critical area can have a substantial impact on overall functioning, as illustrated in Section II. In general, and across age groups developmentally, lesions to the PFC have been associated with memory impairment, impulsivity, attention problems, and disorganization.[37] Damage to the left superior PFC, specifically, has been known to impair divided attention.[37] Unlike the lateral PFC, regions associated with the ventral and medial PFC maintain strong neural connections to the limbic system and amygdala, and as such, are principally responsible for the integration of affective and non-affective information.[36] Given the nature of this relationship, damage to the medial PFC has been linked to impairment in initiation, and individuals with lesions in this particular area typically present as apathetic, flat, and unmotivated.

Specifying unique contributions from one particular cortical area to component aspects of EF remains difficult. Research to date strongly suggests that principal domain controls are best associated with the PFC and its component structures (which will be more fully discussed below), but there remain variabilities that have not been fully delineated. We must continue to seek a better understanding of PFC development and related aspects of emerging EF. Although some research suggests that certain aspects of EF may be associated with specific subregions of the PFC, the majority of this work has been completed with adult and nonhuman samples.[5,10]

It is not known at what age these EF brain–behavior associations are established, and whether these distinctions are relevant for pediatric populations. Preliminary work suggests that children show a broader, less specific recruitment of brain regions during EF performance. For example, when children and adults were assessed with a Go/No-Go task, both groups showed fMRI activation in the ACC, OFC, and inferior and middle frontal gyri.[39] Children demonstrated significantly greater activation in the DLPFC and ACC than did adults. These findings suggest that children recruit more diffuse regions of the PFC during inhibitory tasks when compared to adults.[39,40] In a replication of this study,[41] results further highlighted age-related increases in cortical activation in the left inferior frontal gyrus and OFC, and fMRI data showed that activation within the left superior and middle frontal gyrus and ACC decreased with age.[40,41] In another study using event-related potentials to examine the relationship between cortical activation and conflict resolution in children and adults, findings supported that, as the brain circuitry underlying EF matures, it also becomes more efficient, reflecting the increased specialization of neuroanatomical features over time.[34]

Thus, we provide a brief overview of the primarily adult-based findings for links between subregions of the PFC and specific EF skills, but urge caution, as experience in our field has indicated many times that adult-centered research does not necessarily extend downward to describe children and adolescents. After this brief summary of suggested specificity for subregions of the PFC, we examine functional relations between EF and the PFC.

Subregions of the prefrontal cortex and executive functioning

The *anterior prefrontal cortex* (APFC) is commonly referred to as the frontal pole or rostral frontal cortex. It is an area little understood with regard to its role in EF, although hypotheses have been presented, making use of adult data mostly acquired from neuroimaging studies looking at the broader PFC. In a review of the available literature, Ramnani and Owen have indicated that the APFC is the largest component of PFC proportionally in humans, in comparison with other primate species, and it overlaps significantly with DLPFC in all primates.[42] It has been hypothesized to be primarily engaged in introspective aspects of emotional processing, as well as the identification of and response to internal states. This region has not been examined in either children or adolescents at this time, and its developmental trajectory is unknown.

The *ventrolateral prefrontal cortex* (VLPFC) and *posterior PFC* (including areas in and around the inferior frontal sulcus) have been implicated in rule acquisition, rule switching, inhibition of competing responses, and aspects of WM. Robbins and Roberts have linked the VLPFC to rule acquisition and rule switching.[43] They also report neuroimaging findings, across both humans and monkeys, that indicate a relationship between the posterior areas of the inferior frontal sulcus and attentional set shifting.[43] Spielberg and colleagues have likewise highlighted the posterior region of the middle frontal gyrus as associated with inhibition of competing responses.[44–46] This region also seems to be engaged during WM processes that involve the organization of upcoming action.[35]

The *DLPFC* has been identified in the adult and child-based literature as a particularly important structure for EF, including cognitive set shifting,[37] planning, and response selection in goal-driven behavior,[47] and spatial WM.[26,35,37,48] The DLPFC may be actively involved via anterior attentional circuits in spatial WM and visuospatial problem solving tasks.[49] Although the traditional view of DLPFC function was related directly to spatial WM processing, a two-level hypothesis has since been proposed to account for its relationship with non-spatial WM performance.[50] Within this model, the DLPFC, including the sulcus principalis, receives information from the posterior association areas and is the "locus of the initial interaction of executive processing with STM for modality-specific and multimodal information" [51, p 208]. The DLPFC "that lies above the sulcus principalis, on the other hand, constitutes a second-level interaction with short-term memory when planning and organization – that is, monitoring within working memory – are required" (51, p 208).

Further evidence supporting the relationship between the DLPFC and WM comes from developmental studies examining infant search processes, particularly delayed response tasks.[51] There is considerable research indicating that delayed response tasks are useful measures to assess STM and LTM as early as infancy and continuing across the lifespan.[51] In one study, near-infrared spectroscopy identified increased DLPFC blood flow in infants who reliably searched for objects during a delayed response task compared to those who did not.[51] Notably, those infants who did not search showed decreased total hemoglobin in the PFC relative to baseline.[51]

The *OFC* has been linked to a number of EF skills, including aspects of learning,[43] emotional regulation,[52,53] cognitive and behavioral inhibition,[54] self-awareness,[55] cognitive flexibility,[56] integration,[54] decision making,[36,54] WM,[54] and motivation.[36] The OFC seems to be particularly involved in reversal learning, across species and ages. Across time, the OFC becomes specifically responsible for reward-associated pair learning and the concurrent ability to learn the reverse association tied to the pair.[43] Damage to the OFC in adolescents and adults has been linked to impairment in processing learned associations between situations and emotional responses, and decision-making in a gambling task, perhaps due to ties between the OFC and the limbic system.[36] The links between the OFC and limbic system are also implicated in feelings of euphoria and manic behavior observed after damage to the OFC.[52,53]

Lesion studies, primarily with adults, have suggested that OFC damage is associated with disruptions in cognitive flexibility. Baron-Cohen and colleagues[55] have demonstrated the role of the OFC in recognizing mental state terms, in both adolescent and adult samples, while broader research has associated the OFC with additional executive processes, including integration, inhibition, decision making with feedback, and the frontal WM system.[54] Graham and colleagues urge careful consideration of IQ differences in studies of EF, as they have found a differential impact of IQ on fMRI activation and response strategies,[57] specifically with regard to OFC activation. An area of the frontal lobe known as the gyrus rectus, which can be considered an extension of the cingulate cortex into the OFC, has been linked to the WM system in older adults, specifically inductive reasoning[54]; this has not been replicated in pediatric populations.

Functions of the prefrontal cortex and executive functioning

Inhibitory control has been described as the foundation of EF (see Chapter 2). A number of components of the anterior PFC have been identified as responsible for inhibitory control, which increasingly emerges during toddlerhood, and continues to develop well into adolescence.[35,58] Greene and colleagues have reported that inhibitory processes are largely lateralized to the right hemisphere and dependent on the ventral PFC and parietal lobes;[26] this coordination of the frontal and posterior associative cortices is critical for many EF skills.[21,59] Studies have also linked inhibitory control to the OFC, inferior frontal cortices, ACC, the parietal and temporal cortices, and the gyrus rectus.[32,33,58] Researchers used near-infrared spectroscopy to examine cortical activation during a WM task in a group of normally developing children between the ages of 4 years, 4 months and 6 years, 8 months.[60] Results of multiple regression analyses showed that age, accuracy, and reaction time predicted cortical activation level, with age being the most significant predictor.[60] These results suggest that important morphological and structural changes occur in the PFC and networked brain areas across childhood and into adolescence that impact inhibitory control.

WM has been tied to PFC activation throughout the extant literature, and age-related improvement on WM updating tasks (i.e., the incorporation of new details into a set of information already being held in WM)[33] has been observed, particularly during childhood.[21] Two areas of the PFC, the left middle frontal gyrus and the inferior frontal gyrus, are strongly associated with performance on WM tasks.[44,61] The middle frontal gyrus also plays a role in inhibiting relatively automatic behaviors and competing responses, as well as responding to conflicting emotional information,[44] concurrent with WM. The right middle frontal gyrus has specifically been implicated in WM, as well as the inhibition of a dominant response and the organization of action used to obtain a goal.[44] A cross-sectional study showed a linear increase between the ages of 7 and 22 years in lateral PFC activation during an n-back WM task,[62] illustrating the relationships among development, the PFC, inhibition and WM.

With regard to cognitive *set shifting*, engagement and activation of the PFC is a common finding in the adult literature. Diamond has shown that age-related improvements in attending to and shifting focus, as well as strategy, across information in the environment is directed by several regions of the PFC that are also involved in WM and inhibition.[35] However, differences in regional activation in concordance with set shifting appear to vary across levels of intelligence as well as age. An event-related fMRI study examined youth and adult performance on a cognitive set-shifting task, using IQ as a covariant, and found that individuals with average IQ demonstrated higher activation in both the PFC and ACC during the response selection component.[57] During the feedback condition, participants in the high IQ group demonstrated higher activation in areas associated with more complex reasoning, including the parietal, caudate, fusiform, and occipital regions. The authors suggested that individuals with higher IQ may be more strategic in evaluating feedback and likely experience less response conflict during response selection aspects of the task.

The PFC has also been implicated in the ability to *multi-task*. The PFC clearly plays a role in regulating the ability to hold information online in the presence of interference.[37] This feature is unique in that, unlike inferior temporal neurons, PFC neurons do not stop firing when a new stimulus is presented.[63] This response pattern becomes particularly useful with maturity, when individuals are increasingly forced to interact independently with a complex, changing environment. Consistent with this, Blakemore and Choudhury suggest that adults are significantly better equipped to handle multitasking than children or adolescents.[40] In a study comparing a group of adults (mean age 25) with adolescents (youth aged 11 to 14) and children (aged 6 to 10), they showed that adults employed more efficient strategies than either the adolescents or children when completing a multitask paradigm that drew upon prospective memory.[64] Blakemore and Choudhury suggested that prospective memory emerges during childhood, and continues to develop through adolescence in tandem with development of the PFC.[40] Intact PFC functioning therefore allows us to recall necessary information in order to successfully complete tasks amidst distracting stimuli, as we are required to do in everyday life.

The limbic system

The limbic system, particularly the ACC, is implicated in many aspects of EF, including emotional regulation and processing, inhibition, and directed attention. As mentioned previously, the limbic system is intimately connected with the PFC and broader cortical and subcortical structures, and as a result, is involved in the regulation and support of EF. In particular, the ACC is part of the limbic system and appears to hold a central role in executive aspects of attention and emotion processing.[34] A recent study of early adolescent, late adolescent, and adult performance on an error-monitoring task found that, on average, young adolescents made 11% errors, while the late adolescents made 7% errors, with a further drop in adulthood.[65] Event-related potentials during the task indicated localization in or around the ACC, suggesting that the age-related differences in task performance might be connected to maturation of the ACC. Projections from the ACC to the striatum may influence dopamine (DA) transmission, and thus, performance on inhibitory tasks, further emphasizing a strong role for the ACC and limbic system in regard to EF.[66,67] Older adults with good performance on an inhibition task were found to have larger ACCs on MRI.[53] There has been a suggestion that this finding applies as well to developmentally immature groups, although little research has taken place to test this hypothesis.

There is also evidence to support the relationship between the ACC and the executive control of attention in developing populations.[68] Specifically, the authors describe how attentional tasks that involve conflict, including the Stroop task, have more recently been used to elicit activation in both the ACC and lateral PFC.[68] According to Rueda and colleagues, the ACC is the "[seat of the] network involved in the volitional and controlled aspect of the attentional system."[34] Several mechanisms have been proposed to describe the relationship between the ACC and the PFC during directed attention tasks. One group suggests that the ACC is engaged during tasks that require sustained attentional control and performance monitoring, whereas the PFC is more readily engaged in top-down support of attention maintenance.[69] Others have examined a possible reciprocal relationship between effortful and emotional controls of attention, given the proximity of the ACC to emotion processing regions;[34] this model is supported by the finding that activation in the ACC is associated with the cognitive reappraisal of distressing photographs, thus reducing negative affect.[70]

Parietal and temporal cortices

The temporal and parietal cortices are also important components of the executive network. The temporal cortex is involved in aspects of inhibitory control,[33] and the parietal cortex has been implicated in inhibition, set shifting, initiating, goal-directed behavior, and WM.[33] The superior parietal cortex is supramodal, playing a primary role in task switching regardless of whether the task involves verbal, visual, or spatial information.[33] Other areas of the parietal cortex appear to be primarily responsible for initiating and completing goal-directed activities.[33] Regions of the parietal cortex also appear to be involved in WM updating; although the brain regions activated during such tasks depend largely on the measures and procedures used, they generally include not only the PFC, but also regions of the parietal cortex.[33] Specifically, sustained activity in the left superior parietal region and the frontopolar cortex has been linked with updating tasks, whereas transient activity in the medial frontal gyrus appears to play an inhibitory role.[33]

Cerebellum

An important, but often less considered component of the EF system is the cerebellum. The cerebellum reaches its peak size by about 11 years of age in girls and 15 years of age in boys,[71] and seems important in the coordination of capacities that define EF during the early childhood period.[71] The cerebellum plays a central role in motor control, emotional processing, and higher cognitive functions that mature throughout adolescence.[71] The cortico-ponto-cerebellar network is heavily engaged in aspects of timing and sequencing of such demands as verbal WM and executive aspects of visual and verbal analysis.[72] Research focusing on children with known cerebellar dysfunction suggests that the cerebellum is a modulating influence on affective, cognitive, and regulatory capacities].[73-75] Still, the cerebellum appears to be more a structure of collaboration than direct command, as studies of cerebellar disruption have found that cerebellar lesions alone do not fully explain EdF.[75] When EdF is present in conjunction with cerebellar dysfunction, the functional networks supporting behavior at the cortical level are also disrupted. This suggests that cerebellar dysfunction disrupts the vertically organized regulatory networks of the brain, thus impacting EF.[75]

Subcortical structures

It appears that several subcortical structures are involved in EF, including the basal ganglia, thalamus, and putamen. Brocki and colleagues describe the role of the basal ganglia within the thalamocortical network model, which draw upon GABA-ergic neural connections that serve to coordinate complex actions.[66] They have also linked DA reductions within the striatum to disinhibition,[30] while other research has implicated the thalamus and putamen in tasks of sustained attention.[26]

Differences in basal ganglia thalamocortical circuits have been noted between healthy individuals and those with ADHD, and age-dependent increases in inhibitory control between the ages of 4 and 12 have been attributed, at least in part, to changes within this network.[30] According to Brocki and colleagues, "widely distributed brain systems are slower in gaining the necessary coordination and coherent communication" in children with ADHD, who tend to exhibit more diffuse patterns of brain activity during the performance of cognitive operations (31 p 251). These observations lend credibility to a framework of EF development characterized by initially broad but increasingly localized and coordinated cognitive processes as an individual matures. Furthermore, research by Castellanos and his research group have found lags of up to 5% in whole-brain volume in children with ADHD, particularly with regard to basal ganglia thalamocortical loops.[76] Also highlighted have been findings that describe similar reductions in size of the PFC, caudate, and globus pallidus in ADHD populations.[77–79]

Neurochemical substrates

The relationship between neuroanatomy and EF skill development is not purely structural in nature. Arnsten and Bao-Ming point to potential neurochemical substrates that appear to substantially modulate the role of the PFC on behavioral and emotional regulation, specifically catecholemines.[37] Evaluation of clinical groups such as people with ADHD or schizophrenia also suggests neurochemical disruption in populations with documented EdF. For example, positron emission tomography (PET) imaging has revealed reduced catecholamine inputs to the PFC in children and adults with ADHD.[80] Also, children with ADHD demonstrate enhanced activation of fronto-striato-cerebellar and parieto-temporal attentional networks (relative to healthy controls) when administered a clinical dose of the DA-agonist methylphenidate.[81] Given that many medications used to treat ADHD facilitate DA and norepinephrine (NE) transmission, these findings lend support to a catecholamine hypothesis regarding EF, and suggest the potential impact of selective neurotransmitters on the PFC, and consequently, EF.

A number of studies have associated neurochemical abnormalities observed in schizophrenia with the pattern of EdF seen with that disorder.[82] The current model suggests that reduced levels of N-acetyl-aspartate in the DLPFC are linked with decreased activation of WM neural networks during completion of the WCST in affected individuals.[82] Increased levels of glutamate and glutamine in the left DLPFC are associated with increased WCST perseverative errors in people with schizophrenia relative to healthy controls.[82]

As cautioned in the neuroanatomical underpinnings section, it is important to remember that most of the work regarding neurochemical substrates of EF has been derived from adult and animal models. Very little research to date has occurred with human children; as such, these models proposed are hypothetical and remain in need of direct testing developmentally. Also, most of the studies described below examined neurochemical functioning in the PFC; this reflects a bias in available literature rather than a lack of appreciation for the assumption that neurochemical activity in other brain regions impacts EF.

Dopamine

The role of DA on the PFC has long been studied and is accepted in the literature. The DA-rich ventral tegmental area of the midbrain is responsible for delivery of the neurotransmitter to areas of the PFC, modulating many aspects of EF.[34] The lateral PFC has been shown to be particularly susceptible to DA.[36] Studies have shown that either extreme of catecholamine levels, but specifically DA, can have detrimental effects on PFC functioning in rats, monkeys, and likely humans.[37] Research suggests extreme levels of DA are associated with impairments in WM and attention.[37,83–85] Consistent with these findings, research has indicated that alterations in neurotransmitter availability have a significant impact on WM performance.[85–91]

There is also evidence to support DA's role in attentional set shifting and sustained attention,[43] as well as focusing attention and facilitating judgments. Specifically, Crofts and colleagues have presented results from lesion studies where marmosets that experienced a global depletion of DA throughout the PFC were significantly impaired in their ability to not only acquire, but also maintain attentional set during extradimensional shifts.[92] Granon and colleagues showed that a DA agonist infused into the PFC of rats improved attention during a five-choice task.[84] These findings suggest that aspects of EF, including attention and WM, are highly dependent on the degree of dopaminergic activity in the PFC.[86]

In primate research, DA has been shown to be a stabilizing factor for prefrontal cortical cells that subserve WM representations.[30] Earlier primate research found a reduction in DA level to mirror the effects of PFC lesions on execution function.[87,93] Animal studies have shown that diminished levels of DA in the PFC lead to deficits in spatial WM in delayed response tasks, but do not affect performance in self-ordered searching tasks.[86] Chudasama has suggested that these findings may also hold up in humans.[86] For example, DA depletion in children with phenylketonuria has been associated with impairment in spatial WM during delayed response tasks but not in self-ordered tasks.[86] Greene and colleagues have also described how DA has been implicated in efficient response inhibition.[26] This line of research suggests that DA agonists improve aspects of EF under certain circumstances, whereas the excess release of DA can disrupt EF. Thus, maintaining neurochemical homeostasis in regard to DA appears to be critical when maximizing EF, particularly inhibitory processing.

Animal studies indicate that a rise in DA receptor density in the striatum and PFC occurs in early adolescence, followed by a reduction in dopaminergic activity.[94] The ties between DA and the brain's reward circuitry are generally well known,[53] and suggest that increased reward-seeking behaviors in puberty are particularly tied to increases in DA sensitivity.[95] Performance may be hindered on tasks that involve risk, arousal, or social influence in adolescents, despite appropriate performance on other EF tasks, given alterations in DA availability.[94]

Norepinephrine

NE appears to play a critical role in PFC function, particularly with regard to WM, behavioral inhibition, and protection against distractibility.[37] NE in the PFC has also been linked to attentional set shifting[43] and automatic alerting.[68] Chudasama has presented evidence to suggest that depletions of cortical NE can lead to marked attentional impairment in rats.[86] Similar to DA, NE in low to moderate amounts appears to be advantageous in terms of PFC functioning, and the release of high levels of the neurotransmitter, often in response to stress, appears to hinder PFC responsivity.[86] Elevated levels of NE have been linked to overactivation of protein kinase C (PKC) signaling in the PFC,[86] and have been associated with EdF.[96] PKC signaling has been found to be quite sensitive to certain medications used to treat bipolar disorder and schizophrenia, further complicating the issue of NE balance.[86] Because NE is the pharmaceutical target for some ADHD-related medications (such as guanfacine and atomoxetine), the issue of balance of NE with DA is an important one, in terms of both understanding the presentation of EdF, and with regard to effective pharmacological treatment.[97,98]

Acetylcholine

Alterations in levels of acetylcholine (ACh) in the PFC have a meaningful impact on EF. Chudasama's review of animal (i.e., rat and monkey) studies indicates that decreases in ACh lead to both accuracy and inhibitory deficits during a 5-choice task.[86] Depletions of ACh may also impair WM, as suggested by rat research.[99] Animal studies have found that EdF resulting from diminished levels of ACh can be effectively reversed through administration of physostigmine, a cholinesterase inhibitor.[100] In a five-choice reaction time test, lesion-induced rats experienced decreased choice accuracy that was attributed to attentional deficits. Subsequent treatment with physostigmine was associated with improved accuracy on the task.[100]

Robbins and Roberts have suggested that, while prefrontal ACh does not appear to have a primary role in higher-order attentional set shifting, it may have important implications for reversal learning,[43] across species. As discussed earlier, reversal learning may be a function of the OFC.[86] Preliminary evidence suggests that damage to the cholinergic innervations of the OFC may impair serial reversal learning[43] in rats and non-human primates, although these findings have not been replicated in humans. It also appears that ACh is responsible for modulating orienting behavior in monkeys.[101]

Serotonin

Serotonin's (5-HT) role in emotional and affective regulation is reasonably well established;[102] 5-HT may also be involved in other aspects of EF.[26] There is increasing support in the literature to suggest a link between 5-HT transmission and neuropsychological functioning, as well as data regarding 5-HT as a potential flag of EF vulnerability at the genetic level. Specifically, alterations in gene coding for the serotonin transporter (5HTT) have also been associated with subsequent changes in ACC activation during inhibition tasks in adults.[26] Levels of 5-HT have been associated with levels of impulse control and response inhibition, with possible implication of a polymorphism in 5HTT.[103,104] Other research has considered the effects of a 5HTT polymorphism on ADHD symptoms in the context of an adverse childhood environment.[105] In their sample of young adult males with a history of delinquency, Retz and colleagues found that men with the short allele 5HTT polymorphism who retrospectively reported an adverse childhood environment exhibited a more persistent pattern of ADHD symptoms over time relative to those, with and without the short allele, who did not report childhood adversity.[105]

There is increasing evidence to suggest that 5-HT may be involved in modulating aspects of attention.[86] Chudasama has described how 5-HT levels in the PFC of rats are linked to improved attentional selectivity and decreased impulsivity.[86,106,107] Furthermore, animal studies have associated 5-HT depletion with marked impairment in reversal learning[86] and OFC integrity.[86] These findings suggest that there may be important neuropsychological implications for treatment of EdF with atypical antipsychotic medications and the selective serotonin reuptake inhibitors (SSRIs), both of which target 5-HT receptor sites;[86] further research is warranted.

Genetic influences

In conjunction with neuroimaging methods, a growing body of genetic studies has helped shed light on the relationship between brain structure and higher-order executive processes.[30] Specifically, research has been useful in establishing linkages between certain DA regulation genes (e.g., DAT1 and DRD4) and potential structural and functional changes associated with the caudate, striatum, and PFC, which may pose a risk for the subsequent development of ADHD[30,66] as well as broader forms of EdF. Greene and colleagues and Pennington have both discussed the additive effects of multiple genes in regard to ADHD; in particular, the DA regulation genes may account for approximately 80% of an individual's susceptibility to ADHD.[26,108] Similarly, a longitudinal study demonstrated a brain-derived neurotropic factor polymorphism to be associated with age-related decline on an executive task-switching paradigm in adults.[109] With regard to WM, genetic research has provided heritability estimates for this executive skill to fall between 33% and 49%.[26] While the genetics of EF are not well understood, it has become increasingly evident that a genetic contribution to executive processes is likely present and multifactorial, with impairment involving polygenetic mutations and their interactions with particular environmental factors.[108]

Summary and future directions

The neurodevelopmental foundations of EF, including the neuroanatomical, neurochemical, and genetic correlates, are still emerging. As the findings discussed above are based on studies of animals and human adults, they are not irrefutably extendable to human children and adolescents. Nonetheless, these findings guide us in forming interesting and testable hypotheses regarding the emergence of EF and EdF over time. A significant number of hypotheses have been proposed that could potentially explain the nature of neurocognitive deficits as they relate to the array of neuroanatomical, neurochemical, and genetic factors that unfold across time in humans. Even though top-down control by the PFC is believed central to many cognitive processes, we can be certain that the relationship between neuromodulatory pathways and the PFC is dynamic and ultimately contributes to cognitive plasticity as well as skill acquisition.[43]

There is mounting evidence to suggest that, even though certain cortical regions may be linked to discrete aspects of EF in adults, children have less specificity in their neural representations of EF. Several fMRI studies have demonstrated the involvement of contralateral and neighboring cortical regions in the performance of EF skills in both children and adults.[110,111] While this process depends largely on age, neurological status, and the specific task demands being considered, this finding illustrates that cortical organization with regard to executive and other cognitive processes relies on the activation and coordination of multiple brain regions. Imaging studies examining cortical activation have shown that, while the PFC is involved in Tower of London performance, especially with regard to increased task complexity, multiple areas within the right or bilateral parietal regions are also activated].[112–114] The pediatric literature highlights age-related differences in cognitive functioning across children and adults who have similar PFC lesions at different ages,[37] and reminds us that EdF is as often seen with nonfrontal lesions as not.[4,16] This emphasizes the need for developmental research that might explain the differential impact of such insults, depending on timing[36] and what structures and broader networks they impact.

While the general tendency in the EF literature has historically been an attempt to map certain executive processes to specific cortical regions, it appears that the relationship between these skill sets and their neurocognitive underpinnings is very complex and developmentally intertwined. Brain regions outside the PFC make significant contributions to what are typically considered EF, and these broad regions play an important role in directing and guiding the development of specific EF skills as they emerge, both anatomically and behaviorally. It makes sense to conceptualize the development of EF as an aggregate of maturational and interactive processes. The integration of numerous cognitive elements, and their varied anatomical, chemical, and genetic substrates, ultimately contribute to a diffuse network of brain regions responsible for carrying out higher-order strategic and problem-solving oriented tasks. As we come to better identify and understand the varied neuroanatomical and neurochemical underpinnings of EF and EdF, it is likely that improved approaches to intervention, both behaviorally and pharmacologically, will emerge.

In summary, despite significant improvements in our understanding of the neurobiology of EF over the last several decades, there remain notable gaps in our knowledge of the development and neuroanatomy of EF. Because most of what we know comes from studies of animals and adults, research that more explicitly focuses on the development of EF in human children and adolescents across time is required. Steps have been taken in the neuroimaging literature to address that need; still, it is just a beginning. Longitudinal studies of neuroanatomic and neurochemical correlates of EF will improve our knowledge of both typical and atypical development, and elucidate more directly the factors that affect it. Further, research with children that clarifies the relation between specific subregions of the brain and EF will also meaningfully contribute to our understanding of the interrelationships between internal developmental processes and their transactions with the broader environment. Improved insight into the neuroanatomical development of children and adolescents and the associated neurochemical changes that occur in tandem will inform our approaches to treatment for affective, behavioral, and psychotic disorders; not just in terms of pharmacological approaches, but also those that are cognitive and behavioral. Ultimately, this will contribute to an improved quality of life across the lifespan for all individuals.

References

1. Stuss DT, Alexander MP. Executive functions and the frontal lobes: A conceptual view. *Psychol Res* 2000; 63(3–4): 289–98.

2. Bernstein JH, Waber DP. Executive capacities from a developmental perspective. In Meltzer L, ed. *Executive Function in Education: From Theory to Practice*. New York, NY: Guilford Press; 2007, 39–54.

3. Anderson V. Assessing executive functions in children: Biological, psychological, and developmental considerations. *Neuropsychol Rehabil* 1998; 8(3): 319–49.

4. Anderson P. Assessment and development of executive function during childhood. *Child Neuropsychol* 2002; 8(2): 71–82.

5. Morton JB. Understanding genetic, neurophysiological, and experiential influences on the development of executive functioning: The need for developmental models. *WIREs Cogni Sci* 2010; 1(5): 709–23.

6. De Luca CR, Leventer RJ. Developmental trajectories of executive functions across the lifespan. In Anderson V, Jacobs R, Anderson P, eds. *Executive Functions and the Frontal Lobes: A Lifespan Perspective*. Philadelphia, PA: Taylor & Francis; 2008, 23–56.

7. Stiles J. *The Fundamentals of Brain Development: Integrating Nature and Nurture*. Cambridge, MA: Harvard University Press; 2008.

8. Johnson MH. Functional brain development in infants: elements of an interactive specialization framework. *Child Dev* 2000; 71(1): 75–81.

9. Johnson MH. Development of human brain functions. *Biol Psychiatry* 2003; **54**(12): 1312–16.

10. Anderson V, Anderson P, Jacobs R, Smith MS. Development and assessment of executive function: From preschool to adolescence. In Anderson V, Jacobs R, Anderson P, eds. *Executive Functions and the Frontal Lobes: A Lifespan Perspective.* Philadelphia, PA: Taylor & Francis; 2008, 123–54.

11. Stiles J, Jernigan TL. The basics of brain development. *Neuropsychol Rev* 2010; **20**(4): 327–48.

12. Gogtay N, Giedd JN, Lusk L, *et al.* Dynamic mapping of human cortical development during childhood through early adulthood. *Proc Natl Acad Sci* 2004; **101**(21): 8174–9.

13. Nelson CA, de Haan M, Thomas KM. *Neuroscience of Cognitive Development: The Role of Experience and the Developing Brain.* Hoboken, NJ: John Wiley & Sons, Inc; 2006.

14. Courchesne E, Chisum HJ, Townsend J, *et al.* Normal brain development and aging: quantitative analysis at in vivo MR imaging in healthy volunteers. *Radiology* 2000; **216**(3): 672–82.

15. Sowell ER, Trauner DA, Garnst A, Jernigan TL. Development of cortical and subcortical brain structures in childhood and adolescence: a structural MRI study. *Dev Med Child Neurol* 2002; **44**(1): 4–16.

16. Diamond, A. Normal development of prefrontal cortex from birth to young adulthood: cognitive functions, anatomy, and biochemistry. In Stuss, D.T. & Knight, R.T., eds. *Principles of Frontal Lobe Function.* London, UK: Oxford University Press; 2002, 466–503.

17. Sowell ER, Thompson PM, Leonard CM, Welcome SE, Kan E, Toga AW. Longitudinal mapping of cortical thickness and brain growth in normal children. *J Neurosci* 2004; **24**(38): 8223–31.

18. Sowell ER, Thompson PM, Tessner, Toga AW. Mapping continued brain growth and gray matter density reduction in dorsal frontal cortex: Inverse relationships during postadolescent brain maturation. *J Neurosci* 2001; **21**(22): 8819–29.

19. Huttenlocher PR. Synaptic density in human frontal cortex – developmental changes and effects of aging. *Brain Res* 1979; **163**(2): 195–205.

20. Huttenlocher PR, Dabholkar AS. Regional differences in synaptogenesis in human cerebral cortex. *J Comp Neurol* 1997; **387**(2): 167–78.

21. Tamnes CK, Østby Y, Walhovd KB, Westlye LT, Due-Tønnessen P, Fjell AM. Neuroanatomical correlates of executive functions in children and adolescents: a magnetic resonance imaging (MRI) study of cortical thickness. *Neuropsychologia* 2010; **48**(9): 2496–508.

22. Tsujimoto S. The prefrontal cortex: functional neural development during early childhood. *Neuroscientist* 2008; **14**(4): 345–58.

23. Prencipe A, Kesek A, Cohen J, Lamm C, Lewis MD, Zelazo PD. Development of hot and cool executive function during the transition to adolescence. *J Exp Child Psychol* 2011; **108**(3): 621–37.

24. Fry AF, Hale S. Processing speed, working memory, and fluid intelligence: Evidence for a developmental cascade. *Psychol Sci* 1996; 7(4): 237–41.

25. Bjorklund DF, Harnishfeger KK. The resources construct in cognitive development: Diverse sources of evidence and a theory of inefficient inhibition. *Dev Rev* 1996; **10**(1): 48–71.

26. Greene CM, Braet W, Johnson KA, Bellgrove MA. Imaging the genetics of executive function. *Biol Psychol* 2008; **79**(1): 30–42.

27. Kim Y, Gitelman DR, Nobre AC, Parrish TB, LaBar KS, Mesulam M. The large-scale neural network for spatial attention displays multifunctional overlap but differential asymmetry. *Neuroimage* 1999; **9**(3): 269–77.

28. Kochunov P, Robin DA, Royall DR, Coyle T, Lancaster J, Kochunov V. Can structural MRI indices of cerebral integrity track cognitive trends in executive control

function during normal maturation and adulthood? *Hum Brain Mapp* 2009; **30**(8): 2581–94.

29. Casey BJ, Thomas KM, Welsh TF, *et al.* Dissociation of response conflict, attentional selection, and expectancy with functional magnetic resonance imaging. *Proc Natl Acad Sci USA* 2000; **97**(15): 8728–33.

30. Brocki K, Fan J, Fossella J. Placing neuroanatomical models of executive function in a developmental context: Imaging and imaging-genetic strategies. In Pfaff DW, Kieffer BL, eds. *Molecular and Biophysical Mechanisms of Arousal, Alertness, and Attention*. Malden, MA: Malden Blackwell Publishing; 2008, 246–55.

31. Welsh MC, Pennington BF. Assessing frontal lobe functioning in children: Views from developmental psychology. *Dev Neuropsychol* 1988; **4**(3): 199–230.

32. Lamm C, Zelazo PD, Lewis MD. Neural correlates of cognitive control in childhood and adolescence: disentangling the contributions of age and executive function. *Neuropsychologia* 2006; **44**(11): 2139–48.

33. Collette F, Hogge M, Salmon E, van der Linden M. Exploration of the neural substrates of executive functioning by functional neuroimaging. *Neuroscience* 2006; **139**(1): 209–21.

34. Rueda MR, Posner MI, Rothbart MK. The development of executive attention: contributions to the emergence of self-regulation. *Dev Neuropsychol* 2005; **28**(2): 573–94.

35. Diamond A. The early development of executive functions. In Bialystok E, Craik FIM, eds. *Lifespan Cognition: Mechanisms of Change*. New York, NY: Oxford University Press; 2006.

36. Zelazo PD, Muller U. Executive function in typical and atypical development. In Goswami U, ed. *The Wiley-Blackwell Handbook of Childhood Cognitive Development*. 2nd edn. Oxford, UK: Blackwell Publishing Ltd.; 2011, 574–603.

37. Arnsten AFT, Bao-Ming L. Neurobiology of executive functions: Catecholamine influences on prefrontal cortical functions. *Biol Psychiat* 2005; **57**(11): 1377–84.

38. Isaacs E, Oates J. Nutrition and cognition: Assessing cognitive abilities in children and young people. *Eur J Nutr* 2008; **47**(3): 4–24.

39. Casey BJ, Trainor RJ, Orendi JL, *et al.* A pediatric functional MRI study of prefrontal activation during performance of a Go-No-Go task. *J Cognitive Neurosci* 1997; **9**(6): 835–47.

40. Blakemore S, Choudhury S. Development of the adolescent brain: Implications for executive function and social cognition. *J Child Psychol Psychiatry* 2006; **47**(3–4): 296–312.

41. Tamm L, Menon V, Reiss AL. Maturation of brain function associated with response inhibition. *J Am Acad Child Psychol* 2002; **41**(10): 1231–8.

42. Ramnani N, Owen AM. Anterior prefrontal cortex: insights into function from anatomy and neuroimaging. *Nat Rev Neurosci* 2004; **5**(3): 184–94.

43. Robbins TW, Roberts AC. Differential regulation of fronto-executive function by the monoamines and acetylcholine. *Cereb Cortex* 2007; **17**(Suppl 1): i151–60.

44. Spielberg JM, Miller GA, Engels AS, *et al.* Trait approach and avoidance motivation: lateralized neural activity associated with executive function. *Neuroimage* 2011; **54**(1): 661–70.

45. Kaladjian A, Jeanningros R, Azorin JM, *et al.* Remission from mania is associated with a decrease in amygdala activation during motor response inhibition. *Bipolar Disord* 2009; **11**: 530–8.

46. Liddle PF, Kiehl KA, Smith AM. Event-related fMRI study of response inhibition. *Hum Brain Mapp* 2001; **12**(2): 100–9.

47. Miller EK. The prefrontal cortex and cognitive control. *Nat Rev Neurosci* 2000; **1**(1): 59–65.

48. Shing YLT, Lindenberger U, Diamond A, Li S, Davidson MC. Memory maintenance and inhibitory control differentiate from

early childhood to adolescence. *Dev Neuropsychol* 2010; **35**(6): 679–97.

49. Thomas E, Reeve R, Fredrickson A, Maruff P. Spatial memory and executive functions in children. *Child Neuropsychol* 2011; **17**(6): 599–615.

50. Petrides M. Frontal lobes and behaviour. *Curr Opin Neurobiol* 1994; **4**(2): 207–11.

51. Marcovitch S, Zelazo PD. A hierarchical competing systems model of the emergence and early development of executive function. *Developmental Sci* 2009; **12**(1): 1–25.

52. Fuster JM. *The Prefrontal Cortex: Anatomy, Physiology and Neuropsychology of The Frontal Lobe*, 2nd edn. New York: Raven Press; 1989.

53. Cummings JL. Frontal-subcortical circuits in human behavior. *Arch Neurol* 1993; **50**(8): 873–9.

54. Elderkin-Thompson V, Ballmaier M, Hellemann G, Pham D, Kumar A. Executive function and MRI prefrontal volumes among healthy older adults. *Neuropsychology* 2008; **22**(5): 626–37.

55. Baron-Cohen S, Ring H, Moriarty J, Schmitz B, Costa D, Ell P. Recognition of mental state terms: Clinical findings in children with autism and a functional neuroimaging study of normal adults. *Br J Psychiatry* 1994; **165**(5): 640–9.

56. Murray EA, O'Doherty JP, Schoenbaum, G. What we know and do not know about the functions of the orbitofrontal cortex after 20 years of cross-species studies. *J Neurosci* 2007; **27**(31): 8166–9.

57. Graham S, Jiang J, Manning V, *et al.* IQ-related fMRI differences during cognitive set shifting. *Cereb Cortex* 2010; **20**(3): 641–9.

58. Levin HS, Song J, Ewing-Cobbs L, Roberson G. Porteus maze performance following traumatic brain injury in children. *Neuropsychol* 2001; **15**(4): 557–67.

59. Diamond A, Goldman-Rakic PS. Comparison of human infants and rhesus monkeys on pieagte's AB task: Evidence for dependence on dorsolateral prefrontal cortex. *Exp Brain Res* 1989; **74**(1): 24–40.

60. Tsujimoto S, Yamamoto T, Kawaguchi H, Koizumi H, Sawaguchi T. Functional maturation of the prefrontal cortex in preschool children measured by optical topography. Program No. 196.15. 2003 *Abstract Viewer/Itinerary Planner.* Washington, DC: Society for Neuroscience; 2003.

61. Pochon JB, Levy R, Fossati P, *et al.* The neural system that bridges reward and cognition in humans: An fMRI study. *Proc Natl Acad Sci USA* 2002; **99**(8): 5669–74.

62. Kwon H, Reiss AL, Menon V. Neural basis of protracted developmental changes in visuo-spatial working memory. *Proc Natl Acad Sci USA* 2002; **99**(20): 13336–41.

63. Levy R, Goldman-Rakic PS. Segregation of working memory functions within the dorsolateral prefrontal cortex. *Exp Brain Res* 2000; **133**(1): 23–32.

64. Mackinlay R, Charman T, Karmiloff-Smith A. Remembering to remember: A developmental study of prospective memory in a multitasking paradigm: Biennial Meeting of the Society for Research in Child Development; 2003 Apr 24–27; Tampa, FL.

65. LaDouceur CD, Dahl RE, Carter CS. Development of action monitoring through adolescence into adulthood: ERP and source localization. *Developmental Sci* 2007; **10**(6): 874–91.

66. Brocki K, Clerkin SM, Guise KG, Fan J, Fossella JA. Assessing the molecular genetics of the development of executive attention in children: Focus on genetic pathways related to the anterior cingulate cortex and dopamine. *Neuroscience* 2009; **164**(1): 241–6.

67. Frank MJ, D'Lauro C, Curran T. Cross-task individual differences in error processing: *Neural, electrophysiological, and genetic components. Cogn Affect Behav Neurol* 2007; **7**(4): 297–308.

68. Fan J, McCandliss BD, Sommer T, Raz A, Posner MI. Testing the efficiency and

independence of attentional networks. *J Cogn Neurosci* 2002; **14**(3): 340–7.

69. Osaka N, Osaka M, Kondo H, Morishita M, Fukuyama H, Shibasaki H. The neural basis of executive function in working memory: An fMRI study based on individual differences. *Neuroimage* 2004; **21**: 623–31.

70. Ochsner KN, Bunge SA, Gross JJ, Gabrieli JDE. Rethinking feelings: An fMRI study of the cognitive regulation of emotion. *J Cogn Neurosci* 2002; **14**(8): 1215–29.

71. Giedd JN, Stockman M, Weddle C, *et al.* Anatomic magnetic resonance imaging of the developing child and adolescent brain and effects of genetic variation. *Neuropsychol Rev* 2010; **20**(4): 349–61.

72. Ramnani N, Behrens TE, Johansen-Berg H, *et al.* The evolution of prefrontal inputs to the cortico-pontine system: Diffusion imaging evidence from Macaque monkeys and humans. *Cereb Cortex* 2006; **16**(6): 811–18.

73. Riva D, Giorgi C. The cerebellum contributes to higher functions during development: Evidence from a series of children treated for posterior fossa tumors. *Brain* 2000; **123**(5): 1051–61.

74. Steinlin M. Cerebellar disorders in childhood: Cognitive problems. *Cerebellum* 2008; **7**(4): 607–10.

75. Timmann D, Daum I. Cerebellar contributions to cognitive functions: A progress report after two decades of research. *Cerebellum* 2007; **6**(3): 159–62.

76. Castellanos FX. Neural substrates of attention-deficit hyperactivity disorder. *Adv Neurol* 2001; **85**: 197–206.

77. Castellanos FX, Giedd JN, Marsh WL, *et al.* Quantitative brain magnetic resonance imaging in attention-deficit hyperactivity disorder. *Arch Gen Psychiatry* 1996; **53**: 607–16.

78. Filipek PA, Semrud-Clikeman M, Steingard RJ, Renshaw PF, Kennedy DN, Biederman J. Volumetric MRI analysis comparing subjects having attention-deficit hyperactivity disorder with normal controls. *Neurology* 1997; **48**(3): 589–601.

79. Aylward EH, Reiss AL, Reader MJ, Singer HS, Brown JE, Denckla MB. Basal ganglia volumes in children with attention-deficit hyperactivity disorder. *J Child Neurol* 1996; **11**(2): 112–15.

80. Nigg JT. *What Causes ADHD?: Understanding What Goes Wrong and Why.* New York, NY: The Guilford Press; 2006.

81. Rubia K, Halari R, Cubillo A, Mohammad A, Brammer M, Taylor E. Methylphenidate normalises activation and functional connectivity deficits in attention and motivation networks in medication-naïve children with ADHD during a rewarded continuous performance task. *Neuropharmacology* 2009; **57**(7–8): 640–52.

82. Rüsch N, Tebartz van Elst L, Valerius G, Büchert M, Thiel T, Ebert D, *et al.* Neurochemical and structural correlates of executive dysfunction in schizophrenia. *Schizophr Res* 2008; **99**(1–3): 155–63.

83. Cai JX, Arnsten AFT. Dose-dependent effects of the dopamine D1 receptor agonists A77636 or SKF81297 on spatial working memory in aged monkeys. *J Pharmacol Exp Ther* 1997; **282**(1): 1–7.

84. Granon S, Passetti F, Thomas KL, Dalley JW, Everitt BJ, Robbins TW. Enhanced and impaired attentional performance after infusion of D1 dopaminergic receptor agents into rat prefrontal cortex. *J Neurosci* 2000; **20**(3): 1208–15.

85. Murphy BL, Arnsten AFT, Goldman-Rakic PS, Roth RH. Increased dopamine turnover in the prefrontal cortex impairs spatial working memory performance in rats and monkeys. *Proc Natl Acad Sci USA* 1996; **93**(3): 1325–9.

86. Chudasama Y. Animal models of prefrontal-executive function. *Behav Neurosci* 2011; **125**(3): 327–43.

87. Brozoski TJ, Brown RM, Rosvold HE, Goldman PS. Cognitive deficit caused by regional depletion of dopamine in prefrontal cortex of rhesus monkey. *Science* 1979; **205**(4409): 929–32.

88. Chudasama Y, Robbins TW. Psychopharmacological approaches to

modulating attention in the five-choice serial reaction time task: Implications for schizophrenia. *Psychopharmacology* 2004; **174**(1): 86–98.

89. Floresco SB, Phillips AG. Delay-dependent modulation of memory retrieval by infusion of a dopamine D1 agonist into the rat medial prefrontal cortex. *Behav Neurosci* 2001; **115**(4): 934–9.

90. Sawaguchi T, Goldman-Rakic PS. The role of D1-dopamine receptor in working memory: local injections of dopamine antagonists into the prefrontal cortex of rhesus monkeys performing an oculomotor delayed-response task. *J Neurophysiol* 1994; **71**(2): 515–28.

91. Zahrt J, Taylor JR, Mathew RG, Arnsten AF. Supranormal stimulation of D1 dopamine receptors in the rodent prefrontal cortex impairs spatial working memory performance. *J Neurosci* 1997; **17**(21): 8528–35.

92. Crofts HS, Dalley JW, Collins P, *et al.* Differential effects of 6-OHDA lesions of the prefrontal cortex and caudate nucleus on the ability to acquire an attentional set. *Cereb Cortex* 2001; **11**(11): 1015–26.

93. Goldman-Rakic PS. Prenatal formation of cortical input and development of cytoarchitectonic compartments in the neostriatum of the rhesus monkey. *J Neurosci* 1981; **1**(7): 721–35.

94. Crone EA. Executive functions in adolescence: Inferences from brain and behavior. *Developm Sci* 2009; **12**(6): 825–30.

95. Sisk CL, Zehr JL. Pubertal hormones organize the adolescent brain and behavior. *Front Neuroendocrinol* 2005; **26**: 163–74.

96. Birnbaum SG, Yuan PX, Wang M, *et al.* Protein kinase C overactivity impairs prefrontal cortical regulation of working memory. *Science* 2004; **306**(56–97): 882–4.

97. Arnsten AF. Stimulants: Therapeutic actions in ADHD. *Neuropschyopharmacology* 2006; **31**(11): 2376–83.

98. Arnsten AF, Pliszka SR. Catecholamine influences on prefrontal cortical function: Relevance to treatment of attention deficit/hyperactivity disorder and related disorders. *Phamacol Biochem Behav* 2011; **99**(2): 211–16.

99. Chudasama Y, Dalley JW, Nathwani F, Bouger P, Robbins TW. Cholinergic modulation of visual attention and working memory: dissociable effects of basal forebrain 192-IgG-saporin lesions and intraprefrontal infusions of scopolamine. *Learn Mem* 2004; **11**(1): 78–86.

100. Muir JL, Everitt BJ, Robbins TW. Reversal of visual attentional dysfunction following lesions of the cholinergic basal forebrain by physostigmine and nicotine but not by the 5-HT3 receptor antagonist, ondansetron. *Psychopharmacology* 1995; **118**(1): 82–92.

101. Davidson MC, Marrocco RT. Local infusion of scopolamine into intraparietal cortex slows covert orienting in rhesus monkeys. *J Neurophysiol* 2000; **83**(3): 1536–49.

102. Cools R, Roberts AC, Robbins TW. Serotoninergic regulation of emotional and behavioural control processes. *Trends Cogn Sci* 2008; **12**(1): 31–40.

103. Lesch KP, Bengel D, Heils A, *et al.* Association of anxiety-related traits with a polymorphism in the serotonin transporter gene regulatory region. *Science* 1996; **274**(5292): 1527–31.

104. Lucki I. The spectrum of behaviors influenced by serotonin. *Biol Psychiatry* 1998; **44**(3): 151–62.

105. Retz W, Freitag C, Retz-Junginger P, *et al.* A functional serotonin transporter promoter gene polymorphism increases ADHD symptoms in delinquents: interaction with adverse childhood environment. *Psychiat Res* 2008; **158**(2): 123–31.

106. Passetti F, Dalley JW, Robbins TW. Double dissociation of serotonergic and dopaminergic mechanisms on attentional performance using a rodent five-choice

reaction time task. *Psychopharmacology* 2003; **165**(2): 136–45.

107. Winstanley CA, Chudasama Y, Dalley JW, Theobald DE, Glennon JC, Robbins TW. Intra-prefrontal 8-OH-DPAT and M100907 improve visuospatial attention and decrease impulsivity on the five-choice serial reaction time task in rats. *Psychopharmacology* 2003; **167**(3): 304–14.

108. Pennington BF. *Diagnosing Learning Disorders: A Neuropsychological Framework*, 2nd edn. New York, NY: Guilford Press; 2009.

109. Erickson KI, Kim JS, Suever BL, Voss MW, Francis BM, Kramer AF. Genetic contributions to age-related decline in executive function: A 10-year longitudinal study of COMT and BDNF polymorphisms. *Front Hum Neurosci* 2008; **2**(11): 1–9.

110. Musso M, Weiler C, Kiebel S, Muller S, Balau P, Rijntzes J. Training induced brain plasticity in aphasia. *Brain* 1999; **122**(9): 1781–90.

111. Thulborn KR, Carpenter PA, Just MA. Plasticity of language-related brain function during recovery from stroke. *Stroke* 1999; **30**(4): 749–54.

112. Andreasen NC, Rezai K, Alliger R, *et al.* Hypofrontality in neuroleptic-naïve patients and in patients with chronic schizophrenia: Assessment with Xenon 113 single-photon emission computed tomography and the Tower of London. *Arch Gen Psychiatry* 1992; **49**(12): 943–58.

113. Baker SC, Rogers RD, Owen AM, *et al.* Neural systems engaged by planning: A PET study of the Tower of London task. *Neuropsychologia* 1996; **34**(6): 515–26.

114. Morris RG, Ahmed S, Syed GM, Toone BK. Neural correlates of planning ability: frontal lobe activation during the Tower of London test. *Neuropsychologia* 1993; **31**(12): 1367–78.

Chapter

4

Assessment and identification of executive dysfunction

Elizabeth P. Sparrow

Within an individual evaluation, a child's approach to each task can reveal significant information about executive strengths and weaknesses. Although some tests are explicitly designed to assess aspects of EF, all components of the assessment process provide new information to build, test, support, and/or reject a hypothesis regarding EF and EdF. The recommendations provided in this chapter for record review, observation, interview, questionnaires, and rating scales are good practice for any assessment; however, they are particularly critical when evaluating EF, as subtle aspects of EdF can be difficult to capture with standardized testing. It is important to remember that the presence or absence of EdF is not uniformly diagnostic, although EdF may suggest certain diagnostic considerations (see Section II).

Key issues

1. *Nearly every test involves EF.* EF skills are ubiquitous and it is impossible to exclude them from an evaluation. For example, most standard psychometric measures require some degree of planning, strategy, or inhibition for their completion. The opposite is also true; most tests identified as primary "EF assessment tools" involve other cognitive processes as well. This has been called "task impurity".[1] As a result, other tests (including intellectual functioning and academic achievement) and behavior observations provide information about EF as well (see Table 4.1 for examples). It is important to recognize these elements and their role in assessment and identification.

2. *Standardization may remove aspects of EF.* Ironically, the very structured nature of standardized testing reduces demands for some aspects of EF.[2,3] As Stuss so aptly said, the examiner risks becoming the frontal lobes for the patient.[4] Most standardized tests provide explicit instructions so that they can be reliably administered and scored across sites and examiners. This reduces an examiner's chance to observe EF deficits that are more likely to appear in uncertain or ambiguous situations. Some tests have attempted to create open-ended scenarios with this in mind, although these tests are not yet widely used, due in part to the difficulty that presents in standardizing them. This may partially account for differences in EF scores obtained via tests vs. questionnaires[5] or rating scales.[6] A person may be able to gather sufficient cognitive resources to perform EF tasks for a brief period (like many clinical tasks), but the exertion cannot be sustained over daily activities.[6]

Executive Function and Dysfunction, ed. Scott J. Hunter and Elizabeth P. Sparrow. Published by Cambridge University Press. © Cambridge University Press 2012.

3. *It is challenging to isolate a single EF skill.* Each facet of EF is intertwined with another, making it difficult to isolate a single executive skill or deficit. For example, self-monitoring is part and parcel of inhibition, and vice versa – these skills are different from each other, but are difficult to differentiate as they often occur simultaneously and impact each other. A low score on a test that purports to measure one executive skill could reflect a deficit in a different executive process as well. As discussed in Chapter 1, this murkiness is cited as a criticism of EF as a construct. While it is attractive to imagine that EF can be divided into separate "cubby holes," each with its own label and recommendations, this rarely occurs outside of a laboratory environment, when assessing real people or real-life performances.

4. *EF may vary by setting; gather data from multiple people about multiple places.* When test results show the same deficits as described in everyday performance, interpretation is simple. Unfortunately, when examining EF, there are times when a child may show different patterns of performance across different settings. This might be evident when comparing home with school, comparing different classes, or even when comparing test scores with everyday struggles. It is important in such situations to closely examine all available sources of information in an attempt to dissociate possible contributors to the seeming confusion regarding the child's functioning.

   Some settings may have inherent advantages for a child with EdF, such as a highly structured classroom with immediate, specific, and explicit feedback from the teacher. Some people intuitively increase structure, support, and consistency for a child just when she needs it. Some activities are a perfect match for children with these deficits, such as video games that are interactive, visual, and provide immediate, consistent, and clear consequences or rewards for the child's actions. In such cases, the success of a given setting, person, or activity can suggest optimizing factors that should be considered when developing a treatment plan – but not held as evidence that the child does not have EdF, as can sometimes occur.

   These are among the reasons it is important to gather information about a child's functioning not only from the setting in which she shows the most difficulty, but also from settings where she is successful. These exceptions can provide the very data needed to identify EdF and possible remediation strategies. It is very important to compare and contrast findings in a multi-dimensional way, including home/school, math/science/reading/history, and everyday/laboratory performance, whenever possible.

5. *Some factors exacerbate (or improve) EdF.* There are a number of factors that can exacerbate or even cause EdF. These include self-care factors like fatigue,[7,8] hunger,[7] pain,[9] stress,[10] mood (either positive or negative[11]), or lack of exercise.[12] Overstimulation is also a significant exacerbating factor, including multiple sources of input (e.g., sound, sight, and touch) and the presence of multiple cognitive demands.[13,14] Sudden change in structure and familiarity can cause the appearance of temporary EdF,[15] such as might occur with a new teacher, new class, or new school. These exacerbating factors impact everyone's functioning and are not exclusive in their effect on EdF; however, a child who is already struggling to compensate for EdF typically has fewer cognitive reserves to draw upon. A child with EdF can be more sensitive to the occurrence of any of these factors, and will become quickly overwhelmed when these factors accumulate in their impact. Thus, it is important to proactively monitor these

potential areas of interference and keep them in check. Even young children can learn a checklist for these self-care skills to determine why they are not feeling their best. Of note, research has shown that improved self-care may improve EF.[16,17,18] Therefore, it is always critical to consider these factors in an evaluation and when planning treatment.

6. *Defining the appropriate peer comparison is challenging.* It is important to determine the appropriate peer group to use when considering whether a child has "relative weaknesses" versus "deficits" in EF. This allows for a direct comparison with "typical" expectations, and also provides an important point of contrast should differences be observed. However, it is not always easy to determine the best comparison group, as the appropriate comparison group might be selected based on age, gender, intellectual ability, school grade, or other factors. Consider the case of a child who has average range motor abilities in the context of superior intellectual ability – would this child require occupational or physical therapy to bring his motor skills up to the level of his intellectual skills? Most professionals and parents would say, quite readily, "of course not." But for some reason, many parents and professionals understand this motor skills scenario more readily than the comparison of average EF skills in the context of superior intellect. Perhaps this is the case because many of us know bright people who have succeeded despite below average coordination.

7. *A statistically significant discrepancy between average EF and high IQ is not necessarily a clinical deficit.* There are a range of factors that may lead to EF scores lower than IQ scores.[19,20] A person may simply have average EF, such as the motor functioning example described above.[21] Statistically speaking, when a large number of tests is given, some will be lower than others.[22,23,24] The design of EF tests may limit description of high functioning; although IQ tests were designed to describe both ends of the continuum (above average as well as below average), most neuropsychological tests (including those of EF) were developed to describe deficits rather than strengths.[25] The ceiling of many EF tests may prevent the achievement of "superior" scores commensurate with superior IQ scores.[26] (*Note:* the complex relationships between EF and IQ are examined further in Chapter 20.)

8. *Impairment is an important aspect of EdF.* As with any condition, evaluating presence and degree of impairment is a necessary aspect of examining EdF. If the child does not demonstrate impairment in his everyday life, it will be hard to obtain parent, teacher, or student participation in treatment efforts. It is important to remember that even when a discrepancy between ability and EF scores is absent, a deficit may be evident in the failure to make developmentally expected gains, or in excessive effort and/or time required to meet expectations.

EF deficits clearly impact a number of domains, including academic,[27,28,29,30] emotional,[31] behavioral,[31] social,[30,31,32] and adaptive functioning.[33] Consider multiple aspects of functioning, including social interactions, family relationships, home responsibilities, and community involvement, as well as employment for adolescents and young adults. Adaptive functioning is a key place that EdF can significantly impact a child's success by limiting her ability to function with true independence (i.e., she requires cues, prompts, reminders, or "nags" to complete everyday tasks like dressing, toileting, and bathing). For example, children with ADHD were rated lower than the matched control group for parent- and teacher-completed ratings of adaptive functioning.[33]

It is also important to assess the impact of EdF on intrapersonal functioning and emotional well-being. Consider, for example, a teenaged girl who struggles to integrate information in her English Literature class; she may have the same difficulty integrating and expressing her feelings and thoughts about her emotional and social life. Additionally, her struggles with managing coursework can contribute to increased frustration, anxiety, and lower self-confidence, all issues that can impact her well-being and exacerbate her EdF.

9. *Consider modality and method when collecting data on EF and EdF.* Information about EF can be gathered with multiple modalities, such as record review, observation, interview, questionnaires, and rating scales, in addition to testing. Preliminary research suggests that modality and method of assessment can make a difference in a child's performance. For example, giving adults different colored pens during administration of the ROCF improved performance relative to the traditional examiner flowchart method of administration.[34] It is interesting to ponder the source of this difference; the use of colored pens may draw attention to organizational features of the design, or the prevention of erasure may lead to greater caution and thus more planning. Regardless of the reasons why this difference is found, assessors who prefer using colored pens in administering the ROCF should be certain to reference normative data obtained with that modality of administration.[35] Variation in administration is of particular concern with the proliferation of computerized versions of standard neuropsychological instruments. A computerized version of the WCST produced psychometrically different results than the traditional human-administered version.[36] Several studies have found that children with autism spectrum disorders (ASD) perform better on computerized versions of tasks relative to human-administered tasks, perhaps due to removing the requirement for social interaction.[37,38] Although computer-administered tasks may simplify assessment for an examiner, it is important to also evaluate EF with person-to-person tasks. The world is not always a computer interface (although it is becoming moreso), and results from a computerized EF task may not represent a child's functioning when human interaction is required.

The remainder of this chapter provides an overview of assessment techniques as they pertain to EF, including tests that have been purported to specifically assess executive skill, as well as aspects of other tests that can help describe EF/EdF. Both structured and flexible measures are mentioned (see Appendix 2 for a list of tests referenced in this book; see Appendix 1 for a list of abbreviations used in this book, including test name abbreviations). Although specific tests are used to illustrate points, this chapter does not include an exhaustive review of all published tests that assess EF. Instead, the reader is referred to the following resources for more detailed description of specific tests purported to measure EdF: Baron (2004),[39] Lezak and colleagues (2004),[40] Strauss and colleagues (2006),[41] Golden and Hines (2010),[42] and the Buros reviews.[43] Although the section below describing testing (a.k.a., "Laboratory Performance") is loosely organized by groupings of executive skills, this should not be construed as absolute categorization given the interrelated nature of EF skills.

History, context, and observation

As mentioned earlier, context is critical when assessing for EF and EdF. Test results cannot be interpreted without knowledge of the child's background, current context of successes

Table 4.1. *Examples of executive dysfunction that may be observed during standardized testing*

General purpose of test	Examples of EdF that may be observed during test administration
Intellectual ability	• Disorganized verbal responses; circumlocution; does not identify key facts in responses (e.g., WISC-IV & WPPSI-III Information, Vocabulary, Similarities, Comprehension) • Trial and error approach to problem-solving (e.g., WISC-IV & WPPSI-III Block Design, Matrix Reasoning, Picture Concepts; D-KEFS Sorting, 20 Questions; tower tasks) • Struggles with WM (e.g., WISC-IV Digits Backward significantly worse than Digits Forward)
Academic achievement	• Understands stated facts but misses implied meaning (e.g., some items on WIAT-III Listening Comprehension) • Difficulty grasping the main idea or theme despite intact basic reading skills (e.g., Literal Accuracy higher than Inferential Accuracy on WIAT-III Reading Comprehension) • Spends excessive time on details and does not have time to complete the objective of the task (e.g., WIAT-III Essay Composition) • Poorly organized spoken and written language • Difficulty starting a response, many stops and starts • Does not extract key facts from mathematical word problems (e.g., some items on WIAT-III Applied Problems) • Does not recognize when mathematical operations signs change during a mixed operation worksheet (e.g., WIAT-III Calculation)
Speed of information processing/responding	• Significant decrease in speed as information becomes more complex • Does not seem to automate repeated processes (e.g., WISC-IV Coding)
Attention	• Variable performance over a period of time (e.g., CPTs) • Difficulty sustaining effort (e.g., NEPSY-II Statue)
Learning & memory	• Reliance on rote memory; doesn't use context or past knowledge (e.g., nonsensical errors in story memory, sentence memory) • Limited use of strategies such as clustering (e.g., verbal fluency, list-learning tasks) or organizing materials (e.g., RCFT) • Difficulty with free recall, needs cues to retrieve information • High rates of intrusion and repetition errors (e.g., list-learning and story memory tasks; D-KEFS 20 Questions)
Language	• Disorganized spoken and written language • Difficulty understanding sarcasm, humor, symbolism, body language • Misses implied or abstract information despite intact comprehension of concrete information (e.g., proverbs tasks)

Table 4.1. (cont.)

General purpose of test	Examples of EdF that may be observed during test administration
	• Focuses on one aspect of information or on details (e.g., lists related facts but does not provide the main idea on WISC-IV Vocabulary or Similarities); difficulty integrating multiple aspects (e.g., D-KEFS Word Context) • Becomes louder when asked to work quickly (e.g., RAN/RAS, verbal fluency, Stroop-like tasks) • Impaired sequencing when asked to work quickly (e.g., "square, little red" rather than "little red square" during NEPSY-II Speeded Naming) • Difficulty with understanding complex language that requires more WM (e.g., CELF-4 Concepts & Directions) • Requires repetition and demonstration of instructions
Visual processing	• Overwhelmed by visually complex material • May focus on a less relevant detail (e.g., face recognition tasks) • Difficulty copying complex designs; does not use organizing gestalts (e.g., RCFT, some designs from NEPSY Design Copy or VMI) • Poor organization of visual material (e.g., placement of designs on VMI, writes off the edge of page for Writing Samples)
Sensorimotor functions	• Overflow (oromotor, mirror movements; e.g., NEPSY-II Imitating Hand Positions, pegboards) • Impersistence (e.g., NEPSY-II Statue) • Larger or more exaggerated movements than necessary (e.g., NEPSY-II Manual Motor Sequences, Imitating Hand Positions) • Flailing/uncoordinated movements when required to work quickly (e.g., block assembly, fluency tasks)
Adaptive functioning	• Limited self-initiation; needs prompts and cues • Has knowledge of rules and ability to perform skills, but does not *independently* demonstrate them *when needed* • Low scores on ABAS-II or Conners EC Developmental Milestones that are not due to lack of knowledge or physical ability
Social, emotional, & behavioral functioning	• Impulsive (verbal and motoric; can be seen in blurting out response before question finished, grabbing materials before instructed to do so, turning pages when told not to do so) • Emotional lability or overly restricted affect (may observe as approach more difficult items) • Intrusive, asks inappropriate questions • Difficulty integrating multiple pieces of information (e.g., body language, tone of voice, past knowledge, and word meaning; can sometimes be seen on NEPSY-II Affect Recognition or ToLC; can be recognized in interactions with examiner)

Table 4.1. (cont.)

General purpose of test	Examples of EdF that may be observed during test administration
Other	• Variable performance over course of evaluation • Difficulty with simultaneous processing of multi-modal information (e.g., instructions that are verbal and visual at the same time) • Failure to maintain response set; needs multiple reminders of task instructions; introductory item level instructions may need to be repeated (e.g., forgets to reverse digits in Digit Span Backwards even after successfully completing earlier items) • Difficulty transitioning from one task to the next; misses easier items before getting the "hang" of a test; cannot stop working on a problem when time ends (e.g., WISC-IV Cancellation, Block Design) • Requires frequent queries during testing; has the knowledge but does not always realize when to provide it

and struggles, and functioning in different settings. Key methods for gathering these data include record review, direct observation, interview, questionnaires, and rating scales.

Record review

The assessment of EF begins with a review of the referral question. Because EF deficits impact so many aspects of functioning, there are usually hints of their presence from the very first contact with the child, or in the reporting of concerns from a teacher or parent. The initial referral might include comments such as: "he just can't get his act together," "you never know what to expect with her, she's completely unpredictable," or, "the problem is not how smart he is, it's getting him to do his work."

As past records, including report cards, schoolwork, and progress reports are reviewed, multiple references to potential EdF may emerge. For example, old report cards may include comments about immaturity, difficulty applying concepts, and incomplete assignments. "Poor work habits" such as late or missing assignments, or a consistent failure to "turn work in" can often be a code for EdF. Examples of classwork, homework, and tests can reveal perseveration (e.g., using addition for an entire mixed operations worksheet). Disciplinary records may reveal a pattern of weak inhibition whether expressed verbally (e.g., "smarting off" or "talking back" to the teacher) or physically (e.g., punching students who insult him).

Direct observation

Observation is extremely valuable when assessing EF. As Banich said, " . . . the very nature of executive function makes it difficult to measure in the clinic or the laboratory" (p. 89).[44] It is important to gather observation data from various settings, when possible, as the comparison of the student's functioning across settings will generally reveal aspects of EdF that are not evident in the clinic setting. For example, watching a student in the hallways, lunchroom, or even when walking down the sidewalk may illustrate an "out of control" reaction to less structured situations, in contrast to an ability to show appropriate behavior when in a structured classroom. Some teachers may maintain a traditional, quiet classroom, while others espouse a more experiential, free-flowing learning environment; comments about how the child transitions between these settings or how her response to the different levels of structure varies can be quite informative. Without a doubt, degree of structure is often an important factor in the expression of EdF.

Beyond behavioral self-control, observation can also provide data regarding organizational aspects of EF. Take notice of personal appearance – does the child look disheveled, or neatly put together? When the teacher instructs students to turn to a certain page in the book, does she have difficulty finding the book? Or flip randomly through the book until she comes across the correct page? Does she even have the correct book available for that subject? Additionally, the physical appearance of the student's locker, desk, backpack, and work binders can also provide valuable information about level of organization, planning, and strategy.

In addition to observations outside of the clinical setting, valuable observation data can be collected during formal assessment as discussed below. This is the case, even when specific tests of EF are not being administered. Additional observational data from parents, teachers, and examinees can be gathered through the initial clinical interview, or the completion of standardized behavioral questionnaires and rating scales (see relevant sections in this chapter). Together, these data supplement and extend the behavioral observations made, both during the testing itself and through collateral observation.

Interview

In addition to historical information, an interview offers the evaluator a chance to obtain observational data from parents, teachers, and children (as well as additional direct observation). It is important to engage in active probing of context and concern during the interview rather than just simply recording answers to questions. For example, the report by a parent that her son "does just fine in Mr. Brown's classroom, but all the other teachers say he is out of control," might lead to discussion of course subject matter, time of day, teaching style, classroom features, and the seating chart. Further, in this example, discussion might suggest the need to rule-out possible interference from a specific learning disorder (e.g., Mr. Brown might teach art in a way that does not tax a student with dyslexia) or language disorders (e.g., Mr. Brown might teach science through hands-on demonstration rather than language-intense instruction). Discussion in this example might also reveal that Mr. Brown has a very explicit, structured teaching style, and his classroom has minimal distractions such as wall decorations or windows that overlook the playground. It might be discovered that time of day, which impacts fatigue and hunger, is a factor; Mr. Brown's class may occur right after lunch, when the student is rested and no longer hungry. It is also possible that Mr. Brown might provide immediate, supportive feedback to help keep each student on track, through responding to errors by coaching the student rather than embarrassing him. Perhaps Mr. Brown follows a consistent and predictable routine in his classroom rather than frequently changing the furniture arrangement, agenda, and teaching style. All of this rich information and hypothesis-testing are potentially missed when an interview with the referral source, parent, or teacher is relatively rote and cursory in its explorations, such as when comments by the parent are left unqueried. As such, it is argued that a careful interview is the best approach towards refining both the referral question and directing how to best assess the child.

A key topic to consider when EdF may be part of the differential diagnosis is task completion, such as might be obtained by asking the parents and student to describe a typical homework session. Be attentive to whether the student is a self-starter or requires cues/prompts to get going. Examine how much structure the parent provides within the homework session, and whether this support is *conceptual* (e.g., asking the student clarifying questions about a passage, identifying key themes), *procedural* (e.g., determining order of task completion, breaking long-term projects into smaller pieces), or *physical* (e.g., removing distractions, sitting with the child for the session). Similar information can be obtained by asking about the child's task completion with domestic chores such as cleaning her room, doing the dishes, or helping prepare dinner.

The interview process does not end after the initial diagnostic interview. Other topics may become evident over the course of evaluation and require exploration. Results from parent, teacher, and self-report rating scales may reveal new information or perspectives. Test data may suggest that additional context is needed for interpreting the results. Actual clinic examples of this include a teenager who did extraordinarily well on a tower task despite struggling with all other problem-solving and planning tasks; he revealed in interview that he programmed a tower algorithm as a leisure activity, so the task was certainly not novel. Another true story involved a college student whose performance on a verbal fluency task improved significantly compared to previous evaluation with no known intervention; in a follow-up interview she indicated that she "played word games" with her campers to keep them occupied. For these and many other reasons, it is important to reserve time for a closing interview; this can even be accomplished at the beginning of the feedback session.

Questionnaires

Written questionnaires, whether standardized or more informally constructed, can be a useful way to gather information in advance of meeting with a student, parent, or teacher. They might provide broad background and environmental context for understanding the child, allowing the evaluator to spend more time in hypothesis-testing during the interview. Questionnaires can also include items about specific aspects of EF (e.g., the "Executive Skills Semistructured Interviews"[45] or the "Executive Function Structured Interview"[46] can each be used in a questionnaire format), although this may be better accomplished with standardized rating scales that allow for normative comparisons. It is important to review information from questionnaires and engage in an active discussion to examine the data obtained, as has been described in the Interview section above, in order to maximize an understanding of the context and extent of both difficulties and successes in the EF domain.

Rating scales

In its simplest form, a rating scale is a list of items that are rated to describe the presence, frequency, and/or severity of a behavior, emotion, or thought. Several rating scales have been developed over the past decade to assist in the quantification and description of EdF. In general, results from such rating scales are more predictive of everyday impairment of EF than laboratory testing alone.[47] This may reflect differences in the constructs being assessed by the two types of evaluation. In addition, contextual factors can be protective or exacerbating for the expression of EF and EdF, which may account for some of the variance between standardized test scores obtained in a clinic/laboratory and observation data obtained from home, school, and community settings. Some have suggested that the discrepancies between rating scale results and performance on standardized tests may reflect ecological validity of the rating scales (and implied invalidity of the standardized tests).[47] Given findings that impaired performance on EF tasks is associated with impairment in everyday life,[48] it is unlikely that ecological validity is the best explanation for the discrepancies. Different results from these different approaches to assessment indicate that both are important for understanding the whole story for each child assessed.

Rating scales are found to be most valuable when they have associated normative data, allowing the evaluator to directly compare a person's level of symptoms with what is typically reported for the child's chronological age group and/or grade placement.

When evaluating children, it is crucial to have age-based normative data; smaller age groupings allow more accurate assessment of whether a child's symptoms are developmentally appropriate or more consistent with a pattern of psychopathology (for example, see the comparison of Oppositional Defiant Disorder or ODD symptom frequency for preschoolers vs. older children discussed by Egger and Angold[49]). Normative data also allow the consideration of whether a child has a significant deficit vs. a relative weakness in an EF skill. Numerous studies have demonstrated age-related change for performance on EF tasks over the childhood and adolescence years (see Romine and Reynolds[50] for a summary). While adults show less dramatic change from year to year, it is still meaningful to group data chronologically in order to detect age-related changes, particularly as EF skills typically show deterioration in the later decades. Most statistical analyses of standardization samples for rating scales also indicate significant gender effects, including ratings of EF. Parents and teachers of boys tend to report higher levels of concern about EdF than parents and teachers of girls.[51,52] Some factors seem to show developmental differences not only for sex, but also for age by sex; in other words, girls show a significant change in certain behaviors at a different age than boys do (e.g., on the Inhibit scale of the BRIEF[52]). For this reason, it is helpful to have normative data that is grouped not only by age, but also by gender. This allows for consideration of possible gender-based differences even if a combined gender sample is reported in the final results. Finally, it is useful to have separate normative samples for information obtained from different sources (e.g., parents, teachers, self-report, and other reporters), as research shows variable patterns of reporting between these different observers for some key behaviors.[53,54,55,56]

Rating scales that have been explicitly developed for assessing EF include the Behavior Rating Inventory of Executive Function (BRIEF), which is available for parents and teachers to complete about preschoolers (ages 2 to 5 years, BRIEF-P) and school-aged children (ages 6 to 18 years, BRIEF). There is a self-report form for completion by youth 11 to 18 years old (BRIEF-SR), as well as a group of forms for adults 18 to 90 years old (BRIEF-A). The BRIEF was developed by a group of pediatric neuropsychologists who sought to capture data about real-life EF across the home and school settings. As such, they reference expectations regarding daily adaptive demands and academic success and provide information that makes sense to parents and teachers. Normative data for the BRIEF are somewhat limiting as they were collected from a restricted geographic region and thus may not be representative of the general population as a whole. The BRIEF scores provide summaries of various aspects of EF (e.g., inhibition, WM, self-monitoring) and can help organize a clinician's thoughts about where and why a student is struggling. Interestingly, a recent report found that the BRIEF was more highly correlated with parent and teacher descriptions of impairment than with performance on laboratory tests of EF;[57] this suggests that it may be a good standardized tool for capturing real-world data on a person's EF.

Although not explicitly marketed as an EF assessment tool, the Brown Attention Deficit Disorder Scales for Children and Adolescents (Brown ADD Scales) are based on the theory that attention disorders represent a developmental impairment of EF. These rating scales include such EF skills as organizing, prioritizing/activating, focusing/sustaining/shifting attention, and self-monitoring/self-regulating.

The Conners 3rd edition (Conners 3) is another ADHD-focused rating scale that includes aspects of EF among the domains being assessed. The "Executive Functioning" scale includes initiation, time management, planning, prioritizing, and organization concepts. Other scales on the Conners 3 can also reflect EdF, such as attention/concentration and self-control. Like the Brown ADD Scales and the BRIEF, the information obtained with the Conners 3 can assist in identifying areas requiring greater focus and assessment, as well as guiding intervention efforts.

While broadband rating scales such as the Behavior Assessment System for Children, Second Edition (BASC-2), Conners Comprehensive Behavior Rating Scales (Conners CBRS), and Achenbach System of Empirically Based Assessment (ASEBA) do not explicitly reference EF, data from such rating scales can provide information relevant to a consideration of EdF. Comprehensive rating scales such as these can also help gather information that is relevant to the broader context of issues beyond EF.

Clinical laboratory performance

The evaluation room is truly a laboratory, where hypotheses are developed and tested, and each clinical interaction provides single-case opportunities for assessing how and when EF deficits interfere with functioning. In this laboratory, there are rich opportunities to experiment and test hypotheses about EF and EdF while administering tests, pausing for a break, or cleaning-up materials. This empirical approach forms the basis of clinical assessment, and does not apply exclusively to the completion of research projects alone. While experimenting, it is important to remember that any variation from standardized administration must be noted and can limit use of normative data for comparison. As such, standardized portions of the evaluation should be completed first so that the evaluator can be confident that the experiment will not impact validity of test results.

The observation and interview techniques described above are relevant within the testing session. Some tasks have a constant level of one-to-one interaction (e.g., information subtest on the WISC-IV), while others have less examiner involvement (e.g., computerized continuous performance tests, or CPTs). An examinee's approach to problem-solving can be noted, such as whether he is systematic or random in his efforts to place blocks for WISC-IV Block Design or to produce words for verbal fluency. (See Table 4.1 for other examples of how EF can be observed during standardized test administration.) Neuropsychologists generally examine the process of *how* a score was earned (as well described by Edith Kaplan in her writing about the Boston Process Approach[58,59]) rather than stopping with *what* the score is, by testing the limits to better understand a child's failures as well as her successes. While these observations are not dictated by traditional administration of the tests, they can be implemented without violating standardization. Some tests have added standardized components to evaluate these variables (e.g., WISC-IV-Integrated offers companion tasks that help structure a task or evaluate basic components such as visual perception) or suggested observations that may capture aspects of EF (e.g., NEPSY-II off-task behaviors, oromotor rate change, rule violations, overflow movements).

Once standardized administration is complete, it can be enlightening to ask the examinee how she approached a task, or why she switched strategy mid-stream. When evaluating someone who may need to be tested again in the future, be very cautious about questions or suggestions that could impact future test performance (e.g., by suggesting that the examinee could have remembered more words on a list-learning task by grouping them into semantic categories). But observing how a child demonstrates and describes her approaches to a task provides insight into weaknesses and compensatory strategies she may be using.

As mentioned earlier, there remains a conundrum when developing standardized tools for assessing EF. Standardization typically involves some degree of consistency and structure from the testing environment and examiner; by providing this consistency and structure, some executive demands are significantly diminished or even removed. This is one reason why it is critical to obtain data from observation, interview, and rating scales when assessing for possible EdF. Some efforts have been made to develop less structured tasks, such as the Tinkertoy Test[2] which simply requires the examinee to create something using 50 standard building toy pieces placed on the table. Despite the apparent utility of such a task for capturing "executive" aspects of problem solving, very few studies have employed this task with children, perhaps due to difficulty with standardization and norming. Two studies using the Tinkertoy Test with pediatric samples failed to find significant developmental changes in typical children between 4 and 12 years old, although this test was sensitive to the effects of TBI.[60,61] The BADS-C includes open-ended EF tasks with hands-on items and is well-suited for use with children who have impaired receptive language, but clinical use of this promising tool is limited by a small normative sample from the United Kingdom as well as psychometric concerns.

There are a number of classic paper-pencil tasks that help assess EF, most of which originated in evaluation of people with neurologic insult such as stroke or TBI, and are commonly employed as part of a standard neurological examination. These include repetitive patterns or recurrent series writing (e.g., cursive "m n m n m n" followed by a row of "m m n m m n") and clock-drawing. These tasks provide valuable qualitative information about issues of planning and perseveration. However, apart from a geographically restricted set of pediatric norms for the clock-drawing task,[62] reliable normative data for such pencil and paper tasks are either unavailable or quite limited.

Several test batteries have been developed that are largely (if not exclusively) intended to assess aspects of EF. These include the BADS, BADS-C, CANTAB, CAS, D-KEFS, TEA-Ch, and the Attention and Executive Functioning composite on the NEPSY-II. Specific subtests from these batteries are mentioned as examples in the following sections.

Problem solving, planning, and strategy

Problem solving, planning, and strategy tasks include tower, categorization, 20 questions, and maze tasks. Less complex tasks that reflect strategy formation/use include visual search tasks. Planning can also be evidenced in a child's approach to design copy tasks. Strategy is also used in other tasks discussed in this chapter (e.g., verbal fluency).

The *tower* tasks typically present graduated disks (such as used in the D-KEFS Tower Test, a normed version of the classic Tower of Hanoi) or colored balls (such as used in the NEPSY Tower and TOLDX, normed versions of the classic Tower of London) on a series of pegs, with the requirement that the examinee must rearrange them to reach an end goal.

In the case of the disks, the examinee is told that larger disks cannot go on top of smaller disks, and the goal is to arrange the disks by order of size on a specific peg. In the case of the balls, the examinee is limited by pegs of varying heights, and is given a picture of the desired arrangement. All of the tower tasks require significant planning, particularly with the more complex items. WM is tapped, as the examinee can only move one piece at a time, but must remember his plan for reaching the ultimate goal. The tower tasks become much simpler if the examinee extracts a key underlying principle regarding the opening ploy for an odd versus even number of disks/balls. Self-monitoring is also involved, as some examinees will do and undo the same moves for infinite repetitions as they forget what they have already done and what they desire to do. Nothing is more frustrating than watching a child successfully stack the graduated disks after many torturous moves, only to realize he has stacked them on the wrong peg.

There are several variants of the *categorization* tests. The Wisconsin Card Sorting Test (WCST) requires the examinee to match a single card to one of four choices based on unstated principles. The Category Test and Children's Category Test (CCT) have a similar principle in that the child must decide which of four numbers or colors is suggested by each design. In contrast, the California Sorting Test (now part of the D-KEFS) provides the examinee with a pile of cards and requires her to divide them into groups based on some unspecified feature of the cards. All of these categorization tasks involve determining an unstated category and applying this information to correctly solve each item; for each of these tasks the category shifts multiple times during administration. Children completing the CCT are explicitly told that the rules have changed and that they must figure out the new rule. The D-KEFS Sorting Test is also explicit in that examinees are told to find as many different ways of sorting the cards as possible. The WCST shifts categories without warning – an examinee may be successfully applying one rule, then be startled by the feedback that he is now wrong with his card placement . . . leaving him to decide that he needs to try a new rule.

All of these tasks involve visual reasoning elements; the D-KEFS Sorting task adds a verbal reasoning element in that the examinee gets additional points for explaining the rule for each sorting of the cards (with bonus points for more complete explanations). A nice feature of the D-KEFS Sorting task is that after completing the free sort condition, the examiner completes a structured condition in which the youth is presented with correctly categorized cards and asked to explain how they were grouped. This allows assessment of concept recognition as opposed to initiation/generation involved in the first condition. All of these tasks require the youth to determine a rule, sustain strategy until given feedback to change, shift between response sets, learn from feedback, and inhibit incorrect responses. For the WCST and the CCT, the examinee must also recover from negative feedback ("that is incorrect") and keep trying rather than perseverating on the incorrect response set or the emotional reaction to the error.

The classic *20 questions* task began as a child's game, but was standardized as part of the D-KEFS. In this task, the examinee must ask a series of yes/no questions to determine which picture the examiner has chosen from an array of pictures. High levels of abstraction (e.g., "is it alive?" rather than, "is it the bird?"), planning and sequencing, memory for the strategy, and self-monitoring all contribute toward high scores on this task. Expressive language deficits can have an impact on overall performance.

The *maze* tasks involve visual problem solving and strategy (e.g., the Porteus Mazes or the WPPSI Mazes). Most maze tasks require accurate and rapid completion of the maze.

This involves scanning ahead to determine the best route, memory for the route, and impulse control to avoid taking a wrong turn. Fine motor deficits, slow processing speed, and visual impairment can deflate the score on a maze task. Tasks such as the NEPSY-II Visuomotor Precision task can help dissociate some of these components from the problem-solving aspects of the maze task.

Although simpler than the tasks described above, the classic visual search paradigm can reveal strategy use. Typically, an examinee is asked to quickly find and mark certain items (letters, numbers, pictures, symbols) in a full-page array of items. Relying on the items to pop-out without a strategic search usually results in high omission errors. Strategies might include scanning by rows or columns, or dividing the page into quadrants for review. Examples of visual search tasks include Mesulam's Tests of Directed Attention[63] and NEPSY Visual Search.

Finally, a child's approach to copying designs, whether simple (e.g., Beery–Buktenica's VMI) or complex (e.g., RCFT), can reveal planning deficits. For example, a child who begins by drawing the middle element of a design by the edge of the available space will not have room to accurately copy the design even if his visual perceptual skills and graphomotor skills are intact; his failure to plan for the entire design will limit his performance. This same issue can be observed in where and how a child writes his name at the top of a worksheet, completes a written language task, and performs mathematical calculations (e.g., words crammed onto the end of a line or running off the edge of the paper, calculations obscuring part of the next item).

Fluency

In general, fluency refers to the ability to rapidly and smoothly access stored knowledge. Fluency tasks include verbal fluency and rapid automated naming in the verbal domain, and include design fluency in the visual domain. Academic fluency tasks might also be considered in this category.

Traditionally, *verbal fluency* includes first-letter fluency and semantic fluency. In first letter fluency, the examinee is asked to rapidly produce as many words beginning with a certain letter as she can within the allotted time (often 1 minute). Phonemic fluency is a variation sometimes used with young children, requiring words that begin with the same sound (rather than letter). Semantic fluency is rapid generation of words belonging to the same semantic category (e.g., food, animals). Most commonly, verbal fluency tasks are oral, but there are normative data for written verbal fluency tasks as well. Some standardized versions provide examples to illustrate the point. Most verbal fluency tasks explicitly instruct the examinee to avoid proper nouns (e.g., names of people and places) and to avoid using the same word with different endings (e.g., "say" and "saying"). Some tasks do not allow use of numbers. All of the verbal fluency tasks require the examinee to access his store of verbal knowledge, inhibit related words that do not fit task requirements, and self-monitor to prevent repeating words within the task. Some individuals become fixated on an incorrect word (or a word they feel is inappropriate, such as a swear word), which distracts them from continuing with the task. It is helpful to note the progression of time during verbal fluency tasks, as some examinees begin with a burst of words, but cannot sustain their initial effort over the course of a minute and have no strategy for seeking new words. Methods for noting time include drawing a line in the word list to mark every 15 seconds, or writing the words in a four-block grid, shifting their relative position to reflect whether they were generated at the beginning, middle, or end of each 15-second block. Some individuals will use discernible strategies, such as alphabetical or semantic groupings within first-letter fluency, or grocery aisle groupings for semantic fluency. It is always interesting to note whether an examinee considers environmental cues during this task (e.g., neglecting to say "elephant" when there is an elephant wall-hanging, or adding "airplane" as a jet flies overhead). Once standardized testing is complete, it can be informative to ask the child how he tackled the verbal fluency task, as this may reveal a visual strategy (e.g., picturing co-workers during semantic fluency for names) or another approach.

Rapid automated naming tasks differ from verbal fluency tasks in that they provide stimuli for the examinee to name (rather than requiring generation of the items; standardized examples include the RAN/RAS, NEPSY-II Speeded Naming, and CTOPP Rapid Naming subtests). Common stimuli include colored shapes of varying sizes, although sometimes letters or numbers are used. The examinee is asked to name the items on the page, working quickly and accurately. Different versions vary in whether accuracy or speed are stressed, and whether practice conditions are provided. Some of these tasks have trials for various components before requiring the examinee to integrate all of the elements. For example, the child might complete a "size" condition, then "color" condition, then "shape" condition before being asked to identify size, color, and shape for the stimuli. In a sense, the basic components of a Stroop task (e.g., color naming, word reading) are rapid, automated naming tasks. It is helpful to examine whether these individual components help explain poor performance on the combined condition, particularly when letters or numbers are used. Sometimes examinees become flustered, and block on naming simple things with which they are quite familiar. Errors in the combined condition also include nontraditional sequence of the labels (e.g., "circle, red, little" rather than "little red circle"), effortful rather than fluent labeling, and inconsistent word use (e.g., using "little" on some items, and "small" or "tiny" on others). Even when these error types are not coded for scoring purposes, they can be quite informative in describing the lack of automation for naming, which impacts effort and thus fatigue levels in an everyday setting. Learning disabilities (LD), particularly dyslexia, can impact performance on these tasks. This is true not only for stimuli that are impacted by reversals and rotations (e.g., letters, numbers, and words); people with dyslexia often have a history of difficulty mastering basic labels like color and shape.[64,65]

In the visual domain, *design fluency* (also known as figural fluency; see RFFT, NEPSY-II Design Fluency, and D-KEFS Design Fluency) was designed to parallel verbal fluency. Some design fluency tasks are very unstructured, such as those requiring the examinee to generate many novel doodles on a blank piece of paper; these are more difficult to score in a standardized fashion. More structured design fluency tasks provide multiple grids or dots, and require the examinee to connect the dots to make a number of different designs. The dots may be in a structured array or in a "random" array. When the examinee is given dots to anchor his drawing, it facilitates standardized scoring, but changes the executive demands. Some examinees can be very successful in systematically generating many designs within the dot array, moving from top line to side line to bottom line to diagonal, then every permutation until time is exhausted. This is different from asking an examinee to generate the designs from nothing – a task that can stymie a systematic person. All versions of design fluency tasks share the requirement that the examinee must self-monitor to avoid repetitions.

Most academic achievement batteries include *academic fluency tasks* such as word reading fluency, passage reading fluency, alphabet writing fluency, passage writing fluency, and math calculation fluency (for example, see the academic fluency tasks on the WJ-Ach). These require EF in that they involve rapid access to stored information; however, they are heavily impacted by education. Dysfluency in one of these content areas can be indicative of a learning disability, limiting use of these tasks when examining EF in a person with LD.

Memory

Some memory tasks can be accomplished with very little EF; take for example a person who quickly memorizes large quantities of information without associating any meaning. In most people, though, executive skills can facilitate memory and learning. Developing and using a strategy to process and store information usually improves memory. Some memory tasks explicitly examine strategy use, such as the list-learning and design memory tasks discussed below. Other aspects of memory, such as WM, are generally considered primary EF skills.

List-learning tasks involve asking the examinee to learn a list of words. Most versions offer the examinee several chances to learn the list, assessing his ability to learn from repetition. Some versions ask the examinee to recall the list again after a delay (often 15–30 minutes later). List-learning tasks differ in several ways, including whether an interference trial occurs during the learning of the initial list (i.e., asking the examinee to learn a second list of words, then returning to the first list). Another difference is whether the examinee is explicitly warned that he will be asked to remember the words later in the session. A third difference is whether the words in the list are related. Some tasks, like the CVLT-C and CVLT, provide a score to measure whether the examinee uses a semantic strategy to group and remember words from the list. Researchers have evaluated ways to capture other strategies, such as sequential grouping, with mixed findings.[66] As mentioned with verbal fluency tasks above, visual strategies can aid performance on list-learning tasks. Like many other EF tasks, errors can reflect difficulties with self-monitoring (i.e., repeating words) and filtering (i.e., adding words that were not on the list).

The *Rey Complex Figure Test* (RCFT; also ROCF) is a classic EF task with a memory component. Executive skills are required from the beginning of this task, which requires the examinee to accurately copy a complex design. Using a strategy to organize the picture usually improves the copy condition, whether recognizing the main structural elements or moving systematically from quadrant to quadrant. When an examinee does not strategize, the copy may not resemble the original in many ways. Typically, the examinee copies the figure, then is asked to draw it from memory (either immediately or three minutes later, depending on the version being used). Some versions add a "delayed" recall, asking the examinee to draw the figure again 20 to 30 minutes later. It is useful to examine whether the examinee employs the same approach to drawing the figure across all conditions. Sometimes examinees produce a poor copy, but their reproduction improves by the final recall condition, as if their brain simply needed time to consolidate the design. One version of the task adds a recognition component, allowing the examiner to assess whether the examinee did not remember the design and its elements, or if she simply could not recall the design without prompts.

Working memory tasks share the common element of manipulating information while holding it "on line." Examples include Digit Span Backwards and Number-Letter Sequencing on the Wechsler scales. The classic n-back task (where "n" refers to how far back in a sequence the person must remember) also relies heavily on WM; standardized versions are included in the TEC and TEA-Ch. In a sense, the GDS Vigilance Task, where the button is pressed whenever a 1 is followed by a 9, is a simple n-back (1-back) task. WM tasks are flexible in that difficulty can easily be increased by lengthening the span or increasing the "n."

Inhibition

Although many of the tasks described thus far involve some degree of inhibition (e.g., inhibiting "rule violations" in a Tower or verbal fluency task), there are a group of tasks that focus on assessing inhibition. The "go/no-go" tasks are included in several CPTs as well as other behavioral tasks. The stop-signal tasks have been well-studied, but there are few normed versions.

In its simplest form, the go/no-go task has two conditions; when one type of stimulus appears, the examinee responds (the "go" condition), and when the second type of stimulus appears, the examinee does nothing (the "no-go" condition). There are many variants on this task, but most standardized versions are computerized. Several commercially available *continuous performance tasks (CPTs)* include the go/no-go paradigm (e.g., Conners CPT-II, TOVA, TEC). The "continuous performance" aspect is reflected in that the examinee is expected to perform the task without a break, usually for 10 to 20 minutes. What distinguishes a go/no-go CPT from a vigilance CPT is the proportion of "go" to "no-go" stimuli. In other words, when the examinee is responding at a high rate (i.e., many "go" stimuli), the task is more like a go/no-go task, as opposed to tasks during which the examinee responds infrequently (i.e., few "go" stimuli, many "no-go" stimuli) which is more of a classic vigilance task.

Analyses of go/no-go CPTs typically are based on signal detection theory, and compare proportions of "hits" and "false alarms" (i.e., correct responses with incorrect responses) by means of a discriminability index (d' or d-prime in Conners CPT-II and TOVA). An examinee who responds indiscriminately to every stimulus will produce a low discriminability index, as will the examinee who does not respond to any stimulus. Another statistic that is usually calculated is a bias statistic (beta in Conners CPT-II), which is a way of describing the examinee's bias in the speed-accuracy trade-off; that is, whether the examinee prioritizes speed (which can lead to high rates of commission errors, or impulsivity) or accuracy (which can lead to hesitation and missed items, or high rates of omission errors). Either end of the continuum can indicate impaired inhibition.

Beyond these computerized tests of inhibition, the go/no-go paradigm is represented in some behavioral tasks. For example, the NEPSY uses this paradigm in the Auditory Attention and Response Set. The child is instructed to respond whenever certain words are said, but to show no response to other words. The original version of this task allowed a broader view of inhibition, in that the child had to inhibit her urge to touch the attractive rubber squares until she heard the correct word; the version used in the NEPSY-II is less tempting in that the child simply touches printed color blocks on a page (no manipulatives). This revision helps insure the purity of the task by reducing other distractions, but loses an interesting source of qualitative information about general inhibitory abilities. Stroop-type and card-sorting tasks also require inhibition of the prepotent (but erroneous) response.

The stop-signal task is also a continuous performance task in a manner of speaking, as it requires the person to perform a decision-making task (usually visual) over a period of time; however, the stop-signal task requires the person to simultaneously attend to another signal (either visual or auditory) for a cue to stop responding (the "stop-signal"). The TEA-Ch Walk, Don't Walk subtest is a commercially available variant of the stop-signal task.

Go/No-Go tasks and stop-signal tasks both require inhibition, but research suggests that this inhibition comes at different times in the process. The Go/No-Go task seems to emphasize response selection (or "action restraint," inhibiting a motor response before it starts), whereas the stop-signal task emphasizes response inhibition (or 'action cancellation," stopping a response that has already begun).[67] Electrophysiological, anatomical, and neurochemical data suggest that these aspects of inhibition are separable.[68,69]

Neuromotor

In a sense, some of the neuromotor tasks described here could be subsumed under the Inhibition heading, as they involve the inhibition of neurologic signals beyond the intended motor cortex region. In young human brains, motor signals often are broadcast to groups of body parts, producing more widespread movements than required for the task. This is illustrated when a baby activates his entire body in an effort to reach for a single toy, rather than simply stretching his arm toward the toy and grasping it with his fingers. As the human brain matures, it becomes more adept at isolating signals to specific body parts. Some people with EdF continue showing poor motor inhibition, however.

One type of neuromotor error seen with EdF is *overflow*. Given the cortical map of the motor areas, it is common to see oromotor overflow during manual dexterity tasks (i.e., mouth movements during hand-based tasks). For example, young children often move their tongues and lips while effortfully writing; as children (and their brains) mature, these oromotor movements usually disappear during handwriting tasks. Another type of overflow error is mirror movements (a.k.a., synkinesis; i.e., when only one side of the body is required for a task, but both sides are activated simultaneously); these are usually observed in the hands and fingers. In mirror movements, the executive neural system fails to inhibit the signal from spreading to both sides of the body. In some ways, mirror movements are adaptive in young children (e.g., reaching out with both hands to catch a ball). As children develop, mirror movements should become less frequent. In assessment, tasks like pegboard tasks (e.g., Purdue Pegboard, Grooved Pegboard) and the NEPSY Hand Movements task offer a good chance to observe oromotor overflow and mirror movements, although in severe cases you may not need anything beyond watching the examinee during manipulative tasks (e.g., WISC-IV Block Design, tower tasks) and handwriting tasks. Recent studies suggest that overflow movements typically decrease between 7 to 14 years old, with improvement noted earlier in girls than boys.[70]

Another physical way EdF can be observed is *motor impersistence*. When examining motor impersistence clinically, the examinee is told to take a position and continue it until told otherwise. Common positions include eyes closed, mouth open, sideward gaze, or tongue protruding. People with motor impersistence cannot complete these tasks, or complete them with extreme effort (e.g., squeezing eyes shut tightly, eyelids flickering/ blinking, mouth moving, tongue wavering). The NEPSY Statue task is one standardized method of evaluating motor impersistence.

Shift

The ability to shift is a key aspect of EF, whether shifting from one task to another, shifting response sets, or shifting perspective (e.g., details to big picture and vice versa). Deficits in shifting can include shifting too easily which impacts sustained attention (a.k.a., distractibility). The opposite, difficulty shifting, can result in a child appearing overly rigid or "stuck." (Note the distinction between "directed" attention in this case, which is effortful and involves EF, and "automatic" attention which is an innate stimulus response.[71])

A key assessment tool that involves shifting is the trail-making test (TMT). The shifting component of TMT occurs when the examinee is asked to connect items in order, alternating between two response sets. The response sets are usually numbers and letters, although the Color Trails test (developed for use with non-English speakers and subsequently normed for use with children) may be useful for populations with limited or impaired letter knowledge (such as can occur with LD). This is typically accompanied by other components that help identify contributing factors such as overall slow speed or content-specific deficits (such as might occur with reading disorders). The card-sorting tasks discussed previously also require shifting between response sets, as do some verbal fluency tasks (e.g., D-KEFS Verbal Fluency, switching condition). Other verbal trails tasks include the Oral Trail Making Test (OTMT) and portions of the CMS Sequences subtest.

Although the Posner task has not found its way into the standardized assessment world, this research task was designed to assess shifting abilities. In this research paradigm, the examinee is instructed to watch a central fixation point on the computer monitor, and press the left or right response button when a stimulus appears in the left or right box on the screen. The examinee is given either a valid cue (the box where the stimulus is expected is briefly highlighted) or an invalid cue (the incorrect box is briefly highlighted). The task measures the speed and accuracy with which the examinee responds in both valid and invalid conditions. This task has an extensive research literature, and has merit for clinical use once normative data are made available.

Self-regulation and monitoring

It is critical to self-monitor and regulate one's own behaviors, whether in a social setting or laboratory setting. Although all agree these are essential skills, it is difficult to assess them in a standardized fashion. Within verbal fluency and list-learning tasks, self-regulation and monitoring can be inferred from repetition errors and intrusion errors. The NEPSY-II Visuomotor Precision task can also reveal deficits in these skills, as illustrated by a child's change in speed as she approaches a tight curve in the racetrack.

Organization

Again, this is a difficult task to observe in a quantitative way, but very important to describe. As with other skills described previously, either extreme of organization can pose a problem for a child's functioning, ranging from complete lack of organization to over-organization that interferes with task completion. In a sense, card-sorting tasks involve organization of materials. Written expression and verbal expression tasks such as those on the WIAT-II offer a chance to observe a child's organization of thoughts and language. A child's performance on projective tasks such as the Thematic Apperception Test (TAT) can provide data on his organizational skills, with an interesting contrast between high and low emotional stimulation situations. In the case of less subtle deficits, disorganization of thoughts and language can be observed in responses to short-answer questions, such as those used on the WISC-IV Similarities, Vocabulary, and Comprehension items. Beyond the verbal domain, organization can be observed in the context of a child's approach to copying a design, whether using paper-pencil or blocks.

Summary and future directions

It is important to describe intact aspects of EF when conducting an evaluation, as these strengths may be used to compensate for EdF or other cognitive weaknesses. (In fact, at least one study has reported that good EF can be a protective factor against issues like sleep deprivation).[72] In addition to the specific information gained from standardized tests targeting assessment of EF and EdF, aspects of EF can be observed during administration of most standardized tests, including a standard intellectual assessment. A child's approach to a test, responses to test items, and interaction with the examiner and the environment provide rich information about EF and EdF. Subtle EF deficits can be difficult to quantify in a laboratory setting, so it is critical to consider qualitative sources of data, including records such as report cards and observations from parents, teachers, youth, and other professionals. Examiners must be cautious about assumptions and attributions (by themselves as well as others); expectations about patterns of EF can bias observations and interpretation, suggesting EdF when none exists or missing unanticipated, subtle EdF.

Examination of factors that may be related to EF within more general scales will be helpful (for example, see recent re-analyses of the BASC-2).[73] Additional analyses of when low scores can be interpreted as deficits will guide interpretation of results from standardized testing (such as the work recently published by Crawford and colleagues).[74]

The very structure of standardized testing can reduce opportunities to observe EdF in some cases. Further investigation of assessment techniques that are less structured may lead to clinical tools for observing EdF in the laboratory setting. Possible models for this work might include structured observation systems like the Autism Diagnostic Observation Schedule (ADOS) and Transdisciplinary Play-Based Assessment (TPBA). The features of using certain materials to examine certain behaviors in a less structured assessment environment lend themselves to allowing observations of EF and EdF. Exploration of ways to standardize observations during administration of existing measures may also prove fruitful in capturing subtle EdF.[75]

Several research-based assessment tools have promise for clinical utility, such as the Posner task, the stop-signal task, and elements of the preschool battery developed by Espy and colleagues;[76,77] further development including manuals, standardized forms, and broader normative data would be beneficial. It may also be helpful to develop more companion tools that help assess relative contributions of EF (much like the WISC-IV-Int Coding and Coding Copy partnership helps dissociate graphomotor speed and information processing speed), continuing the initiative shown in parts of the D-KEFS (e.g., the various components that expand traditional TMT-A and TMT-B). Closer examination of similar tasks administered in different modalities (such as written versus oral TMT, or verbal versus figural fluency) may lead to additional insight into EF and EdF. Comparisons of studies with discrepant findings within the same clinical population (such as described in some Section II chapters) may identify key differences in task variations that impact results.

Efforts to identify core components of EF and EdF, including factor analysis[78] may guide which areas need additional measurement instruments. Continued partnership between clinicians and researchers to examine neurologic underpinnings of tasks may guide further refinement of tasks (such as has been initiated with inhibition tasks, comparing go/no-go and stop-signal tasks).

Further research into which aspects of assessment help identify meaningful interventions (such as those described in Chapter 17), measure interval progress, and predict prognosis is critical. Examination of ecological validity for work in EF and EdF is critical. Ultimately, the goal of assessment and identification is not labeling EdF, but leading to ways to make meaningful change to improve the lives of people with EdF.

References

1. Burgess PW. Theory and methodology in executive function research. In Rabbitt P, ed. *Methodology of Frontal and Executive Function*. Hove, England: Psychology Press; 1997, 81–116.

2. Lezak MD. The problem of assessing executive functions. *Int J Psychol*. 1982; 17: 281–97.

3. Bernstein J, Waber D. Developmental neuropsychological assessment: The systemic approach. In Boulton A, Baker G, Hiscock M, eds. *Neuromethods: Neuropsychology*. Clifton, NJ: Humana Press; 1990, 311–71.

4. Stuss DT, Alexander MP. Executive functions and the frontal lobes: a conceptual view. *Psychol Res*. 2000; 63(3–4): 289–98.

5. Biederman J, Petty CR, Fried R, *et al.* Discordance between psychometric testing and questionnaire-based definitions of executive function deficits in individuals with ADHD. *J Atten Disord*. 2008; 12(1): 92–102. Epub 2007 Oct 12.

6. Barkley R, Murphy K. The nature of executive function (EF) deficits in daily life activities in adults with ADHD and their relationship to performance on EF tests. *J Psychopath Behav Assessm*. 2011; 33(2): 137–58.

7. Ståhle L, Ståhle EL, Granström E, Isaksson S, Annas P, Sepp H. Effects of sleep or food deprivation during civilian survival training on cognition, blood glucose and 3-OH-butyrate. *Wilderness Environ Med*. 2011; 22(3): 202–10.

8. Waters F, Bucks RS. Neuropsychological effects of sleep loss: implication for neuropsychologists. *J Int Neuropsychol Soc*. 2011; 4: 1–16. [Epub ahead of print]

9. Abeare CA, Cohen JL, Axelrod BN, Leisen JC, Mosley-Williams A, Lumley MA. Pain, executive functioning, and affect in patients with rheumatoid arthritis. *Clin J Pain*. 2010; 26(8): 683–9.

10. Arnsten AF. The biology of being frazzled. *Science*. 1998; 280(5370): 1711–12.

11. Mitchell RL, Phillips LH. The psychological, neurochemical and functional neuroanatomical mediators of the effects of positive and negative mood on executive functions. *Neuropsychologia*. 2007; 45(4): 617–29. Epub 2006 Sep 7.

12. Chaddock L, Pontifex MB, Hillman CH, Kramer AF. A review of the relation of aerobic fitness and physical activity to brain structure and function in children. *J Int Neuropsychol Soc*. 2011; 17(6): 975–85.

13. Rogers SJ, Ozonoff S. Annotation: what do we know about sensory dysfunction in autism? A critical review of the empirical evidence. *J Child Psychol Psychiatry*. 2005; 46(12): 1255–68.

14. Iarocci G, McDonald J. Sensory integration and the perceptual experience of persons with autism. *J Autism Dev Disord*. 2006; 36(1): 77–90.

15. Suchy Y. Executive functioning: overview, assessment, and research issues for non-neuropsychologists. *Ann Behav Med*. 2009; 37(2): 106–16. Epub 2009 May 20.

16. Tomporowski PD, Davis CL, Miller PH, Naglieri JA. Exercise and children's intelligence, cognition, and academic achievement. *Educ Psychol Rev*. 2008; 20(2): 111–31.

17. Davis CL, Tomporowski PD, McDowell JE, et al. Exercise improves executive function and achievement and alters brain activation in overweight children: a randomized, controlled trial. *Health Psychol.* 2011; **30**(1): 91–8.

18. Barnett AL. Benefits of exercise on cognitive performance in schoolchildren. *Dev Med Child Neurol.* 2011; **53**(7): 580. doi: 10.1111/j.1469-8749.2011.03973.x. Epub 2011 Apr 15.

19. Dodrill CB. Myths of neuropsychology. *Clin. Neuropsychol.* **11**(1), 1997, 1–17.

20. Dodrill CB. Myths of neuropsychology: further considerations. *Clin Neuropsychol.* 1999; **13**(4): 562–72.

21. Zakzanis KK, Jeffay E. Neurocognitive variability in high-functioning individuals: implications for the practice of clinical neuropsychology. *Psychol Rep.* 2011; **108**(1): 290–300.

22. Schretlen DJ, Munro CA, Anthony JC, Pearlson GD. Examining the range of normal intraindividual variability in neuropsychological test performance. *J Int Neuropsychol Soc.* 2003; **9**(6): 864–70.

23. Schretlen DJ, Testa SM, Winicki JM, Pearlson GD, Gordon B. Frequency and bases of abnormal performance by healthy adults on neuropsychological testing. *J Int Neuropsychol Soc.* 2008; **14**(3): 436–45.

24. Binder LM, Iverson GL, Brooks BL. To err is human: "abnormal" neuropsychological scores and variability are common in healthy adults. *Arch Clin Neuropsychol.* 2009; **24**(1): 31–46. Epub 2009 Mar 6.

25. Mahone EM, Hagelthorn KM, Cutting LE, et al. Effects of IQ on executive function measures in children with ADHD. *Child Neuropsychol.* 2002; **8**(1): 52–65.

26. Russell EW. Toward an explanation of Dodrill's observation: High neuropsychological test performance does not accompany high IQs. *Clin Neuropsychol.* 2001; **15**: 423–8.

27. Rabin LA, Fogel J, Nutter-Upham KE. Academic procrastination in college students: the role of self-reported executive function. *J Clin Exp Neuropsychol.* 2011; **33**(3): 344–57. Epub 2010 Nov 25.

28. Bull R, Espy KA, Wiebe SA. Short-term memory, working memory, and executive functioning in preschoolers: longitudinal predictors of mathematical achievement at age 7 years. *Dev Neuropsychol.* 2008; **33**(3): 205–28.

29. Johnson S, Wolke D, Hennessy E, Marlow N. Educational outcomes in extremely preterm children: neuropsychological correlates and predictors of attainment. *Dev Neuropsychol.* 2011; **36**(1): 74–95.

30. Miller M, Hinshaw SP. Does childhood executive function predict adolescent functional outcomes in girls with ADHD? *J Abnorm Child Psychol.* 2010; **38**(3): 315–26.

31. Anderson P. Assessment and development of executive function (EF) during childhood. *Child Neuropsychol.* 2002; **8**(2): 71–82.

32. Rinsky JR, Hinshaw SP. Linkages between childhood executive functioning and adolescent social functioning and psychopathology in girls with ADHD. *Child Neuropsychol.* 2011; **17**(4): 368–90.

33. Harrison PL, Oakland T. *Adaptive Behavior Assessment System, 2nd edn (ABAS-II) Manual.* San Antonio, Texas: The Psychological Corporation; 2003.

34. Ruffolo J Somerville, Javorsky DJ, Tremont G, Westervelt HJ, Stern, RA. A comparison of administration procedures for the Rey-Osterrieth complex figure: flowcharts versus pen switching. *Psychol Assessm.* 2001; **13**(3) 2001:299–305.

35. Bernstein JH, Waber D. *DSS-ROCF: The Developmental Scoring System for the Rey–Osterrieth Complex Figure.* Lutz, FL: Psychological Assessment Resources, Inc., 1996.

36. Steinmetz J-P, Brunner M, Loarer E, Houssemand C. Incomplete psychometric equivalence of scores obtained on the manual and the computer version of the Wisconsin Card Sorting Test? *Psychol Assessm.* 2010; **22**(1): 199–202.

37. Ozonoff S. Reliability and validity of the Wisconsin Card Sorting Test in studies of autism. *Neuropsychology*. 1995; **9**: 491–500.

38. Kenworthy L, Yerys BE, Anthony LG, Wallace GL. Understanding executive control in autism spectrum disorders in the lab and in the real world. *Neuropsychol Rev*. 2008; **18**(4): 320–38. Epub 2008 Oct 28.

39. Baron, IS. *Neuropsychological Evaluation of the Child*. New York: Oxford University Press; 2004.

40. Lezak MD, Howieson DB, Loring DW, Hannay HJ, Fischer J. *Neuropsychological Assessment*. 4th edn. New York: Oxford University Press; 2004.

41. Strauss E, Sherman EMS, Spreen O. *A Compendium of Neuropsychological Tests: Administration, Norms, and Commentary*. 3rd edn. New York: Oxford University Press; 2006.

42. Golden CJ, Hines LJ. Assessment of executive functions in a pediatric population. In Davis A, ed. *Handbook of Pediatric Neuropsychology*. New York, NY: Springer Publ Co; 2011, 261–74.

43. Spies RA, Carlson JF, Geisinger KF (eds). *The 18th Mental Measurements Yearbook*. Lincoln, NE: Buros Institute of Mental Measurements; 2010.

44. Banich MT. Executive function: The search for an integrated account. *Curr Direct Psychol Sci*. 2009; **18**(2): 89–94.

45. Dawson P, Guare R. *Executive Skills in Children and Adolescents: A Practical Guide to Assessment and Intervention*. New York: The Guilford Press; 2004.

46. McCloskey G, Perkins LA, Van Divner B. *Assessment and Intervention for Executive Function Difficulties*. New York: Routledge, Taylor & Francis Group; 2009.

47. Barkley RA, Murphy KR. Impairment in occupational functioning and adult ADHD: the predictive utility of executive function (EF) ratings versus EF tests. *Arch Clin Neuropsychol*. 2010; **25**(3): 157–73. Epub 2010 Mar 2.

48. Burgess PW, Alderman N, Evans J, Emslie H, Wilson BA. The ecological validity of tests of executive function. *J Int Neuropsychol Soc*. 1998; **4**(6): 547–58.

49. Egger H, Angold A. Common emotional and behavioral disorders in preschool children: presentation, nosology, and epidemiology. *J Child Psychol Psychiatry*. 2006; **47**: 313–37.

50. Romine CB, Reynolds CR. A model of the development of frontal lobe functioning: findings from a meta-analysis. *Appl Neuropsychol*. 2005; **12**(4): 190–201.

51. Conners CK. *Conners 3rd Edition (Conners 3) Manual*. Toronto, ON, Canada: Multi-Health Systems, Inc.; 2008.

52. Gioia GA, Isquith PK, Guy SC, Kenworthy L. *BRIEF: Behavior Rating Inventory of Executive Function*. Odessa, Florida: Psychological Assessment Resources; 2000.

53. Achenbach TM, McConaughy SH, Howell CT (1987). Child/adolescent behavioral and emotional problems: Implications of cross-informant correlations for situational specificity. *Psychol Bull*. 1987; **101**: 213–32.

54. De Los Reyes A, Henry DB, Tolan PH, Wakschlag LS. Linking informant discrepancies to observed variations in young children's disruptive behavior. *J Abnorm Child Psychol*. 2009; **37**: 637–52.

55. Hartman CA, Rhee SH, Willcutt EG, Pennington BF. Modeling rater disagreement for ADHD: are parents or teachers biased? *J Abnorm Child Psychol*. 2007; **35**(4): 536–42.

56. Sourander A, Helstelä L, Helenius H. Parent-adolescent agreement on emotional and behavioral problems. *Soc Psychiatry Psychiatry Epidemiol*. 1999; **34**(12): 657–63.

57. McAuley T, Chen S, Goos L, Schachar R, Crosbie J. Is the Behavior Rating Inventory of Executive Function more strongly associated with measures of impairment or executive function? *Journal of the International Neuropsychological Society*. 2010; **16**: 495–505.

58. Milberg WP, Hebben NA, Kaplan E. 'The Boston process approach to neuropsychological assessment'. In Grant I, Adams KM, eds. *Neuropsychological Assessment of Neuropsychiatric Disorders*, 2nd edn. New York: Oxford University Press; 1996, 58–80.

59. White RF, Rose FE. The Boston process approach: A brief history and current practice. In Goldstein G, Incagnoli TM, eds, *Contemporary Approaches to Neuropsychological Assessment: Critical Issues in Neuropsychology*. New York: Plenum Press; 1997, 171–211.

60. Liebermann D. The relation between executive function and motivational orientations via private speech in preschoolers. 2008. Unpublished Dissertation, Accessed 01-12-2011 at http://hdl.handle.net/1828/1318

61. Roberts MA, Franzen KM, Furuseth A, Fuller L. A developmental study of the Tinker Toy test: normative and clinical observations. *Appl Neuropsychol*. 1995; 2(3–4): 161–6.

62. Cohen MJ, Ricci CA, Kibby MY, Edmonds JE. Developmental progression of clock face drawing in children. *Child Neuropsychol*. 2000; 6(1): 64–76.

63. Mesulam MM. *Principles of Behavioral Neurology*. Philadelphia, F.A. Davis; 1985.

64. Denckla MB. Color naming deficits in dyslexic boys. *Cortex* 1972; 8: 164–76.

65. Shaywitz S. *Overcoming Dyslexia*. New York: Vintage Books; 2003.

66. Sparrow EP, Blackburn LB. Performance on list-learning as a predictor of localized brain dysfunction. *JINS: J Int Neuropsychol Soc*. 2000; 6: 130. (Poster presentation at the 28th Annual Meeting of the International Neuropsychological Society, Denver, Colorado).

67. Schachar R, Logan GD, Robaey P, Chen S, Ickowicz A, Barr C. Restraint and cancellation: multiple inhibition deficits in attention deficit hyperactivity disorder. *J Abnorm Child Psychol*. 2007; 35: 229–38.

68. Johnstone SJ, Dimoska A, Smith JL, *et al.* The development of stop-signal and Go/Nogo response inhibition in children aged 7–12 years: performance and event-related potential indices. *Int J Psychophysiol*. 2007; 63(1): 25–38. Epub 2006 Aug 17.

69. Eagle DM, Bari A, Robbins TW. The neuropsychopharmacology of action inhibition: cross-species translation of the stop-signal and go/no-go tasks. *Psychopharmacology (Berl)*. 2008; 199(3): 439–56. Epub 2008 Jun 10.

70. Larson JC, Mostofsky SH, Goldberg MC, Cutting LE, Denckla MB, Mahone EM. Effects of gender and age on motor exam in typically developing children. *Dev Neuropsychol*. 2007; 32(1): 543–62.

71. Posner MI, Dehaene S. Attentional networks. *Trends Neurosci*. 1994; 17: 75–9.

72. Killgore WD, Grugle NL, Reichardt RM, Killgore DB, Balkin TJ. Executive functions and the ability to sustain vigilance during sleep loss. *Aviat Space Environ Med*. 2009; 80(2): 81–7.

73. Garcia-Barrera MA, Kamphaus RW, Bandalos D. Theoretical and statistical derivation of a screener for the behavioral assessment of executive functions in children. *Psychological Assessment*. 2011; 23(1): 64–79.

74. Crawford JR, Garthwaite PH, Sutherland D, Borland N. Some supplementary methods for the analysis of the Delis–Kaplan Executive Function System. *Psychol Assessm* 2011; 23(4): 888–98.

75. Anderson V, Levin H, Jacobs R. Executive functions after frontal lobe injury: A developmental perspective. In Stuss DT, Knight RT, eds. *Principles of Frontal Lobe Function*. 2002, New York: Oxford University Press; 2002, 504–27.

76. Wiebe SA, Espy KA, Charak D. Using confirmatory factor analysis to understand executive control in preschool children: I. Latent structure. *Dev Psychol*. 2008; 44(2): 575–87.

77. Espy KA, Sheffield TD, Wiebe SA, Clark CA, Moehr MJ. Executive control and dimensions of problem behaviors in

preschool children. *J Child Psychol Psychiatry*. 2011; **52**(1): 33–46. doi: 10.1111/j.1469–7610.2010.02265.x.

78. Miyake A, Friedman NP, Emerson MJ, Witzki AH, Howerter A, Wager TD. The unity and diversity of executive functions and their contributions to complex "Frontal Lobe" tasks: A latent variable analysis. *Cogn Psychol*. 2000; **41**(1): 49–100.

Introduction to Section II

Elizabeth P. Sparrow

Many neurodevelopmental and acquired disorders show evidence of EdF. This may reflect the vulnerability of EF given the number of brain areas involved in the executive network, or the extended time frame for the development of EF (see Chapters 2 and 3). The chapters in this section describe the current literature on EF and EdF in a number of disorders that occur in pediatric populations, including clinical presentation and possible neurologic bases.

Although the precise deficits vary by study and by disorder, the disorders discussed in this section share the common element of some degree of EdF being present (although intact aspects of EF are seen as well). Research has identified known genetic links for some of these disorders, like Down Syndrome, and suspected genetic links for others. Neuroimaging has helped identify involvement of multiple aspects of the executive neural network, including white matter tracts, frontal lobes, cerebellum, and/or subcortical areas, for all of these disorders.

There are several recurring themes throughout these disorder-specific chapters. In many cases, comorbidity makes it difficult to determine which disorder is most directly associated with observed EdF, such as is seen with co-occurring ADHD, ODD, and Tourette Syndrome (TS). It can be difficult to determine whether executive deficits are present at greater levels than expected with the pattern of cognitive delays associated with a disorder, such as with some forms of Intellectual Disability (ID). Differences among clinical samples, including age, level of intellectual functioning, sex, SES, and comorbidities can lead to discrepancies among study findings. Age of participants, particularly relative to age of onset/insult, can have a large impact on findings given the developmental sensitivity of EF.

Timing of study can affect results in instances with a waxing and waning course (e.g., TS, depression). Some disorders impact EF through direct as well as indirect mechanisms, as seen with the infectious diseases and TBI. In some instances, treatment for a condition is associated with additional EdF, such as with seizure disorders and pediatric cancers. Many of the disorders described in this section suggest that EdF can lead to additional health risks, such as increased rates of smoking (as seen with ADHD and childhood cancer survivors), dangerous driving (as seen with ADHD and human immunodeficiency virus or HIV), substance use, and poor compliance with treatment.

Most of these chapters describe aspects of EF that are intact, as well as elements of EdF that vary significantly. There are numerous illustrations to support gathering data about real-world functioning, as some aspects of EdF are not captured by widely-used

Executive Function and Dysfunction, ed. Scott J. Hunter and Elizabeth P. Sparrow. Published by Cambridge University Press. © Cambridge University Press 2012.

standardized tests. This is particularly important to consider and helps us remember that the impact of EdF goes beyond academics, and often includes social, emotional, and behavioral functioning. This is clearly supported by research with autism, ID, childhood cancers, and spina bifida, to name just a few of the disorders discussed.

The pervasiveness of EdF and its effect across many aspects of functioning contributes toward the severe impairment that is often observed clinically for children and adolescents with EdF. Many of the chapters in Section II emphasize the need for additional research into effective interventions for people with EdF, particularly interventions that generalize into everyday functioning. It is important to identify prognostic indicators that will help us better predict the outcome for a given person and anticipate her needs as she continues to develop.

Chapter

Executive functions in disruptive behavior disorders

Laura E. Kenealy and Iris Paltin

Attention-deficit/hyperactivity disorder (ADHD) and other disruptive behavior disorders (DBD), including conduct disorder (CD) and oppositional defiant disorder (ODD), are among the most common reasons parents seek mental health treatment for their children. The undercontrolled, impulsive behaviors that characterize these disorders seem, on the surface, to be closely linked to EF skills like self-regulation and inhibitory control. While the topic of EdF has been extensively researched in ADHD, the research into EdF in other DBDs remains at a fairly early stage of development. This chapter reviews the current literature on EdF in these disorders.

Attention-Deficit/Hyperactivity Disorder

The prevalence of ADHD is conservatively estimated at around 5% of school-aged samples,[1] but recently rates closer to 10% have been cited.[2] ADHD is defined by a constellation of difficulties with attention, activity level, impulse control, or a combination of these.[1] Symptoms must begin by age 7, last 6 months or more, be present in more than one setting, and cause impairment. There are three subtypes, including Predominantly Inattentive (ADHD-I), Predominantly hyperactive-impulsive (ADHD-HI), and Combined (ADHD-C). Various prior editions of the DSM have defined subtypes somewhat differently or not at all (for a review, see Barkley).[3] It appears the upcoming DSM-5 will essentially maintain the current subtypes with some additional symptoms for consideration, more flexible age of onset, and possible reductions in number of symptoms required for adult diagnosis.

Executive dysfunction in ADHD

Although the diagnostic criteria for ADHD are organized around the symptom triad of inattention, hyperactivity, and impulsivity, neuropsychological conceptualizations of ADHD have often centered on EF.[4-6] Barkley's detailed theory,[7] which posited a central deficit in behavioral inhibition that then leads to additional EF weaknesses in ADHD, has been the most influential model. Sergeant's cognitive-energetic model[8,9] proposes that individuals with ADHD have difficulties at three levels, including a cognitive level (specific mechanisms of attention), an energetic level (arousal, activation, and effort), and an executive control level (planning, monitoring, etc.). In Sonuga-Barke's dual pathway model,[10-12] ADHD can potentially arise from either a deficit in EF or a motivational style described as delay aversion. The constructs of behavioral disinhibition and delay aversion

Executive Function and Dysfunction, ed. Scott J. Hunter and Elizabeth P. Sparrow. Published by Cambridge University Press. © Cambridge University Press 2012.

appear to be at least somewhat dissociable, and make independent contributions to ADHD symptoms in clinical and community-based samples.[11,13,14]

A voluminous research literature on the nature and extent of EdF in ADHD has unfolded over the past 20 years, and due to space constraints, our discussion will focus primarily on recent findings, meta-analyses, and reviews. Meta-analyses of differences in EF between ADHD and typically-developing control groups show differences in tasks tapping *Inhibition, WM, Vigilance, and Planning.*[15,16] Consistent with theoretical models emphasizing inhibitory control deficits in ADHD, studies have consistently found that children with ADHD have poorer *inhibitory self-regulation* than controls, and, in particular, there is stronger evidence for deficits in ADHD related to suppressing a prepotent response (as on a stop-signal or go/no-go task) than for other types of inhibitory control, such as related to interference control (e.g., on a Stroop-type task).[17,18] In the area of WM, ADHD appears particularly associated with deficits in *spatial WM*, with a meta-analysis showing larger effect sizes when measures required some manipulation rather than simple storage.[19] Zelazo and Mueller have categorized EFs as either "hot" or "cool," and suggest that ADHD is more associated with difficulties on tests of cool *EFs.*[20] These cool EFs are mediated by fronto-striatal brain networks, and involve higher level skills such as planning, WM, and inhibition when it is tested in a way removed from strong affective valence (e.g., Stroop, Go/ No-Go, CPTs). The cool EFs are contrasted with hot EFs that involve stronger affective valence, salient incentives, and motivation (e.g., gambling tasks), and which are mediated by more frontolimbic networks. As Castellanos and colleagues have pointed out,[21] the preponderance of literature on ADHD has focused on tests of "cool" EFs, and they have suggested that while inattention may be related to cool EFs, impulsivity and disinhibition may relate more directly to hot EFs. A recent review by Rubia concluded that this hypothesis is only partly supported by the evidence to date.[22]

It should be noted that most of the subjects in the studies described above were school-aged boys with ADHD-C. There is, however, evidence of similar patterns in girls,[23] and at ages spanning from preschool through adulthood.[24] Indeed, the literature appears to support more similarities than differences across gender, age, and even subtypes of ADHD.[18,24–26] However, there are gaps in the lifespan literature[24] and a need for more longitudinal studies. There are also some major challenges in studying the diagnostic subtypes of ADHD as currently defined. As Diamond has pointed out,[27] ADHD-I tends to be a mixed bag, with some individuals having a subclinical level of hyperactivity and impulsivity, and other individuals having no trace of those qualities. The "pure" form ADHD-I may really represent a different disorder altogether, possibly characterized by a primary deficit in WM.[7,27–29] Indeed, there is at least some evidence that subtypes of ADHD can be distinguished by their EF profiles, with the ADHD-I characterized more by problems in WM, and the ADHD-C by inhibitory deficits.[30]

While there are consistent differences between individuals with ADHD and controls at the group level, there has recently been increasing attention to heterogeneity *within* ADHD. Reviews and meta-analyses of studies using individually-administered tests of EF tend to show only moderate effect sizes[15,16] and significant heterogeneity, with only a portion of individuals with ADHD showing EdF[31] on the commonly-used laboratory and clinical measures of EF included in the reviews (e.g., stop signal tasks, N-back, span tasks, Tower of London, WCST). Thus, some authors have concluded that new models of ADHD must be multifactorial, and account for heterogeneity in the neuropsychological underpinnings of ADHD.[16,31]

Challenges in the measurement of EF may also contribute to the difficulties in reliably capturing EdF in children with ADHD. Brown has suggested that the ability of researchers to identify EdF in ADHD depends on the sensitivity of our neuropsychological tests for EF.[5] As noted elsewhere in this volume (see Chapters 1 and 4 specifically), EF problems that are readily seen in real life can nonetheless be difficult to capture using laboratory or clinical measures.[32] Challenges in identifying EdF with standardized tests include insufficient sensitivity of tests (for example, in terms of their ability to capture more subtle developmental difficulties as opposed to the more frank effects of a major acquired brain insult that the tests were initially designed to measure), the fact that the structure of the testing situation may mask impairments, and the potential that compensatory mechanisms may allow individuals with ADHD to use capabilities in other areas (e.g., strong language skills) to perform adequately on tests of EF.[18,33] It is entirely possible that individuals with ADHD, who are known to display substantial variability in task performance and sensitivity to environmental structure,[3] have deficits in EF that are not reliably captured on laboratory tests.

The neurological basis of executive dysfunction in ADHD

ADHD runs in families (heritability estimates are around 0.76–0.80),[34,35] and molecular genetic studies have implicated dopamine transporter gene variants.[34,36,37] This is particularly interesting, given the positive response of individuals with ADHD to stimulant medications, which largely act on dopamine. Some environmental events, such as maternal smoking during pregnancy or early exposure to lead, also confer some risk of ADHD diagnosis, but reviews have concluded that there is little evidence for shared or common environmental factors (such as general parenting strategies) causing ADHD.[3]

Reviews of the neuroimaging literature in ADHD point to alterations in the PFC, its connections to other areas such as the striatum and cerebellum, and related neural circuitry.[34,35,38,39] Specifically, structural findings show smaller overall cerebral volume in ADHD,[35] with meta-analytic findings indicating the largest differences in cerebellar regions, the splenium of the corpus callosum, total and right cerebral volume, and right caudate.[40] DTI studies indicate abnormalities in white matter tracts that carry information from the frontal lobes to other cortical and subcortical areas.[41] Reviews of functional imaging findings have generally concluded that ADHD involves dysfunction in frontal-striatal areas[34,42] in both adults and children.[43,44] Stimulant medication has been shown to normalize the underactivation in frontal-striatal areas.[45] The overall evidence from both structural and functional imaging research would suggest that brain systems implicated in ADHD include fronto-striatal areas and extend to associated networks and other areas, including cerebellum and parietal lobes.[46]

Oppositional defiant disorder and conduct disorder

The definition of ODD in the DSM-IV-TR is "a recurrent pattern of negativistic, defiant, disobedient, and hostile behavior directed at authority figures that persists for at least 6 months."[1] This is usually observed before the age of 8, and persistent symptoms must be associated with clinically significant impairment. Proposed changes in the DSM-5 involve reorganizing the list of symptoms, adding a severity rating, and possibly including more objective frequency criteria. The definition of CD in the DSM-IV-TR is "a repetitive and persistent pattern of behavior in which the basic rights of others or major age-appropriate societal norms or rules are violated."[1] This includes overt aggression, property destruction, theft, and law breaking. CD is 2–3 times more common in males than females.[47] Changes in the diagnostic criteria are not anticipated in the DSM-5, but a Callous and Unemotional Traits specifier has been proposed.

ODD is the most common comorbid diagnosis in children with ADHD, occurring in up to 60% of the ADHD cohort, with CD co-occurring in about 20% of the cohort.[48] ODD and/or CD occur more in ADHD-C than ADHD-I and are often co-morbid with LD, mood and/or anxiety disorders, and substance use disorders.

Executive dysfunction in ODD and CD

Are ODD and CD associated with EdF beyond what would be expected from comorbid ADHD? The literature related to EdF in ODD is quite limited. One study rather counter-intuitively demonstrated that children with ODD, with or without comorbid ADHD, generally performed *better* on a planning task than other comparison and control groups.[49] While some studies have failed to show EdF in cohorts with pure externalizing disorders,[50] other studies have shown that comorbid ADHD+ODD is associated with more significant deficits than ADHD alone on neuropsychological measures of *attention, inhibition, WM, organization/planning, and self-monitoring*,[51,52] *set shifting* skills,[53] and *global executive functions in daily life* as measured by the BRIEF.[54] Thus, it may be that when ODD presents alone, EF deficits may not be particularly salient, but the combination of ODD+ADHD may confer risk for additional EdF compared to ADHD alone.

Many more studies focus on individuals with CD, which has long been associated with specific EF deficits, including difficulty with *flexibility* (e.g., WCST, TMT-B), *verbal fluency* (e.g., COWAT), *self-monitoring* (e.g., Porteus Maze Test), *inhibition* (e.g., Stroop), *WM* (e.g., WISC-IV Working Memory Index), and *planning* (e.g., RCFT).[55] *Emotional dysregulation* has been proposed as a central deficit in CD.[56] While studies have predominantly focused on males, female cohorts also showed reduced EF, including *verbal fluency, inhibition, planning, and WM*.[57,58] *Motor inhibition*, rather than verbal inhibition or cognitive inhibition, has been specifically identified as an area of impairment in males and females with CD.[59] At the same time, while EF deficits in the domains of flexibility, WM, shifting, and verbal fluency were identified in a CD cohort, these deficits do not always reliably differentiate adolescents with CD from controls when controlling for other aspects of a cognitive profile (e.g., verbal deficits, learning disorders).[60] In a recent review of the literature, however, Rubia concluded that CD is uniquely associated with deficits in hot *EFs* such as impulsive reward-related choice patterns on gambling tasks, and response perseveration due to reduced sensitivity to punishment.[22]

The neurological basis of executive dysfunction in ODD and CD

The biological underpinnings of ODD are not well understood, but a literature is emerging related to CD. Both social and genetic contributions are considered important in the development of the disorder.[56] The short allele of the serotonin transporter gene is likely associated with negative/externalizing behaviors (e.g., impulsivity, aggression, violence), and neural structures (e.g., amygdala), related to dysregulated behaviors like those seen in CD.[22] Androgen receptor genes also appear to play a role in CD.[61]

Neuroimaging studies of CD have rarely examined "pure" samples; comorbid ADHD and mood disorders are common. Structurally, CD appears to be associated with abnormalities in the paralimbic system, including orbitofrontal cortex and associated areas.[22] Consistent with structural findings, functional studies reveal that children with CD (often with comorbid ADHD) evidence abnormal functioning of the paralimbic system, including the ventromedial orbitofrontal temporolimbic system, compared with healthy controls.[22] Thus, the structural and functional abnormalities seen in CD are in brain areas known to regulate motivation and affect and to be associated with the hot EFs.

Summary and future directions

The DBD, including ADHD, CD, and ODD, all appear related to EdF in some respects, and contemporary models almost invariably include some aspect of executive self-regulation in conceptualizing these disorders. Recent research has led to several exciting developments, including an increasingly sophisticated approach to parsing EF skills according to their underlying neural networks, a dramatic increase in structural and functional neuroimaging studies, and increasing attention to heterogeneity within diagnostic categories.

Several challenges face future studies of EF and EdF in ADHD, ODD, and CD. Many studies use traditional, individually administered tests of EF that may lack ecological validity and appropriate sensitivity to developmental deficits. Studies sometimes use one test to measure a broad EF construct, and different studies may use different measures to assess the same function. Important covariates such as IQ, gender, and socio-economic variables may not be adequately controlled for, and in addition to the problem of comorbid ADHD/CD/ODD in samples, other common comorbidities (LD, mood disorder) are usually not addressed. ODD remains understudied compared to CD and especially ADHD. Lastly, longitudinal studies are needed to better understand developmental trajectories of EF in the disruptive behavior disorders.

References

1. American Psychiatric Association. *Diagnostic and Statistical Manual of Mental Disorders.* Revised 4th edn. Washington DC: Author; 2000.

2. Centers for Disease Control and Prevention. Increasing prevalence of parent-reported attention-deficit/hyperactivity disorder among children – United States, 2003 and 2007. *MMWR* 2010; 50(44): 1439–43.

3. Barkley RA. *Attention-deficit Hyperactivity Disorder: A Handbook for Diagnosis and Treatment.* 3rd edn. New York: Guilford; 2006.

4. Pennington BF, Ozonoff S. Executive functions and developmental psychopathology. *J Child Psychol Psychiatry* 1996; 37(1): 51–87.

5. Brown TE. Executive functions and attention deficit hyperactivity disorder: implications of two conflicting views. *Int J Disabil Dev Educ* 2006; 53(1): 35–46.

6. Denkla MB. Executive function: Binding together the definitions of attention-deficit/hyperactivity disorder and learning disabilities. In Meltzer L, ed. *Executive Function in Education.* New York: Guilford; 2007, 5–18.

7. Barkley RA. *ADHD and the Nature of Self-control.* New York: Guilford; 1997.

8. Sergeant JA, Oosterlaan J, van der Meere J. Information processing and energetic factors in attention-deficit/hyperactivity disorder. In Quay HC, Hogan AE, eds. *Handbook of Disruptive Behavior Disorders.* New York: Plenum; 1999, 75–104.

9. Sergeant, JA. Modeling attention-deficit/hyperactivity disorder: a crucial appraisal of the cognitive-energetic model. *Biol Psychiatry* 2005; 57: 1248–55.

10. Sonuga-Barke EJS. Psychological heterogeneity in AD/HD: a dual pathway model of behaviour and cognition. *Behav Brain Res* 2002; 130: 29–36.

11. Sonuga-Barke EJS. The dual pathway model of AD/HD: an elaboration of neuro-developmental characteristics. *Neurosci Biobehav Rev* 2003; **27**: 593–604.

12. Sonuga-Barke EJS, Sergeant JA, Nigg J, Willcutt E. Executive dysfunction and delay aversion in attention deficit hyperactivity disorder: nosologic and diagnostic implications. *Child Adolesc Psychiatr Clin N Am* 2008; **17**(2): 367–84.

13. Dalen L, Sonuga-Barke EJS, Hall M, Remington B. Inhibitory deficits, delay aversion and preschool AD/HD: implications for the dual pathway model. *Neural Plast* 2004; **11**(1–2): 1–11.

14. Solanto MV, Abikoff H, Sonuga-Barke EJS, *et al*. The ecological validity of delay aversion and response inhibition as measures of impulsivity in AD/HD: a supplement to the NIMH multimodal treatment study of AD/HD. *J Abnorm Child Psychol* 2001; **29**(3): 215–28.

15. Wilcutt EG, Doyle AE, Nigg JT, Faraone SV, Pennington BF. Validity of the executive function theory of Attention Deficit/ Hyperactivity Disorder: a meta-analytic review. *Biol Psychiatry* 2005; **57**: 1336–46.

16. Willcutt EG, Attention-deficit/ hyperactivity disorder. In Yeates KO, Ris MD, Taylor HG *et al*., eds. *Pediatric Neuropsychology: Research, Theory and Practice*. New York: Guilford; 2010, 393–417.

17. Nigg JT. Is ADHD a disinhibitory disorder? *Psychol Bull* 2001; **127**(5): 571–98.

18. Doyle AE. Executive functions in attention-deficit/ hyperactivity disorder. *J Clin Psychiatry* 2006; **67** Suppl 8: 21–6.

19. Martinussen R, Hayden J, Hogg-Johnson S, Tannock R. A meta-analysis of working memory impairments in children with attention deficit/ hyperactivity disorder. *J Am Acad Child Adolesc Psychiatry* 2005; **44**(4): 377–84.

20. Zelazo PD, Mueller U. Executive function in typical and atypical development. In Goswami U, ed. *The Blackwell Handbook of Childhood Cognitive Development*. Malden, MA: Blackwell; 2002, 445–69.

21. Castellanos FX, Sonuga-Barke EJS, Milham MP, Tannock R. Characterizing cognition in ADHD: beyond executive dysfunction. *Trends Cogn Sci* 2006; **10**: 117–23.

22. Rubia K. "Cool" inferior frontostriatal dysfunction in attention-deficit/ hyperactivity disorder versus "hot" ventromedial orbitofrontal-limbic dysfunction in conduct disorder: a review. *Biol Psychiatry* 2011; **69**: e69–e87.

23. Miller M, Hinshaw SP. Does childhood executive function predict adolescent functional outcomes in girls with ADHD? *J Abnorm Child Psychol* 2010; **38**: 315–26.

24. Seidman LJ. Neuropsychological functioning in people with ADHD across the lifespan. *Clin Psychol Rev* 2008; **26**: 466–85.

25. Geurts HM, Verte S, Oosterlaan J, Roeyers H, Sergeant JA. ADHD subtypes: do they differ in their executive functioning profile? *Arch Clin Neuropsychol* 2005; **20**: 457–77.

26. Martel M, Nikolas M, Nigg JT. Executive function in adolescents with ADHD. *J Am Acad Child Adolesc Psychiatry* 2007; **46**(11): 1437–44.

27. Diamond A. Attention-deficit disorder (attention-deficit hyperactivity disorder without hyperactivity): a neurobiologically and behaviorally distinct disorder from attention-deficit/ hyperactivity disorder (with hyperactivity). *Dev Psychopathol* 2005; **17**: 807–25.

28. Goodyear P, Hynd GW. Attention-deficit disorder with (ADD/H) and without (ADD/WO) hyperactivity: Behavioral and neuropsychological differentiation. *J Child Clin Psychol* 1992; **21**: 273–305.

29. Barkley RA. The inattentive type of ADHD as a distinct disorder: What remains to be done. *Clin Psychol-Sci Pr* 2001; **8**: 489–93.

30. Gioia GA, Isquith PK, Kenworthy L, Barton, R. Profiles of everyday executive function in acquired and developmental disorders. *Child Neuropsychol* 2002; **8**(2): 121–37.

31. Nigg JT, Willcutt EG, Doyle AE, Sonuga-Barke, EJS. Causal heterogeneity in attention-deficit/hyperactivity disorder: do

we need neuropsychologically impaired subtypes? *Biol Psychiatry* 2005; **57**: 1224–30.

32. Cripe LI. The ecological validity of executive function testing. In Sbordone RJ, Long CI, eds. *Ecological Validity of Neuropsychological Testing*. Delray Beach, FL: GR Press/ St Lucie Press; 1996, 71–202.

33. Doyle AE, Faraone SV, Seidman LJ, *et al.* Are endophenotypes based on measures of executive functions useful for molecular genetic studies of ADHD? *J Child Psychol Psychiatry* 2005; **46**(7): 774–803.

34. Biederman J, Faraone SV. Attention-deficit hyperactivity disorder. *Lancet* 2005; **366**: 237–48.

35. Kieling C, Goncalves RRF, Tannock R, Castellanos FX. Neurobiology of attention deficit hyperactivity disorder. *Child Adolesc Psychiatr Clin N Am* 2008; **17**: 285–307.

36. Mick E, Faraone SV. Genetics of attention deficit hyperactivity disorder. *Child Adolesc Psychiatr Clin N Am* 2008; **17**: 261–84.

37. Kirley A, Hawi Z, Daly G, *et al.* Dopamine system genes in ADHD: toward a biological hypothesis. *Neuropsychopharmacology* 2002; **27**(4): 607–19.

38. Arnsten AFT. Fundamentals of attention-deficit/hyperactivity disorder: circuits and pathways. *J Clin Psychiatry* 2006; **67** Suppl 8: 7–12.

39. Roth RM, Saykin AJ. Executive dysfunction in attention deficit/ hyperactivity disorder: cognitive and neuroimaging findings. *Psychiatr Clin N Am* 2004; **27**: 83–96.

40. Valera EM, Faraone SV, Murray KE, Seidman LJ. Meta-analysis of structural imaging findings in attention-deficit/ hyperactivity disorder. *Biol Psychiatry* 2007; **61**: 1361–9.

41. Liston C, Cohen MM, Teslovich T, Levenson D, Casey BJ. Atypical prefrontal connectivity in attention-deficit/ hyperactivity disorder: pathway to disease or pathological endpoint? *Biol Psychiatry* 2011; **69**: 1168–77.

42. Bush G, Valera EM, Seidman LJ. Functional neuroimaging of attention-deficit/ hyperactivity disorder: a review and suggested future directions. *Biol Psychiatry* 2005; **57**: 1273–84.

43. Cubillo A, Halari R, Smith A, Taylor E, Rubia K. A review of fronto-striatal and fronto-cortical brain abnormalities in children and adults with attention deficit hyperactivity disorder (ADHD) and new evidence for dysfunction in adults with ADHD during motivation and attention. *Cortex* 2012; **48**(2): 194–215.

44. Dickstein SG, Bannon K, Castellanos FX, Milham MP. The neural correlates of attention deficit hyperactivity disorder: an ALE meta-analysis. *J Child Psychol Psychiatry* 2006; **47**(10): 1051–62.

45. Rubia K, Halari R, Cubillo A, *et al.* Methylphenidate normalizes fronto-striatal underactivation during interference inhibition in medication-naïve boys with attention-deficit hyperactivity disorder. *Neuropsychopharmacology* 2011; **36**: 1575–86.

46. Cherkasova MV, Hechtman L. Neuroimaging in attention-deficit hyperactivity disorder: Beyond the frontostriatal circuitry. *Can J Psychiatry* 2009; **54**(10): 651–64.

47. Moffitt T, Caspi A, Rutter M, Silva P. *Sex Differences in Antisocial Behavior: Conduct Disorder, Delinquency, and Violence in the Dunedin Longitudinal Study*. Cambridge: Cambridge University Press; 2001.

48. Connor DF, Steeber J, McBurnett K. A review of attention-deficit/hyperactivity disorder complicated by symptoms of oppositional defiant disorder or conduct disorder. *J Dev Behav Pediatr* 2010; **31**(5): 427–40.

49. Klorman R, Hazel-Fernandez LA, Shaywitz, SE, *et al.* Executive functioning deficits in attention-deficit/hyperactivity disorder are independent of oppositional defiant or reading disorder. *J Am Acad Child Adolesc Psychiatry* 1999; **38**(9): 1148–55.

50. Clark C, Prior M, Kinsella GJ. Do executive function deficits differentiate between adolescents with ADHD and Opposition Defiant/Conduct Disorder? A neuropsychological study using the Six

Elements Test and Hayling Sentence Completion Test. *J Abnorm Child Psychol* 2000; **28**(5): 403–14.

51. Youngwirth SD, Harvey EZ, Gates EC, *et al.* Neuropsychological abilities of preschool-aged children who display hyperactivity and or oppositional-defiant behavior problems. *Child Neuropsychol* 2007; **13**(5): 422–43.

52. Giancola PR, Mezzich AC, Tarter RE. Executive cognitive functioning, temperament, and antisocial behavior in Conduct-Disordered adolescent females. *J Abnorm Psychol* 1998; **107**(4): 629–41.

53. Van Goozen S, Cohen-Kettenis PT, Snoek H, *et al.* Executive functioning in children: a comparison of hospitalized ODD and ODD/ADHD children and normal controls. *J Child Psychol Psychiatry* 2004; **45**(2): 284–92.

54. Qian Y, Shuai L, Cao Q, *et al.* Do executive function deficits differentiate between children with attention deficit hyperactivity disorder (ADHD) and ADHD comorbid with oppositional defiant disorder? A cross-cultural study using performance-based tests and the Behavior Rating Inventory of Executive Function. *Clin Neuropsychol* 2010; **24**(5): 793–810.

55. Moffitt T. The neuropsychology of Conduct Disorder. *Dev Psychopathol* 1993; **5**: 135–51.

56. Cappadocia MC, Desrocher M, Pepler D, *et al.* Contextualizing the neurobiology of Conduct Disorder in an emotion dysregulation framework. *Clin Psychol Rev* 2009; **29**(6): 506–18.

57. Giancola PR, Mezzich AC. Executive cognitive functioning mediates the relation between language competence and antisocial behavior in Conduct-Disordered adolescent females. *Aggressive Behav* 2000; **26**: 359–75.

58. Pajer K, Chung J, Leininger L, *et al.* Neuropsychological function in adolescent girls with conduct disorder. *J Am Acad Child Adolesc Psychiatry* 2008; **47**(4): 416–25.

59. Herba CM, Tranah T, Rubia K, *et al.* Conduct problems in adolescence: Three domains of inhibition and effect of gender. *Dev Neuropsychol* 2006; **30**(2): 659–95.

60. Närhi V, Lehto-Salo P, Ahonen T, *et al.* Neuropsychological subgroups of adolescents with conduct disorder. *Health Disabil* 2010; **51**: 278–84.

61. Comings DE, Gade-Andavolu T, Gonzalez, *et al.* Mulivariate analysis of associations of 42 genes in ADHD, ODD and Conduct Disorder. *Clin Genet* 2000; **58**: 31–40.

Chapter

Executive functions in autism spectrum disorders

Lauren Kenworthy, Laura Gutermuth Anthony, and Benjamin E. Yerys

Autism is a neurodevelopmental disorder that is behaviorally defined by the presence of a triad of behavioral impairments affecting social abilities, communication skills, and rigid, repetitive behaviors and interests.[1] The DSM-IV-TR divides autism, or in its terminology, Pervasive Developmental Disorders, into diagnostic subcategories, including Asperger's Disorder, Autistic Disorder, and Pervasive Developmental Disorder–Not Otherwise Specified (PDD-NOS; a category for individuals who do not meet full criteria for autism). The application of these subcategories is inconsistent across clinics in the United States, however, and there is confusion about associated features and additional diagnoses, such as ADHD.[2] The proposed criteria for a new category, Autism Spectrum Disorder (ASD), in the DSM-5 include dropping all subcategories of diagnosis and utilizing a dimensional approach to complement the single categorical label of ASD. This dimensional approach would allow for the designation of associated features as qualifiers, such as intellectual or language difficulties and ADHD.[3] The term "ASD" is used throughout this chapter to describe research findings for Asperger's Disorder, Autistic Disorder, and PDD-NOS.

Executive dysfunction in ASD

Damasio and Maurer[4] first linked ASD to EdF when they described behavioral similarities between individuals with ASD and those with frontal lesions, including lack of social motivation, poor communication, and perseverative behavior. Although EdF has not been demonstrated as a causal factor in ASD,[5] it has been related to symptoms that define ASD,[6–8] as well as to lower adaptive functioning in ASD.[9] Findings of EdF are robust in school age children with ASD,[5,10–12] who show specific impairment with tasks that require cognitive flexibility[13–14] and organization.[15] Reviews also highlight numerous studies where children with ASD demonstrate an impaired ability to plan on tasks such as the Tower of London.

Our understanding of EF in ASD has evolved over the last 20 years. In their extensive review, Pennington and Ozonoff[11] reported larger effect sizes associated with cognitive inflexibility and poor planning in ASD than for any EF measures in other developmental disorders (i.e., ADHD, CD, and Tourette Syndrome or TS). Inhibition and WM, on the other hand, were considered mostly intact in ASD. Hill's[10] review supported the argument for significant planning and cognitive flexibility deficits in individuals with ASD, as well as suggesting difficulties with inhibiting a pre-potent response (i.e., response inhibition), and generativity. Kenworthy and colleagues[5] reviewed positive evidence for EF

Executive Function and Dysfunction, ed. Scott J. Hunter and Elizabeth P. Sparrow. Published by Cambridge University Press. © Cambridge University Press 2012.

deficits in inhibition and spatial WM, but found that multiple recent investigations of performance on *computerized* measures of planning[16] and flexibility[17-18] failed to replicate the robust findings of deficits on the planning and flexibility tasks that are administered by a human being. This discrepant finding across administration formats supports the hypothesis that multi-step EF tasks are most difficult when individuals with ASD must adhere to arbitrary, socially presented rules or feedback.[19] Difficulty with using internal speech to guide behavior may contribute to impaired EF performance for individuals with ASD.[20-25] Related to the possibility that EF deficits in ASD arise from "real world" demands to be flexible, organized and planful in socially-mediated settings, informant report measures of EF (e.g., the BRIEF and The Behavior Flexibility Rating Scale-Revised (BFRS-R);[26]) consistently show impairment in ASD groups.

The implications of our still evolving understanding of EdF in ASD for clinical practice include:

1. It is important to assess EF, particularly in high-functioning school age children with ASD, in whom deficits are common.

2. Complex EF tasks that tap several discrete processes and are administered by a human being, such as the Tower tasks, the WCST and the ROCF are sensitive to impairments in ASD.

3. Assessing spatial WM is also recommended. Williams and colleagues[27-28] found WRAML Finger Windows to be sensitive to deficits in ASD.

4. It is important to sample multiple EF subdomains. Several processes underlying EF are purportedly impaired in ASD, although the heterogeneity within this diagnostic category may confound efforts to identify specific EF profiles. Furthermore, comorbidity between ASD and ADHD, obsessive-compulsive disorder (OCD), and other conditions linked to EdF may impact EF profiles[29] Thus developing a test battery that assesses core EF processes – flexibility, planning/organization, verbal and spatial WM, and inhibition – is important.

5. Informant report measures, such as the BRIEF and BFRS, and other ecologically valid tools are useful compliments to laboratory tasks when attempting to characterize EdF in ASD.[30]

The neurological basis of executive dysfunction in ASD

Neuroimaging literature in ASD has progressed substantially over the last 20 years, with early results highlighting changes in brain structure, and more recent studies examining brain function and connectivity. PFC, striatum, and parietal cortex are considered critical brain structures for EF.[31-33] The PFC develops atypically, with early excessive growth in gray matter in children with ASD[34-35] and reduced gray matter in adulthood.[36] Neuropathology studies show narrowed and more densely packed minicolumns in dorsal PFC.[37] Structural studies have also highlighted atypical development of the striatum[36,38-39] and gray matter in the parietal cortex,[40-42] although this is not a consistent finding.[43-44] White matter structures (e.g., corpus callosum, uncinate) relevant for connectivity within and across the PFC have also been identified as atypical in ASD.[45] In particular, cross-sectional structural studies using DTI techniques in children with ASD show atypical development of white matter in the PFC[46-48] and volumetric studies have shown abnormal white matter volumes, particularly in boys with ASD.[49-50]

In addition to structural neuroimaging studies of brain regions critical for EF, there is a small fMRI literature on set-shifting/cognitive flexibility, planning, WM, and inhibition in individuals with ASD. fMRI measures changes in hemodynamic response (i.e., blood flow) while an individual is completing a task, and this serves as a proxy for brain activity. With respect to cognitive flexibility, there are a handful of studies showing adolescents/young adults with ASD demonstrate altered hemodynamic responses in key prefrontal regions like the DLPFC, ACC, and mesial/inferior parietal cortex relative to age- and IQ-matched controls[51–53] Furthermore, these differences in function have been correlated with gray matter abnormalities reported in the same sample's structural images.[51] In another study of set shifting, hemodynamic response in the ACC correlated negatively with reported repetitive behavior symptoms,[52] such that hemodynamic response decreased as lifetime occurrence of symptoms increased. In a study of WM,[54] adults with ASD were reported to perform similarly to controls, but to have increased hemodynamic responses in right prefrontal and parietal cortices relative to controls. Reduced hemodynamic response in PFC, ACC, and other posterior regions was seen in an inhibition/inhibition+WM task.[55]

A major advancement in the study of ASD has been the use of functional connectivity methods that have shown atypical synchronization among brain regions that comprise a network.[45] Functional connectivity methods can briefly be described as investigating correlations between two brain regions' hemodynamic response during a task or while individuals are engaged in a resting state. This correlation is speculated to represent the efficiency of synchronous activity between the two brain regions. An example of this technique's benefit is seen in an fMRI study of planning that employed a forced-choice version of the Tower of London task and reported no differences in task performance or the hemodynamic response between ASD and control groups,[56] but did find reduced correlations between brain regions in the ASD group relative to the matched controls. This reduced correlation has also been reported in EF studies of ASD where group differences exist in standard fMRI analyses. In the WM and inhibition studies discussed above, factor analyses also revealed altered functional connectivity in ASD relative to controls, including greater within hemisphere connectivity in the ASD group during a WM task.[54] A separate study found that the inhibition network was less integrated in ASD relative to controls.[55] There is also evidence suggesting that lateral inferior PFC may have reduced functional connectivity with striatal and parietal regions across age.[57]

Summary and future directions

In summary, EF is an important area to assess in ASD. Multiple EF subdomains should be sampled, using complex EF tasks (e.g., WCST, tower tasks, ROCF), which although non-specific, are useful for assessing the global coordination of EF, as well as measures of WM and inhibition. Use of real-world informant report measures (e.g., BRIEF) to complement the data acquired from cognitive tasks administered in the clinic or laboratory is important to capture the full presentation of EdF, which is most evident in unstructured settings where task demands are not explicitly stated. At the same time, it is important to recognize that there is clear evidence for a biological basis for EdF in ASD, highlighting EdF as a potential core feature. Abnormalities in the development of gray and white matter structure in the brain and differences in functional activity and connectivity have been documented and correlated in some cases with the severity of autism symptoms.

Disentangling the complex interrelationships between social, language and EF demands in ASD and in EF assessment tools is a thorny problem for the future. Reconciling evidence of ASD-related impairment on human-administered tower and card sorting tasks, but generally intact performance on similar computer-administered tasks[58] requires careful parsing of the multiple language, social, and executive demands inherent in these tasks. The clinician is sometimes able to do this by virtue of comparisons in an individual's performance on a variety of tasks, by looking for patterns across neuropsychological domains, and differences in performance on tasks with overlapping demands.[59] Meanwhile, researchers have their work cut out for them in the attempt to disambiguate the complex and interrelated developmental trajectories of social and non-social cognition in ASD.[60]

Integrating disparate findings on laboratory EF tasks and real-world EF measures is another challenge for the future. Real-world EF tasks are less able to disentangle social, language and EF demands than laboratory tasks, but they are better at capturing essential aspects of EF, which requires the execution of multiple step plans in *unstructured* settings.[61–62] See Kenworthy and colleagues[5] for a detailed discussion of this problem in ASD.

There is also work to be done on recognizing and measuring variability in ASD. Hill[10,63] has identified the powerful role that variability in IQ and performance on cognitive tasks plays in our understanding of EF in ASD. High comorbidity with other disorders associated with EdF, such as ADHD and OCD[29] further complicates the problem. Larger sample sizes and the proposed DSM-5 revision to permit the comorbid diagnosis of ADHD in ASD will allow future research to investigate variability of performance as an independent variable of interest and also to compare ASD groups with and without key comorbid disorders such as ADHD.[64–65]

The specific methods used to analyze functional neuroimaging data to support the "general underconnectivity" hypothesis of ASD[66] may significantly affect the type of results generated (for reviews and empirical demonstration of how analysis methods affect functional connectivity results see Jones and colleagues[67] and Muller and colleagues).[68] This raises the question of whether the observed differences are true or driven by data analysis methods. Future research will aim to refine the analysis methods to reduce bias, and this will offer us a clearer window into the neural function of individuals with ASD relative to other clinical groups and typically developing individuals.

While we continue to study the mechanisms and measurement of EF in ASD, it is also imperative that we develop innovative interventions that target EF and enhance the everyday lives and independence of individuals with ASD. There have been several promising starts at interventions improving EF in children with ASD.[69–71] We are currently testing a new contextually based intervention[72] that builds upon this work and the Ylvisaker and Feeney[73–74] intervention for children with TBI. Future research is needed to identify effective EF supports, such as technology and apps, develop interventions that are appropriate for different ages and functioning levels, and personalize interventions for children and adults.

References

1. American Psychiatric Association. (2000). *Diagnostic and Statistical Manual of Mental Disorders (4th ed., Text Revision).* Arlington, VA: American Psychiatric Publishing.

2. Lord C. Epidemiology: how common is autism? *Nature* 2011; **474**: 166–8.

3. Happé F. Criteria, categories, and continua: autism and related disorders in DSM-5. *J Am Acad Child Adolesc Psychiatry* 2011; **50**: 540–2.

4. Damasio AR, Maurer RG (1978). Neurological model for childhood autism. *Arch Neurol* 1978; **35**: 777–86.

5. Kenworthy LE, Yerys BE, Anthony LG, Wallace GL. Understanding executive control in autism spectrum disorders in the lab and in the real world. *Neuropsychol Rev* 2008; **20**: 320–38.

6. Lopez BR, Lincoln AJ, Ozonoff S, Lai Z. Examining the relationship between executive functions and restricted repetitive symptoms of autistic disorder. *J Autism Dev Disord* 2005; **35**: 445–60.

7. Reed P, Watts H, Truzoli R. Flexibility in young people with autism spectrum disorders on a card sort task. *Autism* 2012; **345**(11): 33–42.

8. South M, Ozonoff S, McMahon WM (2007). The relationship between executive functioning, central coherence, and repetitive behaviors in the high-functioning autism spectrum. *Autism* 2007; **11**: 437–51.

9. Gilotty L, Kenworthy L, Sirian L, Black DO, Wagner AE. Adaptive skills and executive function in autism spectrum disorders. *Child Neuropsycho* 2002; **8**: 241–8.

10. Hill EL. Executive dysfunction in autism. *Trends in Cogn Sci* 2004; **8**: 26–32.

11. Pennington BF, Ozonoff S (1996). Executive functions and developmental psychopathology. *J Child Psychol Psychiatry* 1996; **37**: 51–87

12. Seargant JA, Geurts H, Oosterlaan J. How specific is a deficit of executive functioning for attention-deficit/hyperactivity disorder? *Behav Brain Res* 2002; **130**: 3–28.

13. Gioia GA, Isquith P K, Kenworthy L, Barton RM. Profiles of everyday executive function in acquired and developmental disorders. *Child Neuropsych* 2002; **8**: 121–37.

14. Hughes C, Russell J, Robbins TW. Evidence for executive dysfunction in autism. *Neuropsychologia*, 1994; **32**: 477–92.

15. Kenworthy LE, Black DO, Wallace GL, Ahluvalia T, Wagner AE, Sirian LM (2005). Disorganization: The forgotten executive dysfunction in high-functioning autism (HFA) spectrum disorders. *Dev Neuropsychol* 2005; **28**: 809–27.

16. Ozonoff S, Cook I, Coon H, *et al.* Performance on Cambridge Neuropsychological Test Automated Battery subtests sensitive to frontal lobe function in people with autistic disorder: evidence from the Collaborative Programs of Excellence in Autism Network. *J Autism Dev Disord* 2004; **34**: 135–50.

17. Geurts HM, Verté S, Oosterlaan J, Roeyers H, Sergeant JA. How specific are executive function deficits in attention deficit hyperactivity disorder and autism? *J Child Psychol Psychiatry* 2004; **45**: 836–54.

18. Landa R, Goldberg MC. Language, social, and executive functions in high-functioning autism: a continuum of performance. *J Autism Dev Disord* 2005; **35**: 557–73.

19. Bíró S, Russell J. The role of arbitrary procedures in means-end behavior in autism. *Dev Psychopathol* 2001; **13**: 96–108.

20. Joseph RM, McGrath LM, Tager-Flusberg H. Executive dysfunction and its relation to language ability in verbal school-age children with autism. *Dev Neuropsychol* 2005; **27**: 361–78.

21. Joseph RM, Steele SD, Meyer E, Tager-Flusberg H. Self-ordered pointing in children with autism: Failure to use verbal mediation in the service of working memory? *Neuropsychologia* 2005; **43**: 1400–11.

22. Russell J, Jarrold C, Hood B. Two intact executive capacities in children with autism: Implications for the core executive dysfunctions in the disorder. *J Autism Dev Disord* 1999; **29**: 103–12.

23. Wallace GL, Silvers JA, Martin A, Kenworthy LE. Brief report: further evidence for inner speech deficits in autism spectrum disorders. *J Autism Dev Disord* 2009; **39**: 1735–9.

24. Wallace GL, Dankner N, Kenworthy L, Giedd J, Martin A. Age-related temporal and parietal cortical thinning in autism spectrum disorders. *Brain* 2010; **133**: 3745–54.

25. Whitehouse AJO, Maybery MT, Durkin K. Inner speech impairments in autism. *J Child Psychol Psychiatry* 2006; **57**: 857–65.

26. Peters-Scheffer N, Didden R, Green VA, *et al.* The behavior flexibility rating scale-revised (BFRS-R): Factor analysis, internal consistency, inter-rater and intra-rater reliability, and convergent validity. *Rese Dev Disab* 2008; **29**: 398–407.

27. Williams DL, Goldstein G, Carpenter, PA, Minshew NJ. Verbal and spatial working memory in autism. *J Autism Dev Disord* 2005; **35**: 747–56.

28. Williams DL, Goldstein G, Carpenter PA, Minshew NJ. The profile of memory function in children with autism. *Neuropsychology* 2006; **20**: 21–9.

29. Leyfer OT, Folstein SE, Bacalman S, *et al.* Comorbid psychiatric disorders in children with autism: interview development and rates of disorders. *J Autism Dev Disord* 2006; **36**: 849–61.

30. Geurts HM, Corbett B, Solomon M. The paradox of cognitive flexibility in autism. *Trends Cogn Sci* 2009; **13**: 74–82.

31. Goldman-Rakic PS. Regional and cellular fractionation of working memory. *Proc Nat Acad Sci USA* 1996; **93**: 13473–80.

32. Hazy TE, Frank MJ, O'Reilly RC. Towards an executive without a homunculus: computational models of the prefrontal cortex/basal ganglia. *Phil Trans Roy Soc B-Biol Sci* 2007; **362**: 1601–13.

33. Miller EK, Cohen JD. An integrative theory of prefrontal cortex function. *Ann Rev Neurosci* 2001; **24**: 167–202.

34. Belmonte MK, Allen G, Beckel-Mitchener A, Boulanger LM, Carper RA, Webb SJ. Autism and abnormal development of brain connectivity. *J Neurosci* 2004; **24**: 9228–31.

35. Courchesne E, Pierce K, Schumann CM, *et al.* (2007). Mapping early brain development in autism. *Neuron* 2007; **56**: 399–413.

36. Rojas DC, Peterson E, Winterrowd E, Reite ML, Rogers SJ, Tregellas JR. Regional gray matter volumetric changes in autism associated with social and repetitive behavior symptoms. *BioMed Centr Psychiatry* 2006; **6**: 56.

37. Buxhoeveden DP, Semendeferi K, Buckwalter J, Schenker N, Switzer R, Courchesne E. Reduced minicolumns in the frontal cortex of patients with autism. *Neuropathol Appl Neurobiol* 2006; **32**: 483–91.

38. Haznedar MM, Buschbaum MS, LiCalzi EM, Cartwright C, Hollander E. Volumetric analysis and three-dimentional glucose metabolic mapping of the striatum and thalamus in patients with autism spectrum disorders. *J Am Psychiatry* 2006; **163**: 1252–63.

39. Langen M, Schnack HG, Nederveen H, *et al.* Changes in the development trajectories of striatum in autism. *Eur Neuropsychopharmacol* 2009; **19**: S678–9.

40. Brieber S, Neufang S, Bruning N, *et al.* Structural brain abnormalities in adolescents with autism spectrum disorder and patients with attention deficit/hyperactivity disorder. *J Child Psychol Psychiatry Allied Discipl* 2007; **48**: 1251–8.

41. Eckeret C, Marquand A, Mourao-Miranda J, *et al.* Ascribing the brain in autism in five dimensions – Magnetic resonance imaging-assisted diagnosis of autism spectrum disorder using a multiparameter classification approach. *J Neurosci* 2010; **32**: 10612–23.

42. Schumann CM, Bloss CS, Barnes CC, *et al.* Longitudinal magnetic resonance imaging study of cortical development through early childhood in autism. *Journal of Neurosci* 2010; **30**: 4419–27.

43. Hardan AY, Muddasani S, Vemulapalli M, Keshavan MS, Minshew NJ. An MRI study of increased cortical thickness in autism. *Am J Psychiatry* 2006; **163**: 1290–2.

44. Hazlett HC, Poe MD, Gerig G, Smith RG, Piven J. Cortical gray and white brain tissue volume in adolescents and adults with autism. *Biol Psychiatry* 2006; **59**: 1–6.

45. Müller RA. The study of autism as a distributed disorder. *Ment Retard Dev Disab Res Rev* 2007; **13**: 85–95.

46. Barnea-Goraly N, Kwon H, Menon V, Eliez S, Lotspeich L, Reiss AL. White matter

disruption in autism: preliminary evidence from diffusion tensor imaging. *Biol Psychiatry* 2004; **55**: 326.

47. Ben Bashat D, Kronfeld-Duenias V, Zachor DA, *et al.* Accelerated maturation of white matter in young children with autism: a high B value DWI study. *Neuroimage* 2007; **37**: 40–7.

48. Sundaram SK, Kumar A, Makki MI, Behen ME, Chugani HT, Chugani DC. Diffusion tensor imaging of frontal lobe in autism spectrum disorder. *Cereb Cortex* 2008; **18**: 2659–65.

49. Herbert MR, Ziegler DA, Deutsch CK, *et al.* (2003). Dissociations of cerebral cortex, subcortical and cerebral white matter volumes in autistic boys. *Brain* 2003; **126**: 1182–92.

50. Herbert MR, Ziegler DA, Makris N, *et al.* Localization of white matter volume increase in autism and developmental language disorder. *Ann Neurol* 2004; **55**: 530–40.

51. Schmitz N, Rubia K, Daly E, Smith A, Williams S, Murphy DGM. Neural correlates of executive function in autistic spectrum disorders. *Biol Psychiatry* 2006; **59**: 7–16.

52. Shafritz KM, Dichter GS, Baranek GT, Belger A. The neural circuitry mediating shifts in behavioral response and cognitive set in autism. *Biol Psychiatry* 2008; **63**: 974–80.

53. Solomon M, Ly S, Yoon JH, Carter CS. Neural correlates of the development of cognitive controls in adolescents with autism spectrum disorders. *Biol Psychiatry* 2009; **65**: 148S–9S.

54. Koshino H, Carpenter PA, Minshew NJ, Cherassky VL, Keller TA, Just MA. Functional connectivity in an fMRI working memory task in high-functioning autism. *Neuroimage* 2005; **24**: 810–21.

55. Kana RK, Keller TA, Minshew NJ, Just MA. Inhibitory control in high-functioning autism: decreased activation and underconnectivity in inhibition networks. *Biol Psychiatry* 2007; **62**: 198–206.

56. Just MA, Cherkassky VL, Keller TA, Kana RK, Minshew NJ. Functional and anatomical cortical underconnectivity in autism: evidence from an fMRI study of an executive function task and corpus callosum morphometry. *Cereb Cortex* 2007; **17**: 951–61.

57. Lee PS, Yerys BE, Della Rosa A, *et al.* Functional connectivity of the inferior frontal cortex changes with age in children with autism spectrum disorders: a fcMRI study of response inhibition. *Cereb Cortex* 2009; **19**: 1787–94.

58. Ozonoff S. Reliability and validity of the Wisconsin card sorting tests in studies in autism. *Neuropsychology* 1995; **9**: 491–500.

59. Denckla MB. The behavior rating inventory of executive function: commentary. *Child Neuropsychology* 2002; **8**: 304–6.

60. Pellicano E. The development of core cognitive skills in autism: a 3-year prospective study. *Child Dev* 2010; **81**: 1400–16.

61. Gioia GA, Isquith PK. Ecological assessment of executive function in traumatic brain injury. *Dev Neuropsychol* 2004; **25**: 135–58.

62. Bernstein JH, Waber DP. Developmental neuropsychological assessment: the systemic approach. In Boulton AA, Baker GB, Hiscock M, eds. *Neuropsychology: Neuromethods* Vol. **17**. Clifton, NJ: Humana; 1990.

63. Hill EL, Bird CA. Executive processes in Asperger syndrome: Patterns of performance in a multiple case series. *Neuropsychologia* 2000; **44**: 2822–35.

64. Sinzig J, Morsch D, Bruning N, Schmidt MH, Lehmkhuhl G. Inhibition, flexibility, working memory, and planning in autism spectrum disorders with and without comorbid ADHD symptoms. *Child Adolesc Psychiatry Ment Hlth* 2008; **2**: 4.

65. Yerys BE, Wallace GL, Sokoloff JL, Shook DA, James JD, Kenworthy LE. Attention deficit/hyperactivity disorder symptoms moderate cognition and behavior in children with autism spectrum disorders. *Autism Res* 2009; **2**: 322–33.

66. Just MA, Cherkassky VL, Keller TA, Minshew NJ. Cortical activation and synchronization during sentence

comprehension in high-functioning autism: evidence of underconnectivity. *Brain* 2004; **127**: 1811–21.

67. Jones TB, Bandettini PA, Kenworthy L, *et al.* Sources of group differences in functional connectivity: An investigation applied to autism spectrum disorder. *Neuroimage* 2010; **49**: 401–14.

68. Müller RA, Shih P, Keehn B, Deyoe JR, Leyden KM, Shukla DK. Underconnected, but how? A survey of functional connectivity MRI studies in autism spectrum disorders. *Cereb Cortex* 2011; **21**(10): 2233–43.

69. Calhoun JA. Executive functions: A discussion of the issues facing children with autism spectrum disorders and related disorders. *Semin Speech Lang* 2006; **27**: 60–72.

70. Fisher N, Happé F. A training study of theory of mind and executive function in children with autistic spectrum disorders. *J Autism Dev Disord* 2005; **35**: 757–71.

71. Solomon M, Goodwin-Jones B, Anders T. A social adjustment enhancement intervention for high functioning autism, Asperger syndrome, and Pervasive Developmental Disorder NOS. *J Autism Dev Disord* 2004; **34**: 649–68.

72. Cannon L, Kenworthy L, Alexander K, Werner M, Anthony LG. *Unstuck and On Target!: An Executive Function Curriculum to Improve Flexibility and Goal Directed Behavior for Children with ASD*. Baltimore: Paul H. Brookes Publishing Co; 2011.

73. Feeney T, Ylvisaker M. Context-sensitive cognitive behavioral supports for young children with TBI. *J Positive Behav Intervent* 2008; **10**: 115–28.

74. Ylvisaker M, Feeney T. Helping children without making them helpless: facilitating development of executive self-regulation in children and adolescents. In Anderson V, Jacobs R, Anderson P eds. *Executive Functions and the Frontal Lobes: A Lifespan Perspective*. London, UK: Taylor and Francis; 2008, 409–38.

Chapter

7

Executive functions in intellectual disability syndromes

Kelly Janke and Bonnie Klein-Tasman

Intellectual disability (ID) is characterized as intellectual functioning falling significantly below population norms, accompanied by difficulties with day-to-day tasks (i.e., adaptive functioning), that is first observed during childhood. The DSM-IV-TR relies on the level of intellectual functioning (i.e., IQ) to denote severity, as intelligence is the most clearly defined component of ID. A practical alternative approach to classifying severity used by the American Association on Intellectual and Developmental Disabilities (AAIDD)[1] is to consider the level of support the individual requires. A clearer conceptualization of adaptive functioning and a classification system no longer based on IQ are among the proposed changes for DSM-5.

Some of the most common known causes of ID are genetic syndromes, which have distinct etiologies and are often associated with characteristic cognitive and behavioral phenotypes. Although ID syndromes are by definition associated with a general decline in intellectual functioning, there is variation in their specific cognitive profiles which is not adequately captured by an overall IQ score. Hence, a primary goal of research with these populations is to clarify unique patterns in cognitive and adaptive functioning. Both cognitive and adaptive functioning are impacted by EdF;[2] therefore, investigation of neurocognition in genetic syndromes helps elucidate genetic and neural mechanisms underlying EdF in ID. To illustrate the role of EdF in a range of genetic disorders associated with ID, this chapter focuses on EF in four of the most common ID syndromes with genetic etiologies: Down syndrome, Fragile X syndrome, Williams syndrome, and phenylketonuria. Summaries of EdF in other neurodevelopmental disorders commonly associated with ID are also provided for reference in Table 7.1.

Down syndrome

Down syndrome (DS) is the most common genetic cause of ID, affecting 1 in 600 to 1000 live births. In addition to cognitive delays, DS is associated with characteristic facial features (depressed nasal bridge, slanting palpebral fissures, epicanthic folds, tongue protrusion), congenital heart malformations, gastrointestinal defects, hearing and vision impairment, delayed motor function, language impairments, accelerated aging, and an increased risk for early-onset Alzheimer's disease. DS results from the presence of extra genetic material on chromosome 21, and three types of chromosome errors have been described.[3,4] Variability in the etiology of DS is useful for specifying genotype–phenotype relations. Current

Executive Function and Dysfunction, ed. Scott J. Hunter and Elizabeth P. Sparrow. Published by Cambridge University Press. © Cambridge University Press 2012.

Table 7.1. *Summary of EF-related findings in ID syndromes*

Syndrome/disorder	EF-related neuropsychological and neurological findings
22q11.2 deletion syndrome	• Deficits are consistently observed in EF, WM, and motor organization compared to standardized norms and sibling controls.[80] Parent-reported EF difficulties correlate with social skills deficits.[81] Impairment on a card sort task was found to correlate with schizophrenia-prodrome symptoms in adolescents.[82] • EdF may be related to abnormal prefrontal-basal ganglia circuitry.[83]
*Down syndrome (DS)	• EF deficits are seen in childhood, and there may be age-related changes that correspond with brain pathology.[11] EdF is seen in the preclinical stages of early onset Alzheimer's disease in DS.[15] • Reduced volumes of the PFC and cerebellum may contribute to EdF.[17]
*Fragile X syndrome (FraX)	• Deficits are seen across many EF measures, even when controlling for intellectual functioning.[26,29] • Brain abnormalities are consistently seen in the caudate nucleus, cerebellum, and frontal lobe.[36] These anatomical changes are related to FMRP levels.[38]
Idiopathic ID	• Relations between impaired cognitive and motor control have been observed in children with idiopathic ID, and there is evidence that inhibitory control deficits underlie ADHD symptoms and repetitive behaviors.[73,84] WM difficulties are also present, particularly with the phonological loop.[85,86] • Some of the most prevalent brain anomalies that disrupt cognitive processes like EF include enlargement of the body/frontal horn of the lateral ventricles and white matter abnormalities such as corpus callosal dysgenesis.[87]
Migration Disorders	• The literature on EF in neuronal migration disorders is limited. Deficits in planning, cognitive flexibility and problem solving were observed in a young girl with subcortical band heterotopia (SBH). WM deficits were seen in a small sample of children with SBH.[88,89] Difficulties with WM and set-shifting have also been seen in adults with schizencephaly and periventricular nodular heterotopia.[90,91] EdF is also associated with cerebellar agenesis/dysgenesis.[92]
Neurofibromatosis-1 (NF-1)	• Difficulties with inhibition, planning, and cognitive flexibility are seen across childhood; however, findings are somewhat mixed regarding if EdF is in excess of expectations based on level of intellectual functioning.[93–96] Functional EF deficits are reported by parents.[97] • T2-weighted hyperintensities are often seen in the cerebellum and subcortical white matter, which may disrupt circuits important for EF.[98]
*Phenylketonuria (PKU)	• Difficulties with inhibitory control, cognitive flexibility, planning, attention, and WM have been observed in children and adolescents.[58] Inhibitory control deficits are observed early in childhood, whereas other EF deficits may become more pronounced with age.[63,64]

Table 7.1. (cont.)

Syndrome/disorder	EF-related neuropsychological and neurological findings
	• Phenylalanine build-up disrupts dopaminergic pathways and myelin production, which likely contribute to frontal lobe dysfunction[65,70]
Prader–Willi syndrome	• Deficits are seen in response inhibition and cognitive flexibility, even when controlling for intellectual functioning.[99,100] Task switching difficulties appear related to repetitive behavior problems and difficulty adapting to changes in routine.[101] • Children with Prader-Willi syndrome show less frontal activation during a switching task than typically developing controls.[102] Abnormal functioning of the orbitofrontal cortex in particular may be related to difficulties with satiety and emotion regulation.[103,104]
Tuberous sclerosis	• Global intellectual impairment is seen in about 50% of people with tuberous sclerosis. Specific deficits in EF and attention are prevalent in children and adults who do not show global impairment.[105] • Tubers appear most frequently in the frontal lobe. Individuals with tuberous sclerosis show decreased cerebral volumes, particularly in the frontal lobe, and increased cerebellar white matter volumes.[106] Verbal/spatial WM deficits are related to abnormalities of fronto-striatal circuits.[107]
Turner syndrome	• Girls with Turner syndrome show more difficulty with inhibitory control, planning, and organization than controls matched for age and intellectual functioning.[108] Studies have also found some evidence for deficits in cognitive flexibility and verbal fluency.[109] • Structural changes of the cerebellum and frontal regions have been consistently observed.[110–112] Decreased activation of frontal-parietal regions has been seen during math tasks.[113]
*Williams syndrome (WS)	• Relative strengths are seen in verbal WM and verbal fluency, and a significant weakness in visuospatial WM.[47] Inhibition difficulties contribute to the hypersociability that is characteristic of WS.[9] • Findings of abnormal frontal-striatal connectivity suggest some degree of overlap between the WS and ADHD profiles.[50,55]

* Summaries of disorders included in the text.

research is aimed at elucidating specific gene segments that are linked to the neuroanatomical and neuropsychological profile observed in DS.

Executive dysfunction in DS

Delayed cognitive development, typically falling in the mild to moderate range of ID is very common in DS; however, severe ID is also found and individuals with a mosaic genotype may have intellectual abilities in the average range. Specific weaknesses in expressive language, verbal STM and explicit LTM are often seen in addition to these general delays, but visuospatial skills are a relative strength.[5]

Most researchers have found evidence for significant EdF in DS, though others have found EF skills to be at the level expected for mental age. Deficits in response inhibition during play, sustained attention, and motor planning have been observed during early childhood.[6-8] Although children with DS struggle to initiate and maintain conversations due to language difficulties, they are more likely than typically developing children to approach strangers; this hypersociability may be related to poor response inhibition.[9] Adolescents with DS performed at a level expected for their intellectual functioning on measures of inhibition, WM, verbal and nonverbal fluency, and planning;[10] in contrast, two other studies found that both adolescents and adults performed poorer on tasks assessing inhibition, sustained attention, WM, planning, cognitive flexibility, and fluid reasoning than controls matched for mental age.[11,12] This discrepancy in findings may reflect differences in mental age across studies.[11] Longitudinal studies are needed to examine the trajectory of EF skills across the lifespan for individuals with DS.

Elevated rates of dementia, particularly Alzheimer's disease, have been found in DS. It is hypothesized that early frontal lobe abnormalities weaken tolerance to age-related brain changes (i.e., reserve capacity) and make individuals with DS more vulnerable to frontal lobe pathology.[13] Evidence that EdF occurs in the preclinical stages of dementia in DS, and that reported changes in personality and behavior are predictive of performance on EF tasks[14,15] suggest that EF tasks and personality/behavior inventories are necessary elements when evaluating an adult with DS as they may help identify risk for early onset dementia. These tools should also be included when assessing adolescents and young adults with DS to determine baseline abilities, allowing changes in functioning to be identified.

The neurological basis of executive dysfunction in DS

Although nearly all adults with DS show brain pathology, brain development is relatively normal at birth.[16] Signs of microcephaly emerge in infancy and remain throughout the lifespan. Findings regarding specific neuroanatomical abnormalities during early childhood are not all encompassing, but there is evidence for delayed myelination, a smaller brainstem and cerebellum, reduced frontal lobe growth, and a larger third ventricle, which is likely due to abnormal development of the thalamus and hypothalamus.[17,18] In addition to the reduced cerebellar and PFC volumes seen in childhood, many adolescents and adults with DS also have a smaller hippocampus, corpus callosum, and temporal lobe after controlling for total brain volume.[19,20] Reduced cerebellar volumes may account for some of the EdF seen with DS. A gradual deterioration of the frontal lobes, cerebellum, hippocampus, and temporal lobe is seen with age,[10,19,21] which corresponds with the decline in cognitive functioning that is typically observed in adults with DS.

Fragile X syndrome

Fragile X syndrome (FraX) is a sex-linked single gene disorder, affecting 1 in 4000 males and 1 in 8000 females. FraX is caused by unstable repetitions of the CGG trinucleotide on the long arm of the X chromosome. A full mutation reduces production of fragile X mental retardation protein (FMRP), which is vital for brain development. In addition to being the most prevalent cause of *inherited* ID, FraX is also associated with impairment across many neuropsychological domains, emotion regulation difficulties, self-injurious behaviors, and high rates of comorbid autism and ADHD.[22] Physical features characteristic of FraX (e.g., elongated face, macrocephaly, prominent jaw and ears) generally do not become noticeable until later in childhood, so developmental delays are often the first indication of this syndrome. As a result, early identification of FraX (rather than a more general ID diagnosis) can be challenging; however, research indicates that motor skills deficits and social avoidance can be used to distinguish preschoolers with FraX from children with idiopathic developmental delays.[23]

Executive dysfunction in FraX

Due to the X-linked transmission of FraX, males are affected more severely than females. Males with FraX generally have IQ scores in the moderate to severe range and a decline is seen with age. Females with FraX have IQ scores in the mild to moderate range of ID, and may show average range IQ with discrete learning difficulties.[17] Age-related decline in IQ is not typically seen in females. The cognitive profile for FraX includes relative strengths in vocabulary, recognition memory, and selective attention, and relative weaknesses in sustained attention, EF, visuospatial construction, and linguistic processing.[24,25]

EdF is particularly pervasive in the FraX population, even after controlling for IQ. Research has consistently shown that boys with FraX have significant difficulty with verbal fluency, cognitive flexibility, planning, WM, and inhibitory control relative to controls matched for mental age, including boys with DS.[26-28] Persistent deficits in WM and inhibitory control have been observed in girls with FraX even after controlling for IQ.[29-32] Findings have demonstrated that some components of EF (e.g., inhibition, motor planning) are relatively independent of developmental level once a threshold is reached, whereas other components such as cognitive flexibility and WM are not.[26,33] It is noteworthy that a large percentage of these samples were unable to complete some of the more complex tasks assessing cognitive flexibility and WM, highlighting that some EF tasks require a particular threshold of intellectual functioning. Further evidence of EdF in FraX is provided by difficulties with mathematics and sequential processing, tasks which have a significant WM component.[17,34] Behavior problems including high rates of inattention, disinhibition, repetitive behaviors, emotion regulation difficulties, and social skills deficits are also indicative of EdF.

The neurological basis of executive dysfunction in FraX

Given that FMRP is crucial for dendritic spine maturation and pruning, reduced levels of this regulator result in structural and functional brain changes. The most consistent abnormalities have been seen in brain regions important for EF. Enlargement of the caudate nucleus has been observed in FraX across the lifespan.[35,36] The caudate nucleus, which is part of the basal ganglia, is thought to serve as a filter of information to the frontal lobes and to therefore play a role in motor planning and attention shifting. Studies have demonstrated a negative relation between caudate nucleus volume and both FMRP levels and intellectual functioning.[36,37] Reduced volume of the cerebellar vermis has also been observed in both males and females across the lifespan.[38] Research indicates that cerebellar size is positively related to FMRP levels, intellectual functioning, visuospatial abilities and EF in children and adolescents with FraX.[36,38] Gothelf and colleagues[36] found that together, caudate nucleus and vermis volumes accounted for approximately one third of the variation in IQ scores. Functional studies have demonstrated decreased frontal lobe activation during EF tasks, including measures of WM and inhibitory control.[29,30] Other brain abnormalities observed in FraX include greater hippocampal volumes, reduced amygdala and temporal lobe volumes, and ventricular enlargement.[39]

Williams syndrome

Williams syndrome (WS) is a particularly useful ID syndrome for examining brain-behavior relations because individuals with WS generally experience milder forms of ID compared with those with other genetic syndromes. WS is a rare genetic neurodevelopmental disorder (1 in 7500 births) caused by a hemizygous microdeletion on chromosome 7q11.23. WS is associated with a characteristic cognitive and personality profile, including developmental delay, profound visuospatial construction difficulties, relatively preserved language and verbal STM, hypersociability, anxiety, and attention problems. Individuals with WS also exhibit common physical/medical features that are often identified at birth, including dysmorphic facial features (e.g., broad brow, upturned nose, small jaw, prominent lips and earlobes), stunted growth, and cardiovascular disease.[40,41] Genetic discoveries in WS have included evidence that the elastin gene is involved in the connective tissue abnormalities, and GTF2, a general transcription factor gene, is related to lower cognitive abilities and craniofacial features.[42–44] As with DS, further genetic findings in WS may eventually be associated with variations in cognitive functioning, including EdF.

Executive dysfunction in WS

A wide range of intellectual functioning has been observed for children with WS, although most function in the mild range of ID. General developmental delays are accompanied by a characteristic cognitive phenotype of profound weaknesses in visuospatial construction and fine motor coordination and relative strengths in verbal STM, oral fluency, and language.[45,46]

Consistent with this cognitive profile, children with WS perform better on verbal WM tasks and worse on visuospatial WM tasks than IQ-matched individuals with DS or idiopathic ID.[47] Similarly, studies have shown that children with WS perform better on verbal fluency measures than controls matched for mental age;[46,48,49] however, some authors noted that low frequency words (e.g., crane, newt) were often generated, suggesting unusual semantic organization. Difficulty with response inhibition may contribute to the hypersociability that is quite characteristic of WS.[9]

Findings of abnormal frontal–striatal connectivity and pervasive difficulties with sustained attention, attentional set-shifting, inhibition, and WM suggest that the WS and ADHD phenotypes may overlap. A study of WS and ADHD (samples matched for verbal abilities) found the WS group did not significantly differ from the ADHD group on parent ratings of attention and impulsivity; both groups had means in the clinical range.[50] Significant differences on measures of planning and WM were observed, with typically developing children showing the best performance and children with WS having the most difficulty. These results suggest that treatments used for ADHD may be useful for reducing inattention and impulsivity in WS.

The neurological basis of executive dysfunction in WS

Studies have consistently observed a reduction in overall brain volume in WS, with relative sparing of cerebellar and frontal lobe volume.[17] Cerebral white matter is reduced in WS,[51] while gray matter is relatively preserved other than parietal gray matter which is significantly reduced.[52–54] Functional neuroimaging studies have reduced activity in the DLPFC, striatum, and dorsal ACC during an inhibition task relative to typically developing controls.[55] Abnormal connectivity between the PFC and amygdala may underlie social difficulties often seen in WS.[56]

Phenylketonuria

Phenylketonuria (PKU) is an autosomal recessive metabolic disorder that affects one in 10 000 to 20 000 live births. A mutation in the PAH gene on chromosome 12 disrupts the conversion of phenylalanine to tyrosine, and subsequently causes a build-up of phenylalanine in the blood.[57] Early identification and dietary treatment can prevent severe deficits in cognitive and behavioral functioning; however, subtle neurocognitive sequelae are still observed.

Executive dysfunction in PKU

In a recent meta-analysis, DeRoche and Welsh[58] compared individuals with early-treated PKU to unaffected controls and found a moderate effect size for overall IQ scores. Significant relations between intellectual functioning and blood phenylalanine levels have been demonstrated.[59] In addition to this decline in overall intellectual functioning, the neurocognitive profile for PKU includes visuospatial and visuomotor integration difficulties, slowed processing speed, global processing difficulties, and EdF. DeRoche and Welsh[58] observed large effect sizes for measures of inhibitory control and cognitive flexibility, and medium effect sizes for measures of planning and WM. Other recent studies have observed difficulties with sustained attention, inhibition, divided attention, planning, and self-monitoring.[60–62] There is some indication that EF deficits in PKU may become more pronounced with age.[63,64]

The neurological basis of executive dysfunction in PKU

Research indicates that a build-up of phenylalanine indirectly produces neuropsychological deficits by disrupting brain function.[65] One possible mechanism is dysfunction of the PFC and dopaminergic pathways. Dopaminergic neurons in the PFC are quite sensitive to the decrease in tyrosine that occurs in PKU. This model is supported by numerous findings that performance is impaired on measures thought to involve frontal lobe functioning.[60,66,67] Phenylalanine also inhibits myelination, so researchers have hypothesized that white matter abnormalities may impair processing speed and therefore overall cognitive function. Findings regarding the relations between white matter abnormalities and neuropsychological functioning have been somewhat mixed;[68,69] however, meta-analytic reviews have found support for this model overall.[57,60] Joseph and Dyer[70] found that myelin production is a better regulator of dopamine synthesis than tyrosine, suggesting that white matter abnormalities influence frontal lobe functioning.

Summary and future directions

In addition to a shared deficit in intellectual functioning, there is evidence for EdF in each of the ID syndromes described above. There is not, however, a universal response to the question of whether the EF difficulties seen in children with ID are above and beyond what would be expected based on their intellectual impairments. Some studies find specific EF deficits even after controlling for IQ, particularly for individuals with FraX,[11,28] but it is less clear for the other ID syndromes. Further, it may be that specific components of EF are affected above and beyond deficits in intellectual functioning, whereas others components are not.[26] While some EF components may be more highly correlated with measures of intelligence,[71] specific executive skills should be examined with measures appropriate for developmental level, given that many commonly used measures of EF require a particular intellectual threshold to be able to complete the task. The use of appropriate control groups is also important when conducting research with children with ID. Many studies use controls matched for mental age; however, the construct of mental age is statistically problematic, and the mental ages yielded depend heavily on the nature of the measure used (see[72] for a discussion).

The neurodevelopmental disorders discussed here also differ in their profile of specific executive skills, the course of EdF, and the functional impairment or behavioral presentation associated with the EdF. Psychological evaluations for children with ID should therefore focus on identifying each child's unique pattern of strengths and weaknesses, level of functioning, and needed support so that recommendations can be tailored to specific needs. Some studies have found relations between EF and other neuropsychological skills such as motor control or language abilities (e.g.,[73,74]). It is possible that early motor or language deficits contribute to later EdF, and conversely, that early EdF contributes to cognitive and academic difficulties.[75,76] Additional research is needed to clarify such relations and the interventions that can strengthen foundational skills and prevent subsequent difficulties.

Unlike the focal deficits associated with neurological insult in adults, developmental disabilities disrupt neural organization both pre- and post-natally, and may dramatically impact the expected gene–brain-behavior relations. Subtle differences at an early age can increase over time and create very different developmental trajectories.[77,78] It is therefore important to consider the neural substrates that are required for the development of a particular domain, and how a disorder may limit the availability of reserve capacities.[79] Longitudinal research would clarify whether gains in EF follow a similar trajectory as seen for typically developing children, or if there is deviation from typical EF development. Such work is required to predict outcomes for specific neurodevelopmental disorders associated with ID, and to design the most appropriate interventions.

References

1. Schalock RL, Borthwick-Duffy SA, Bradley VJ, et al. *Intellectual Disability: Definition, Classification, and Systems of Supports. 11th edn.* American Association on Intellectual and Developmental Disabilities; 2010.

2. Ozonoff S, Schetter PL. Executive dsyfunction in autism spectrum disorders: From research to practice. In Meltzer L, ed. *Executive Function in Education: From Theory to Practice.* New York: Guilford Press; 2007. 133–60.

3. Merrick J, Kandel I, Vardi G. Adolescents with down syndrome. *Int J Adolesc Med Hlth* 2004; **16**(1): 13–19.

4. Sherman SL, Allen EG, Bean LH, Freeman SB. Epidemiology of down syndrome. *Ment Retard Dev Disab Res Revi* 2007; **13**(3): 221–7.

5. Davis AS. Children with down syndrome: Implications for assessment and intervention in the school. *School Psychol Quart* 2008; **23**(2): 271–81.

6. Brown JH, Johnson MH, Paterson SJ, Gilmore R, Longhi E, Karmiloff-Smith A. Spatial representation and attention in

toddlers with williams syndrome and down syndrome. *Neuropsychologia* 2003; **41**(8): 1037–46.

7. Fidler DJ, Hepburn S, Rogers S. Early learning and adaptive behaviour in toddlers with down syndrome: evidence for an emerging behavioural phenotype? *Down's Syndr, Res Pract: J Sarah Duffen Centre/ Univ Portsmouth* 2006; **9**(3): 37–44.

8. Kopp CB The growth of self-monitoring among young children with down syndrome. In Cicchetti D, Beeghly M, Cicchetti D, Beeghly M, eds. *Children with Down Syndrome: A Developmental Perspective*. New York, NY US: Cambridge University Press; 1990, 231–51.

9. Porter MA, Coltheart M, Langdon R. The neuropsychological basis of hypersociability in williams and down syndrome. *Neuropsychologia* 2007; **45**(12): 2839–49.

10. Pennington BF, Moon J, Edgin J, Stedron J, Nadel L. The neuropsychology of down syndrome: Evidence for hippocampal dysfunction. *Child Dev* 2003; **74**(1): 75–93.

11. Lanfranchi S, Jerman O, Dal Pont E, Alberti A, Vianello R. Executive function in adolescents with down syndrome. *J Intell Disab Res* 2010; **54**(4): 308–19.

12. Rowe J, Lavender A, Turk V. Cognitive executive function in down's syndrome. *Br J Clin Psychol Br Psychol Soc* 2006; **45**(1): 5–17.

13. Adams D, Oliver C. The relationship between acquired impairments of executive function and behaviour change in adults with down syndrome. *J Intell Disab Res* 2010; **54**(5): 393–405.

14. Ball SL, Holland AJ, Treppner P, Watson PC, Huppert FA. Executive dysfunction and its association with personality and behaviour changes in the development of alzheimer's disease in adults with down syndrome and mild to moderate learning disabilities. *Br J Clin Psychol/Br Psychol Soc* 2008; **47**(1): 1–29.

15. Ball SL, Holland AJ, Watson PC, Huppert FA. Theoretical exploration of the neural bases of behavioural disinhibition, apathy

and executive dysfunction in preclinical alzheimer's disease in people with down's syndrome: potential involvement of multiple frontal-subcortical neuronal circuits. *J Intell Disab Res* 2010; **54**(4): 320–36.

16. Nadel L. Down syndrome in cognitive neuroscience perspective. In Tager-Flusberg H, Tager-Flusberg H, eds. *Neurodevelopmental Disorders*. Cambridge, MA, USA: MIT Press; 1999, 197–221.

17. Pennington BF, McGrath LM, Peterson RL. Intellectual disability. In Pennington BF, ed. *Diagnosing Learning Disorders*. 2nd edn. New York: Guilford Press; 2008, 182–226.

18. Schimmel MS, Hammerman C, Bromiker R, Berger I. Third ventricle enlargement among newborn infants with trisomy 21. *Pediatrics* 2006; **117**(5): E928–31.

19. Teipel SJ, Alexander GE, Schapiro MB, Moller HJ, Rapoport SI, Hampel H. Age-related cortical grey matter reductions in non-demented down's syndrome adults determined by MRI with voxel-based morphometry. *Brain* 2004; **127**: 811–24.

20. Fidler DJ, Nadel L. Education and children with down syndrome: Neuroscience, development, and intervention. *Ment Retard Dev Disab Res Rev* 2007; **13**(3): 262–71.

21. Beacher F, Daly E, Simmons A, et al. Brain anatomy and ageing in non-demented adults with Down's syndrome: An in vivo MRI study. *Psychol Med* 2010; **40**(4): 611–19.

22. Schwarte AR. Fragile X syndrome. *School Psychol Quart* 2008; **23**(2): 290–300.

23. Kau AS, Reider EE, Payne L, Meyer WA, Freund L. Early behavior signs of psychiatric phenotypes in fragile X syndrome. *Am Jo Ment Retard* 2000; **105**(4): 286–99.

24. Cornish KM, Turk J, Wilding J, et al. Annotation: deconstructing the attention deficit in fragile X syndrome: a developmental neuropsychological approach. *J Child Psychol Psychiatry, Allied Discipl* 2004; **45**(6): 1042–53.

25. Cornish KM, Munir F, Cross G. Differential impact of the FMR-1 full mutation on memory and attention functioning: a neuropsychological perspective. *J Cogn Neurosci* 2001; **13**(1): 144–50.

26. Hooper SR, Hatton D, Sideris J, et al. Executive functions in young males with fragile X syndrome in comparison to mental age-matched controls: baseline findings from a longitudinal study. *Neuropsychology* 2008; **22**(1): 36–47.

27. Moore CJ, Daly EM, Schmitz N, et al. A neuropsychological investigation of male premutation carriers of fragile X syndrome. *Neuropsychologia* 2004; **42**(14): 1934–47.

28. Wilding J, Cornish K, Munir F. Further delineation of the executive deficit in males with fragile-X syndrome. *Neuropsychologia* 2002; **40**(8): 1343–9.

29. Tamm L, Menon V, Johnston CK, Hessl DR, Reiss AL. fMRI study of cognitive interference processing in females with fragile X syndrome. *J Cogn Neurosci* 2002 15; **14**(2): 160–71.

30. Kwon H, Menon V, Eliez S, et al. Functional neuroanatomy of visuospatial working memory in fragile X syndrome: Relation to behavioral and molecular measures. *Am J Psychiatry* 2001; **158**(7): 1040–51.

31. Kirk JW, Mazzocco MM, Kover ST. Assessing executive dysfunction in girls with fragile X or turner syndrome using the contingency naming test (CNT). *Dev Neuropsychol* 2005; **28**(3): 755–77.

32. Bennetto L, Pennington BF, Porter D, Taylor AK, Hagerman RJ. Profile of cognitive functioning in women with the fragile X mutation. *Neuropsychology* 2001; **15**(2): 290–9.

33. Loesch DZ, Bui QM, Grigsby J, et al. Effect of the fragile X status categories and the fragile X mental retardation protein levels on executive functioning in males and females with fragile X. *Neuropsychology* 2003; **17**(4): 646–57.

34. Rivera SM, Menon V, White CD, Glaser B, Reiss AL. Functional brain activation during arithmetic processing in females with fragile X syndrome is related to FMR1 protein expression. *Hum Brain Mapping* 2002; **16**(4): 206–18.

35. Hazlett HC, Poe MD, Lightbody AA, et al. Teasing apart the heterogeneity of autism: same behavior, different brains in toddlers with fragile X syndrome and autism. *J Neurodev Disord* 2009; **1**(1): 81–90.

36. Gothelf D, Furfaro JA, Hoeft F, et al. Neuroanatomy of fragile X syndrome is associated with aberrant behavior and the fragile X mental retardation protein (FMRP). *Ann Neurol* 2008; **63**(1): 40–51.

37. Hoeft F, Lightbody AA, Hazlett HC, Patnaik S, Piven J, Reiss AL. Morphometric spatial patterns differentiating boys with fragile X syndrome, typically developing boys, and developmentally delayed boys aged 1 to 3 years. *Arch Gen Psychiatry* 2008; **65**(9): 1087–97.

38. Lightbody AA, Reiss AL. Gene, brain, and behavior relationships in fragile X syndrome: *evidence from neuroimaging studies. Dev Disab Res Revi* 2009; **15**(4): 343–52.

39. Schneider A, Hagerman RJ, Hessl D. Fragile X syndrome – from genes to cognition. *Dev Disab Res Rev* 2009; **15**(4): 333–42.

40. Mervis CB. Williams syndrome: 15 years of psychological research. *Dev Neuropsychol* 2003; **23**(1–2): 1–12.

41. Morris CA, Mervis CB. Williams syndrome. In Goldstein S, Reynolds CR, Goldstein S, Reynolds CR, eds. *Handbook of Neurodevelopmental and Genetic Disorders in Children*. New York, NY, USA: Guilford Press; 1999, 555–90.

42. Morris CA, Mervis CB, Hobart HH, et al. GTF2I hemizygosity implicated in mental retardation in williams syndrome: genotype–phenotype analysis of five families with deletions in the williams syndrome region. *Am J Med Genet A.* 2003 15; **123A**(1): 45–59.

43. Ewart AK, Morris CA, Atkinson D, et al. Hemizygosity at the elastin locus in a

developmental disorder, williams syndrome. *Nat Genet* 1993; **5**(1): 11–16.

44. Tassabehji M, Hammond P, Karmiloff-Smith A, *et al.* GTF2IRD1 in craniofacial development of humans and mice. *Science* 2005; **310**(5751): 1184–7.

45. Mervis CB, Robinson BF, Bertrand J, Morris CA, Klein-Tasman B, Armstrong SC. The williams syndrome cognitive profile. *Brain Cogn* 2000; **44**(3): 604–28.

46. Volterra V, Capirci O, Pezzini G, Sabbadini L. Linguistic abilities in italian children with williams syndrome. *Cortex: a J Devoted Study Nerv Syst Behav* 1996; **32**(4): 663–77.

47. Rowe ML, Mervis CB. Working memory in williams syndrome. In Alloway TP, Gathercole SE, Alloway TP, Gathercole SE, eds. *Working Memory and Neurodevelopmental Disorders*. New York, NY, USA: Psychology Press; 2006, 267–93.

48. Temple CM, Almazan M, Sherwood S. Lexical skills in williams syndrome: A cognitive neuropsychological analysis. *J Neurolinguistics* 2002; **15**(6): 463–95.

49. Wang PP, Bellugi U. Williams syndrome, down syndrome, and cognitive neuroscience. *Am J Dis Child* 1993; **147**(11): 1246–51.

50. Rhodes SM, Riby DM, Matthews K, Coghill DR. Attention-deficit/hyperactivity disorder and williams syndrome: Shared behavioral and neuropsychological profiles. *J Clin Exp Neuropsychol* 2011; **33**(1): 147–56.

51. Martens MA, Wilson SJ, Reutens DC. Research review: Williams syndrome: a critical review of the cognitive, behavioral, and neuroanatomical phenotype. *J Child Psychol Psychiatry* 2008; **49**(6): 576–608.

52. Boddaert N, Mochel F, Meresse I, *et al.* Parieto-occipital grey matter abnormalities in children with williams syndrome. *Neuroimage* 2006 15; **30**(3): 721–5.

53. Eckert MA, Hu D, Eliez S, *et al.* Evidence for superior parietal impairment in williams syndrome. *Neurology* 2005; **64**(1): 152–3.

54. Meyer-Lindenberg A, Kohn P, Mervis CB, *et al.* Neural basis of genetically determined visuospatial construction deficit in williams syndrome. *Neuron* 2004; **43**(5): 623–31.

55. Mobbs D, Eckert MA, Mills D, *et al.* Frontostriatal dysfunction during response inhibition in williams syndrome. *Biol Psychiatry* 2007; **62**(3): 256–61.

56. Meyer-Lindenberg A, Hariri AR, Munoz KE, *et al.* Neural correlates of genetically abnormal social cognition in williams syndrome. *Nat Neurosci* 2005; **8**(8): 991–3.

57. Welsh M, DeRoche K, Gilliam D. Neurocognitive models of early-treated phenylketonuria: insights from meta-analysis and new molecular genetic findings. In Nelson CA, Luciana M, Nelson CA, Luciana M, eds. *Handbook of Developmental Cognitive Neuroscience*, 2nd edn. Cambridge, MA, USA: MIT Press; 2008, 677–89.

58. DeRoche K, Welsh M. Twenty-five years of research on neurocognitive outcomes in early-treated phenylketonuria: Intelligence and executive function. *Dev Neuropsychol* 2008; **33**(4): 474–504.

59. Waisbren SE, Noel K, Fahrbach K, *et al.* Phenylalanine blood levels and clinical outcomes in phenylketonuria: A systematic literature review and meta-analysis. *Mol Genet Metab* 2007; **92**(1–2): 63–70.

60. Moyle JJ, Fox AM, Arthur M, Bynevelt M, Burnett JR. Meta-analysis of neuropsychological symptoms of adolescents and adults with PKU. *Neuropsychol Rev* 2007; **17**(2): 91–101.

61. Araujo GC, Christ SE, Steiner RD, *et al.* Response monitoring in children with phenylketonuria. *Neuropsychology* 2009; **23**(1): 130–4.

62. Gassió R, Artuch R, Vilaseca MA, *et al.* Cognitive functions in classic phenylketonuria and mild hyperphenylalaninaemia: experience in a paediatric population. *Dev Med Child Neurol* 2005; **47**(7): 443–8.

63. White DA, Nortz MJ, Mandernach T, Huntington K, Steiner RD. Age-related working memory impairments in children with prefrontal dysfunction associated with

phenylketonuria. *J Int Neuropsychol Soc* 2002; **8**(1): 1–11.

64. Christ SE, Steiner RD, Grange DK, Abrams RA, White DA. Inhibitory control in children with phenylketonuria. *Dev Neuropsychol* 2006; **30**(3): 845–64.

65. Waisbren SE. Phenylketonuria. In Goldstein S, Reynolds CR, Goldstein S, Reynolds CR, eds. *Handbook of Neurodevelopmental and Genetic Disorders in Children*, 2nd edn. New York, NY, USA: Guilford Press; 2011, 398–424.

66. Diamond A, Prevor MB, Callender G, Druin DP. Prefrontal cortex cognitive deficits in children treated early and continuously for PKU. *Monogr Soc Res Child Dev* 1997; **62**(4): 1–205.

67. Huijbregts S, de Sonneville L, Licht R, Sergeant J, van Spronsen F. Inhibition of prepotent responding and attentional flexibility in treated phenylketonuria. *Dev Neuropsychol* 2002; **22**(2): 481–99.

68. Channon S, Mockler C, Lee P. Executive functioning and speed of processing in phenylketonuria. *Neuropsychology* 2005; **19**(5): 679–86.

69. Jones SJ, Turano G, Kriss A, Shawkat F, Kendall B, Thompson AJ. Visual evoked potentials in phenylketonuria: Association with brain MRI, dietary state, and IQ. *J Neurol Neurosurg Psychiatry* 1995; **59**: 260–5.

70. Joseph B, Dyer CA. Relationship between myelin production and dopamine synthesis in the PKU mouse brain. *J Neurochem* 2003; **86**(3): 615–26.

71. Friedman NP, Miyake A, Corley RP, Young SE, DeFries JC, Hewitt JK. Not all executive functions are related to intelligence. *Psychol Sci* 2006; **17**(2): 172–9.

72. Mervis CB, Klein-Tasman B. Methodological issues in group-matching designs: α levels for control variable comparisons and measurement characteristics of control and target variables. *J Autism Dev Disord* 2004; **34**(1): 7–17.

73. Hartman E, Houwen S, Scherder E, Visscher C. On the relationship between motor performance and executive functioning in children with intellectual disabilities. *J Intell Disab Res* 2010; **54**(5): 468–77.

74. Willner P, Bailey R, Parry R, Dymond S. Evaluation of executive functioning in people with intellectual disabilities. *J Intellect Disabil Res* 2010; **54**(4): 366–79.

75. Samango-Sprouse C. Frontal lobe development in childhood. In Miller BL, Cummings JL, Miller BL, Cummings JL, eds. *The Human Frontal Lobes: Functions and Disorders*. New York, NY, USA: Guilford Press; 1999, 584–603.

76. Maehler C, Schuchardt K. Working memory in children with learning disabilities: rethinking the criterion of discrepancy. *Int J Disab, Dev Educ* 2011; **58**(1): 5–17.

77. Waber DP. *Rethinking Learning Disabilities: Understanding Children Who Struggle in School*. New York, NY, USA: Guilford Press; 2010.

78. Karmiloff-Smith A. Trajectories of development and learning difficulties. In Cooper CL, Field J, Goswami U, *et al*, eds. *Mental Capital and Wellbeing*. Wiley-Blackwell; 2010, 867–73.

79. Bernstein JH. Developmental models in pediatric neuropsychology. In: Donders J, Hunter SJ, eds. *Principles and Practice of Lifespan Developmental Neuropsychology*. New York: Cambridge; 2010, 17–40.

80. Campbell LE, Azuma R, Ambery F, *et al*. Executive functions and memory abilities in children with 22q11.2 deletion syndrome. *Aust N Z J Psychiatry* 2010; **44**(4): 364–71.

81. Kiley-Brabeck K, Sobin C. Social skills and executive function deficits in children with the 22q11 deletion syndrome. *Appl Neuropsychol* 2006; **13**(4): 258–68.

82. Rockers K, Ousley O, Sutton T, *et al*. Performance on the modified card sorting test and its relation to psychopathology in adolescents and young adults with 22q11.2 deletion syndrome. *J Intell Disab Res* 2009; **53**(7): 665–76.

83. Sobin C, Kiley-Brabeck K, Daniels S, *et al.* Neuropsychological characteristics of children with the 22q11.2 deletion syndrome: a descriptive analysis. *Child Neuropsychol* 2005; **11**(1): 39–53.

84. Burbidge C, Oliver C, Moss J, *et al.* The association between repetitive behaviours, impulsivity and hyperactivity in people with intellectual disability. *J Intell Disab Res* 2010; **54**(12): 1078–92.

85. Henry L, Winfield J. Working memory and educational achievement in children with intellectual disabilities. *J Intell Disab Res* 2010; **54**(4): 354–65.

86. Schuchardt K, Gebhardt M, Mäehler C. Working memory functions in children with different degrees of intellectual disability. *J Intell Disab Res* 2010; **54**(4): 346–53.

87. Spencer MD, Gibson RJ, Moorhead TWJ, *et al.* Qualitative assessment of brain anomalies in adolescents with mental retardation. *Am J Neurol Res* 2005; **26**: 2691–7.

88. Jacobs R, Anderson V, Harvey AS. Neuropsychological profile of a 9-year-old child with subcortical band heterotopia or 'double cortex.' *Dev Med Child Neurol* 2001; **43**(9): 628–33.

89. Spencer-Smith M, Leventer R, Jacobs R, De Luca C, Anderson V. Neuropsychological profile of children with subcortical band heterotopia. *Dev Med Child Neurol* 2009; **51**(11): 909–16.

90. Allen BJ, Reid-Arndt S, Rolan T. Neuropsychological functioning in a young adult case of schizencephaly. *Clin Neuropsychol* 2010; **24**(5): 827–40.

91. Chang BS, Ly J, Appignani B, *et al.* Reading impairment in the neuronal migration disorder of periventricular nodular heterotopia. *Neurology* 2005; **64**(5): 799–803.

92. Tavano A, Fabbro F, Borgatti R. Language and social communication in children with cerebellar dysgenesis. *Folia Phoniatr Logop* 2007; **59**(4): 201–9.

93. Levine TM, Materek A, Abel J, O'Donnell M, Cutting LE. Cognitive profile of neurofibromatosis type 1. *Semin Pediatr Neurol* 2006; **13**(1): 8–20.

94. Rowbotham I, Pit-ten Cate IM, Sonuga-Barke E, Huijbregts SCJ. Cognitive control in adolescents with neurofibromatosis type 1. *Neuropsychology* 2009; **23**(1): 50–60.

95. Hyman SL, Shores A, North KN. The nature and frequency of cognitive deficits in children with neurofibromatosis type 1. *Neurology* 2005; **65**(7): 1037–44.

96. Roy A, Roulin JL, Charbonnier V, *et al.* Executive dysfunction in children with neurofibromatosis type 1: a study of action planning. *J Int Neuropsychol Soc* 2010; **16**(6): 1056–63.

97. Payne JM, Hyman SL, Shores EA, North KN. Assessment of executive function and attention in children with neurofibromatosis type 1: relationships between cognitive measures and real-world behavior. *Child Neuropsychol* 2011; **17**(4): 313–29.

98. North KN. *Neurofibromatosis Type I in Childhood.* 1st edn. London: MacKeith Press; 1997.

99. Woodcock KA, Oliver C, Humphreys GW. A specific pathway can be identified between genetic characteristics and behavior profiles in Prader–Willi syndrome via cognitive, environmental and physiological mechanisms. *J Intell Disabil Res* 2009; **53**(6): 493–500.

100. Stauder JEA, Boer H, Gerits RHA, Tummers A, Whittington J, Curfs LMG. Differences in behavioural phenotype between parental deletion and maternal uniparental disomy in Prader–Willi syndrome: An ERP study. *Clin Neurophysiol* 2005; **116**(6): 1464–70.

101. Woodcock KA, Oliver C, Humphreys GW. The relationship between specific cognitive impairment and behavior in Prader–Willi syndrome. *J Intell Disab Res* 2011; **55**(2): 152–71.

102. Woodcock KA, Humphreys GW, Oliver C, Hansen PC. Neural correlates of task switching in paternal 15q11–q13 deletion Prader–Willi syndrome. *Brain Res* 2010; 1.

103. Ogura K, Shinohara M, Ohno K, Mori E. Frontal behavioral syndromes in

Prader–Willi syndrome. *Brain Dev* 2008; **30**(7): 469–76.

104. Walley RM, Donaldson MDC. An investigation of executive function abilities in adults with prader-willi syndrome. *J Intell Disab Res* 2005; **49**(8): 613–25.

105. Prather P, de Vries PJ. Behavioral and cognitive aspects of tuberous sclerosis complex. *J Child Neurol* 2004; **19**(9): 666–74.

106. DiMario, Francis J., Jr. Brain abnormalities in tuberous sclerosis complex. *J Child Neurol* 2004; **19**(9): 650–7.

107. Ridler K, Suckling J, Higgins NJ, *et al.* Neuroanatomical correlates of memory deficits in tuberous sclerosis complex. *Cereb Cortex* 2007; **17**(2): 261–71.

108. Romans SM, Roeltgen DP, Kushner H, Ross JL. Executive function in girls with turner's syndrome. *Dev Neuropsychol* 1997; **13**(1): 23–40.

109. Hong D, Kent JS, Kesler S. Cognitive profile of turner syndrome. *Dev Disab Res Rev* 2009; **15**(4): 270–8.

110. Holzapfel M, Barnea-Goraly N, Eckert MA, Kesler SR, Reiss AL. Selective alterations of white matter associated with visuospatial and sensorimotor dysfunction in turner syndrome. *J Neurosci* 2006; **26**(26): 7007–13.

111. Brown WA, Kesler SR, Eliez S, *et al.* Brain development in turner syndrome: A magnetic resonance imaging study. *Psychiatry Res: Neuroimaging* 2002; **116**(3): 187–96.

112. Cutter WJ, Daly EM, Robertson DMW, *et al.* Influence of X chromosome and hormones on human brain development: A magnetic resonance imaging and proton magnetic resonance spectroscopy study of turner syndrome. *Biol Psychiatry* 2006; **59**(3): 273–83.

113. Kesler SR, Menon V, Reiss AL. Neurofunctional differences associated with arithmetic processing in turner syndrome. *Cereb Cortex* 2006; **16**(6): 849–56.

Executive functions in pediatric movement and motor control disorders

8

Emily J. Helder and Tory L. Larsen

Several childhood movement disorders have frequently been linked to EdF due to involvement of the fronto-subcortical circuits affecting both motor and cognitive functions. The current chapter includes discussion of involuntary movement disorders (i.e., Tourette syndrome, PANDAS, and Sydenham's Chorea) and motor control disorders (i.e., cerebral palsy).

Tourette syndrome

Tourette Syndrome (TS; a.k.a. Tourette's Disorder) is a child-onset neurodevelopmental condition characterized by the presence of chronic motor and vocal tics that may wax and wane over time. Tics are defined as "sudden, rapid, recurrent, nonrhythmic motor movements or vocalizations".[1] TS has a prevalence of approximately 1% and occurs more frequently in boys as compared to girls, at a ratio of approximately 4:1.[2] Onset of symptoms generally occurs in early childhood with possible worsening of symptoms during adolescence. Tics may decline or remit in adulthood, though approximately 20% of individuals experience persisting tics into adulthood.[3] TS commonly co-occurs with a variety of conditions, particularly ADHD and OCD, with comorbidity estimates of 35%[4] and 41%,[3] respectively.

Executive dysfunction in Tourette syndrome

Studies examining the neuropsychological profile of individuals with TS have reported significant variability, with some individuals with TS having no significant areas of deficit.[5] Common deficits include difficulties with visuospatial processing,[6] visual memory,[7] and a variety of EF tasks.[8] However, this research is complicated by high levels of comorbidity with conditions such as ADHD and OCD, resulting in disagreement about whether EdF in TS is due to comorbid conditions[9] or is independent of comorbidity.[10]

A small study of EF (including inhibitory control, multitasking, rule following, and set shifting) in TS with various comorbidities (including children with TS only, TS + ADHD, TS + OCD, and a healthy control group) found the TS + ADHD group had the greatest degree of EdF, performing worse than controls on several measures of inhibitory control and multi-tasking.[11] In comparison, the TS only group performed worse than controls on only one measure of inhibition. A larger study examined the impact of comorbidity (including samples of children with TS only, TS + ADHD, ADHD only, and healthy control group) on sustained attention (Conners' CPT-II) and impulse control (Stroop

Executive Function and Dysfunction, ed. Scott J. Hunter and Elizabeth P. Sparrow. Published by Cambridge University Press. © Cambridge University Press 2012.

task).[12] The ADHD only and TS + ADHD groups had more errors of omission and greater reaction time variability than the controls; the TS only group did not differ from controls. On the Stroop task, the ADHD only group showed deficits relative to controls; the TS only and TS+ADHD groups did not differ from controls. Research utilizing parent report has reached similar conclusions. For example, Mahone[13] found that children with TS + ADHD and ADHD only had more parent-reported difficulties with behavioral regulation and metacognition on the BRIEF when compared with children with TS only and healthy controls. These studies suggest that EdF in TS may be secondary to comorbid conditions rather than primary for TS alone.

Summarizing the literature on EdF in TS, Eddy and colleagues[8] suggested that conclusive evidence was lacking for the presence of WM, verbal fluency, planning, and cognitive flexibility deficits in individuals with TS only. However, in TS + ADHD, WM, planning, and inhibitory deficits were consistently seen across several studies. Additionally, cognitive flexibility deficits appeared more commonly in TS + OCD. Eddy and colleagues[8] and others[14] have suggested that impairments in inhibitory control may be a core EF deficit in "pure" TS. Intact performance has been reported on less sensitive inhibitory tasks (i.e., Stroop, Go/No-Go) though consistent deficits are observed on the Hayling task even in "pure" TS.[11] Eddy and colleagues[8] outlined a number of factors that contribute to disagreement between studies examining EF in TS, including sensitivity of the chosen measure, waxing and waning of tics and cognitive symptoms, age of participants, and lack of control of factors such as medication use and comorbid conditions.

The neurological basis of executive dysfunction in Tourette syndrome

TS has been linked to a variety of brain abnormalities (see review Rickards[15]). Reduced volume and functional activity of basal ganglia regions (particularly on the left side) have been reported[16-17] in contrast to increased activity in frontal regions. Abnormalities in the cortico-striato-thalamo-cortical circuits resulting in reduced inhibitory control may underlie both the tics seen in TS and some of the cognitive deficits described above.[8] Interestingly, some functional imaging studies have reported increased activation in frontal regions during inhibitory tasks in TS compared with non-patient controls,[18-19] which may reflect a compensatory mechanism. Additional brain regions, such as the corpus callosum and cerebellum have also been implicated as contributing to cognitive deficits in TS.[15,20] Similar to studies examining cognitive deficits in TS, neuroimaging studies are also influenced by inclusion of patients with and without comorbidities. Behen and colleagues[17] examined serotoninergic functioning in TS utilizing PET. Their results revealed different patterns of tryptophan metabolism in the basal ganglia and thalamus among subgroups of patients (TS only, TS + ADHD, TS + OCD) included in the study, as compared to controls.

Pediatric autoimmune neuropsychiatric disorder associated with streptococcal infection and Sydenham's Chorea

Pediatric autoimmune neuropsychiatric disorder associated with streptococcal infection (PANDAS) and Sydenham's Chorea are neuropsychiatric conditions caused by abnormal immune reactions to group A β-hemolytic streptococcal (GABHS) infection. The autoimmune reaction in PANDAS and Sydenham's Chorea may alter neuronal signaling.[21] Overlap in clinical presentation and proposed etiological mechanisms makes diagnostic differentiation between these two syndromes difficult.

Criteria for PANDAS include the presence of OCD and/or tic disorder, onset in childhood, episodic course of symptoms (abrupt onset or dramatic waxing of symptoms), temporal association with GABHS infection, and neurological abnormalities (such as choreiform movements) present during periods of symptom exacerbation.[22] It is suspected that the propensity to develop this auto-immune response following GABHS infection may be genetically mediated. Neuropsychiatric symptoms of Sydenham's Chorea include chorea (primarily in the face, feet, and hands), other motor symptoms (ballismus, gait disturbance, hypotonia), obsessive-compulsive symptoms, cognitive deficits (attention and EF), and mood disturbance (depression, anxiety). Average age of onset is 8 years,[23] with duration of approximately 1 year, though symptoms may persist.

Executive dysfunction in PANDAS and Sydenham's Chorea

Common behavioral associations in PANDAS include hyperactivity, impulsivity, distractibility, and emotional lability.[24] A recent study of PANDAS found urinary urgency, hyperactivity, impulsivity, and deterioration in handwriting were more prevalent in PANDAS-related OCD than non-PANDAS OCD.[25] Common psychiatric comorbidies include ADHD, major depression, separation anxiety, and enuresis.[22]

Given the low incidence of PANDAS, few studies exist that examine the neuropsychological profile in a large group of patients. One study of children with PANDAS found decreased response accuracy on a research-based attention and impulse control task for the PANDAS groups relative to healthy controls, with no significant differences on the WCST or Tower of Hanoi;[26] however, these findings may have reflected comorbidity. Specifically, the PANDAS + tics group (with comorbid TS or OCD) performed worse than the PANDAS + OCD only (no tics) group on the attention and impulse control task, and the PANDAS + ADHD group had slower reaction times on the sustained attention task than those without comorbid ADHD. These findings suggest that PANDAS alone may not be associated with specific EdF, but that comorbid tics and/or ADHD may lead to EF deficits.

Researchers examining children with Sydenham's Chorea in comparison to healthy controls have reported deficits in divided attention, planning deficits on the Tower of Hanoi,[27-28] and decreased phonemic fluency in the context of spared semantic fluency.[29] Differences were not observed between patients and controls on the WCST or simple reaction time.[27-28] In a study examining adults with Sydenham's Chorea, results revealed EdF (verbal fluency, inhibition, planning ability) in the context of a general sparing of intellectual functioning.[30] Patients with persisting Sydenham's Chorea were reported to have more significant EdF in comparison to those with remitting Sydenham's chorea. Deficits, such as increased response latencies on basic visual tasks,[31] and difficulties with attention, WM, and speeded information processing[32] have been reported in a subset of adults with histories of Sydenham's Chorea in childhood.

The neurological basis of executive dysfunction in PANDAS and Sydenham's Chorea

MRI studies in individuals with PANDAS have reported enlargement of basal ganglia regions.[33] The antibodies produced in the PANDAS autoimmune reaction are thought to specifically attack basal ganglia regions.[21] Similarly, neuroimaging studies have revealed abnormalities in the basal ganglia in Sydenham's Chorea, with increased blood flow to the basal ganglia and larger volumes of the caudate, putamen, and globus pallidus[34–35] during acute symptomatic periods.

Cerebral palsy

Cerebral palsy (CP) designates a group of non-progressive neurodevelopmental disorders of movement and posture which result from pre-, peri-, or post-natal insult to the brain.[36] Subtypes of CP are classified according to the clinical motor presentation (spastic, dyskinetic, hypotonic), and the topographical presentation (diplegic, hemiplegic, etc.).[37] Key risk factors for CP include low birthweight, intrauterine infections, and multiple gestation. Children with CP often also present with epilepsy, especially those with spastic CP.[38–39] Although exact figures are not known, the incidence of CP is reported to be between 2–4 per 1000 live births.[37–39]

Executive dysfunction in cerebral palsy

Although variability exists among the current literature examining EF in children with CP, a review of the subject reported that impairments are likely to be found within the domains of focused and sustained attention, inhibitory control, and WM.[40] Tasks of dichotic listening seem to be sensitive to problems of attentional shifting in children with hemiplegia,[41–42] and deficits on NEPSY's sustained attention task have been reported, again in children with hemiplegia.[43] Bottcher and colleagues[44] also reported deficits in both divided and sustained attention on the TEA-Ch.

A small study of children with bilateral spastic CP found children with CP performed worse than matched controls in both the control and incongruent conditions of the Stroop task, made significantly more errors in the incompatible condition of a stimulus–response reversal task, and made more errors in both conditions of an antisaccade task.[45] Warschausky and colleagues[46] found that children with CP made more perseverative errors on the WCST than children with acquired cerebral lesions (e.g., TBI), although another study found differences in *non*-perseverative errors relative to healthy controls on the same task.[47] Inhibitory deficits have also been reported on NEPSY's inhibition task,[43] simple switching tasks, and teacher reports of behavior.[44]

Literature examining WM in children with CP is scarce and inconsistent in its findings; one study of memory span reported deficits[43] relative to healthy controls, while others found no such differences.[48–49] One study evaluated WM and inhibitory control in elementary school-aged children with CP and found a significant effect for educational placement; those who were receiving special education performed significantly worse on WM tasks and a Stroop-like shifting-naming task relative to healthy peers, whereas children with CP who were in mainstream education were not impaired relative to healthy peers.[50] Furthermore, set-shifting and components of WM were strong predictors of arithmetic ability in students with CP;[50] although not all children with CP struggle with arithmetic, children with CP who also have deficits in shifting and WM are more likely to develop arithmetic problems.

Extenuating factors such as lesion location (i.e., lateralized vs. diffuse) may further complicate reported EdF findings. Although not every study on CP reports lesion information, those that do often find differences for those with left hemisphere, right hemisphere, and bilateral lesions. For example, Kolk and Talvik[43] found that sustained attention and inhibitory control were significantly more impaired in children with right hemisphere lesions; WM performance was similarly affected by lesion location, but the trend was not significant. Other studies have found that focused attention might be more vulnerable when left hemisphere lesions are present,[42] and that inhibitory control may be more affected by diffuse rather than unilateral lesions,[44] although the latter was only a statistical trend. Collectively, these findings imply that lesion location may play a role in determining the severity and type of EdF in children with CP. Finally, children with CP had elevated teacher ratings on the BRIEF;[44] these everyday deficits in EF (in addition to the challenges of motor impairment) may further obstruct children with CP from engaging in social relationships and learning academic and social skills.

The neurological basis of executive dysfunction in cerebral palsy

A variety of abnormalities have been observed in imaging studies of CP, including periventricular leukomalacia (PVL), a condition involving the dilation of the ventricles and reduction of white matter; brain malformations; intracranial hemorrhage; and asphyxia-related brain injury.[36,51] These abnormalities affect motor regions and white matter pathways that underlie the movement and posture difficulties in CP.[52] They may also disrupt the cortico-striato-thalamo-cortical circuits and/or frontal, parietal, and basal ganglia regions resulting in EdF, such as difficulties with attention, WM, and inhibition.[40,53]

Summary and future directions

Involvement of the fronto-subcortical circuits not only affects motor functioning in certain childhood movement disorders, but also cognitive functioning. EF, in particular, seems to be affected in TS, PANDAS, Sydenham's Chorea, and CP, although some variability exists within the literature.

Are the EdF observed in the movement and motor control disorders primary, or are they related to common comorbidities? Reviews of the TS research literature suggest that reported deficits, with the exception of inhibitory control, are better accounted for by comorbid conditions (ADHD and OCD) instead of TS alone.[8] Future research should carefully control for comorbidity, age, medication, and waxing/waning of tics, as well as employ measures that allow for assessment of component skills. Some of the EdF reported in individuals with PANDAS and Sydenham's Chorea may be related to associated comorbidities (ADHD, etc.). It is less clear in these disorders, however, if deficits exist apart from comorbidities due to the scarcity of research. More research in general is needed to examine EdF associated with these disorders in children, as well as to tease out the influence of comorbidities on observed deficits. Finally, core EF deficits do appear to be present in individuals with CP, with inhibitory difficulties being reported most consistently.[45] Again, more research is warranted, particularly into reasons for the variability found in EF dimensions such as WM. It will be helpful to examine possible associations between lesion location and the different types of CP (i.e., spastic vs. dyskinetic) with the extent and nature of EdF in CP. Finally, longitudinal research of EF in adolescents with movement disorders will elucidate if EF develop differently in this population relative to the general population or other clinical populations with EdF.

References

1. American Psychiatric Association. *Diagnostic and Statistical Manual of Mental Disorders IV-TR* 2000. Washington, DC: Author.

2. Robertson M. The prevalence and epidemiology of Gilles de la Tourette syndrome. Part 1: The epidemiology and prevalence studies. *J Psychosom Res* 2008; **65**: 461–72.

3. Bloch MH, Peterson BS, Scahill L, *et al.* Adulthood outcome of tic and obsessive-compulsive symptom severity in children with Tourette syndrome. *Arch Pediatr Adolesc Med* 2006; **160**: 65–9.

4. Erenberg G. The relationship between Tourette syndrome, attention deficit hyperactivity disorder, and stimulant medication: a critical review. *Semin Pediatr Neurol* 2005; **12**: 217–21.

5. Bornstein RA. Neuropsychological performance in children with Tourette syndrome. *Psychiatry Res* 1990; **33**: 73–81.

6. Osmon DC, Smerz JM. Neuropsychological evaluation in the diagnosis and treatment of Tourette Syndrome. *Behav Mod* 2005; **29**: 746–83.

7. Lavoie ME, Thibault G, Stip E, O'Connor KP. Memory and executive functions in adults with Gilles de la Tourette syndrome and chronic tic disorder. *Cog Neuropsychol* 2007; **12**: 165–81.

8. Eddy CM, Rizzo R, Cavanna AE. Neuropsychological aspects of Tourette syndrome: a review. *J Psychosom Res* 2009; **67**: 503–13.

9. Denckla MB. Attention deficit hyperactivity disorder: the childhood co-morbidity that most influences the disability burden in Tourette syndrome. *Adv Neurol* 2006; **99**: 17–21.

10. Crawford S, Channon S, Robertson M. Tourette Syndrome: performance on tests of behavioral inhibition, working memory and gambling. *J Child Psychol Psychiatry* 2005; **46**: 1327–36.

11. Channon S, Pratt P, Robertson M. Executive function, memory, and learning in Tourette Syndrome. *Neuropsychology* 2003; **17**: 247–54.

12. Sukhodolsky DG, Landeros-Weisenberger A, Scahill L, Leckman JF, Schultz RT. Neuropsychological functioning in children with Tourette syndrome with and without Attention-Deficit/Hyperactivity disorder. *J Am Acad Child Adolesc Psychiatry* 2010; **49**: 1155–64.

13. Mahone EM. *Behavior Rating Inventory of Executive Function ratings in children with Tourette Syndrome.* 2000: Unpublished raw data.

14. Pennington BF, Ozonoff S. Executive functions and developmental psychopathology. *J Child Psychol Psychiatry* 1996; **37**: 51–87.

15. Rickards H. Functional neuroimaging in Tourette syndrome. *J Psychosom Res* 2009; **67**: 575–84.

16. Singer HS, Reiss AL, Brown JE, *et al.* Volumetric MRI changes in basal ganglia of children with Tourette's syndrome. *Neurology* 1993; **43**: 950.

17. Behen ME, Chugani HT, Juhasz C, *et al.* Abnormal brain tryptophan metabolism and clinical correlates in Tourette syndrome. *Mov Disord* 2007; **22**: 2256–62.

18. Marsh R, Zhu H, Wang Z, Skudlarski P, Peterson BS. A developmental fMRI study of self-regulatory control in Tourette's syndrome. *Am J Psychiatry* 2007; **164**: 955–66.

19. Eichele H, Eichele T, Hammar A, Freyberger HJ, Hugdahl K, Plessen KJ. Go/nogo performance in boys with Tourette syndrome. *Child Neuropsychol* 2010; **16**: 162–8.

20. Plessen KJ, Lundervold A, Gruner R, *et al.* Functional brain asymmetry, attention modulation, and interhemispheric transfer in boys with Tourette syndrome. *Neuropsychologia* 2007; **45**: 767–74.

21. Kirvan CA, Swedo SE, Heuser JS, Cunningham MW. Mimicry and autoantibody-mediated neuronal cell signaling in Sydenham chorea. *Nat Med* 2003; **9**: 914–20.

22. Swedo SE, Leonard HL, Garvey M, et al. Pediatric autoimmuneneuropsychiatric disorders associated with streptococcalinfections: clinical description of the first 50 cases. Am J Psychiatry 1998; 155: 264–71.

23. Dewey D, Tupper D E, Bottos S. Involuntary motor disorders in childhood. In Dewey D, Tupper DE, eds. Developmental Motor Disorders: A Neuropsychological Perspective. New York: Guilford Press; 2004, 197–210.

24. Schneider RK, Robinson MJ, Levenson JL. Psychiatric presentations of non-HIV infection diseases. Pediatr Clin N Am 2002; 25: 1–16.

25. Bernstein GA, Victor AM, Pipal AJ, Williams KA. Comparison of clinical characteristics of PANDAS infections and childhood obsessive-compulsive disorder. J Child Adolesc Psychopharmacol 2010; 20: 333–40.

26. Hirschtritt ME, Hammond CJ, Luckenbaugh D, et al. Executive and attention functioning among children in the PANDAS subgroup. Child Neuropsychol 2009; 15: 179–94.

27. Casey BJ, Vauss, YC, Chused A, Swedo SE. Cognitive functioning in Sydenham's chorea: Part 2. Executive functioning. Dev Neuropsychol 1994a; 10(2): 89–96.

28. Casey BJ, Vauss YC, Swedo SE. Cognitive functioning in Sydenham's chorea: Part 1. Attentional processes. Dev Neuropsychol 1994b; 10(2): 75–88.

29. Cunningham MC, Maia DP, Teixeira AL, Cardoso F. Sydenham's Chorea is associated with decreased verbal fluency. Parkinsonism Relat Disord 2006; 12(3): 165–7.

30. Beato R, Maia DP, Teixeira AL, Cardoso F. Executive functioning in adult patients with Sydenham's chorea. Mov Disord 2010; 25: 853–7.

31. Cairney S, Maruff P, Currie J, Currie B. Increased anti-saccade latency is an isolated lingering abnormality in Sydenham Chorea. J Neuro-Ophthalmol 2009; 29: 143–5.

32. Cavalcanti A, Hilario MO, dos Santos FH, Bolognani SAP, Bueno OFA, Len CA. Subtle cognitive deficits in adults with a previous history of Sydenham's Chorea during childhood. Arthritis Care Res 2010; 62(8): 1065–71.

33. Giedd JN, Rapoport JL, Garvey MA, Perlmutter S, Swedo SE. MRI assessment of children with obsessive-compulsive disorder or tics associated with streptococcal infection. Am J Psychiatry 2000; 157: 281–3.

34. Goldman S, Amrom D, Szliwowski HB, et al. Reversible striatal hypermetabolism in a case of Syndenham's chorea. Mov Disord 1993; 8: 355–8.

35. Giedd JN, Rapoport JL, Kruesi MJP, et al. Sydenham's chorea: magnetic resonance imaging of the basal ganglia. Neurology 1995; 45: 2199–202.

36. Straub K, Obrzut JE. Effects of cerebral palsy on neuropsychological function. J Dev Phys Disab 2009; 21: 153–67.

37. Hunter SJ. Pediatric movement disorders. In Hunter SJ, Donders J, eds. Pediatric Neuropsychological Intervention. Cambridge: Cambridge University Press; 2007, 314–37.

38. Fennell EB, Dikel TN. Cognitive and neuropsychological functioning in children with cerebral palsy. J Child Neurol 2001; 16(1): 58–63.

39. Odding E, Roebroeck ME, Stam HJ. The epidemiology of cerebral palsy: Incidence, impairments and risk factors. Disab Rehab 2006; 28(4): 183–91.

40. Bottcher L. Children with spastic cerebral palsy, their cognitive functioning, and social participation: A review. Child Neuropsychol 2010; 16: 209–28.

41. Hugdahl K, Carlsson G. Dichotic-listening and focused attention in children with hemiplegic cerebral-palsy. J Clini Exp Neuropsychol 1994; 16: 84–92.

42. Korkman M, Von Wendt L. Evidence of altered dominance in children with congenital spastic hemiplegia. J Int Neuropsychol Soc 1995; 1: 261–70.

43. Kolk AK, Talvik T. Cognitive outcomes of children with early-onset hemiparesis. *J Child Neurol* 2000; **15**: 581–7.

44. Bottcher L, Flachs EM, Uldall P. Attentional and executive impairments in children with spastic cerebral palsy. *Dev Med Child Neurol* 2009; **52**: e42–7.

45. Christ SE, White DA, Brunstrom JE, Abrams Ra. Inhibitory control following perinatal brain injury. *Neuropsychol* 2003; **17**(1): 171–8.

46. Warschausky S, Argento AG, Hurvitz E, Berg M. Neuropsychological status and social problem solving in children with congenital or acquired brain dysfunction. *Rehab Psychol* 2003; **48**: 250–4.

47. Nadeau L, Routhier ME, Tessier R. The performance profile on the Wisconsin Card Sorting Test of a group of children with cerebral palsy aged between 9 and 12. *Devel Neurorehab* 2008; **11**(2): 134–40.

48. White D, Craft S, Hale D, Schatz J, Park TS. Working memory following improvements in articulation rate in children with cerebral palsy. *J Int Neuropsychol Soc* 1995; **1**: 49–55.

49. White D, Craft S, Hale S, Park TS. Working memory and articulation rate in children with spastic diplegic cerebral palsy. *Neuropsychol* 1994; **8**: 180–6.

50. Jenks KM, De Moor J, Van Leishout E. Arithmetic difficulties in children with cerebral palsy are related to executive function and working memory. *J Child Psychol Psychiatry* 2009; **50**(7): 824–33.

51. Prasad R, Verma N, Srivastava A, Das BK, Mishra OP. Magnetic resonance imaging, risk factors and co-morbidities in children with cerebral palsy. *J Neurol* 2011; **258**(3): 471–8.

52. Yoshida S, Hayakawa K, Yamamoto A, *et al*. Quantitative diffusion tensor tractography of the motor and sensory tract in children with cerebral palsy. *Dev Med Child Neurol* 2010; **52**(10): 935–40.

53. Korzeniewski S, Birbeck G, DeLano MC, Potchen MJ, Paneth N. A systematic review of neuroimaging for cerebral palsy. *J Child Neurol* 2008; **23**(2): 216–27.

Chapter

9

Executive functions in learning disorders

Laura A. Barquero, Lindsay M. Wilson, Sabrina L. Benedict, Esther R. Lindström, Heather C. Harris, and Laurie E. Cutting

Growing evidence supports the involvement of EF in academic performance and, consequently, EdF in learning disorders (commonly known as learning disabilities or LD). Often, the first indicator of LD is low academic achievement in areas of reading, math, or writing.[1–4] The terminology used to describe different LD conditions varies by field and includes dyslexia and reading disorder/disability, dyscalculia and mathematics disorder/disability, and disorder of written expression/writing disability. Comorbidity among these learning disorders is common, as is the co-occurrence of LD with ADHD.[5,6]

Recent US data indicate that almost 2.5 million public school students received special education and related services for LD in 2008, and 43% of all public school students receiving special education and related services were identified as having a specific learning disability.[7] Federal guidelines[8] used in educational settings indicate that a child may have a specific LD if, in the absence of any other disability or limiting condition and despite appropriate instruction and experiences, the child does not adequately achieve for age or state standards in one of the following eight academic areas: oral expression, listening comprehension, written expression, basic reading skills, reading fluency skills, reading comprehension, mathematics calculation, or mathematics problem solving. The DSM-IV-TR indicates diagnosis of specific disorders of reading, math, and written expression based on lower than expected performance on standardized tests "given the person's chronological age, measured intelligence, and age-appropriate education."[9] The proposed changes for DSM-5 include defining these disorders based on low performance on standardized measures without requiring a significant discrepancy between measured intelligence and achievement. The proposed changes are more consistent with IDEA guidelines and reflect research findings that discredit IQ-achievement discrepancy as a defining characteristic of Reading Disorder (RD).[10–13] Exactly how the diagnosis of LD is operationalized varies from state to state, and currently includes demonstrating a child's lack of response to instruction in his/her area of academic weakness, though the IQ-achievement discrepancy criterion remains in use.[14] In contrast to these ways of operationalizing LD, researchers typically define difficulty in an academic area as age-based performance at or below the 10th–25th percentile on one or more individually administered standardized measures of that construct.[3,15–21]

Executive dysfunction in LD

Students with LD who have difficulty in planning, initiating work, organizing thoughts and materials, self-monitoring actions and progress, inhibiting unproductive impulses, or

Executive Function and Dysfunction, ed. Scott J. Hunter and Elizabeth P. Sparrow. Published by Cambridge University Press. © Cambridge University Press 2012.

shifting from one activity to another do not learn as efficiently as those who are adept at these EF skills.[22] Though EdF and LD often present concurrently, the relationship between EdF and LD has still not been fully established. A central question is whether there are particular types of EdF that are salient features of difficulty in specific academic domains. A larger related question is the degree to which EdF *itself* is considered a LD, even in the absence of any academic weaknesses. Since the focus of the current chapter is on EdF as related to LDs in specific academic areas, such as reading, writing, and math, defining the construct of EdF and its overall relationship to LD is important. Ongoing studies that characterize the relation of EdF and LD will provide insight that hopefully will lead to better diagnosis and treatment for individuals with EdF and LD, and clarify the relationship between EdF and LD.

Reading disorder

Though phonological deficits are implicated as the largest contributor to reading difficulties,[23] EdF accounts for additional variance in reading.[24] A recent study showed that children with developmental dyslexia produced fewer words than typical readers during a semantic fluency task, and completed fewer categories on the WCST.[25] In addition, meta-analyses of the literature on EF in RD show that children with RD perform lower than typically achieving peers on tests of EF. For example, a meta-analysis of 48 studies comparing typically developing readers to children with RD resulted in a moderate overall mean effect size of 0.57 (Hedges' g) for EF tasks (including WISC-IV Coding, WCST, Tower of Hanoi, MFFT, Stroop, and TMT), with different EF measures moderating the magnitude of the effect size.[15] WISC-IV Coding was found to be most accurate in differentiating participants with RD from typically developing peers (mean effect size of +1.83). Similarly, a meta-analysis of 13 studies comparing children with RD to typically developing readers indicated a moderate overall effect size for EF as measured by the WCST, Tower of London, and other tests of planning, organizing, strategizing, attention to detail and remembering details ($g = -0.595$).[3] Verbal WM showed much larger effect sizes than visual WM, although effect sizes for both types were robust (Verbal: $g = -0.920$; Visual: $g = -0.637$). This WM gap between RD and typical readers appears to increase with age.[20] Overall, findings suggest a strong association between RD and EdF.

Some studies have explored EdF in RD subtypes. In particular, researchers have contrasted word reading difficulties with isolated reading comprehension difficulties. For example, in one study adolescents were categorized as having word-reading difficulties, isolated reading comprehension difficulties, or typical reading achievement; WM and planning significantly contributed to reading comprehension but not word recognition (when controlling for attention, decoding, fluency, and vocabulary).[19] The findings of planning deficits (Tower of London; WISC-IV-Int Elithorn mazes) in adolescents with isolated reading comprehension difficulties persisted even after controlling for comorbid ADHD and phonological processing ability.[17,18] In contrast, adolescents with word-reading difficulties showed EdF in verbal WM (Digit Span Backward) and response inhibition (more errors on Conflicting Motor Response), but these findings were not significant after controlling for comorbid ADHD and phonological processing ability.[17] Although LD often presents comorbidly with ADHD, these studies indicate EdF can occur in individuals with reading comprehension difficulties in the absence of ADHD, and that strategic planning difficulties are closely linked with reading comprehension difficulties.

Another recent study of isolated reading comprehension difficulties revealed differences from typically achieving readers in WM and response to proactive interference (as assessed by WM updating span, categorization, numerical updating, intrusion errors in numerical updating and intrusions in a proactive interference task).[26] Interestingly, meta-analysis did not find significant differences in EdF when comparing studies of word-reading difficulties and isolated reading comprehension difficulties groups, yet it is possible that power of the analysis was limited by unequal sample sizes (42 studies vs. 6 studies).[15] Further research is needed to clarify differences in these findings.

Mathematics disorder

EF also correlates with math achievement scores, although there is comparatively less research on the topic. Longitudinal studies have shown that preschoolers' EF task performance is predictive of later math achievement. In one recent study, performance on set shifting, inhibition, and EF composite score at age 4 (as assessed by a combination of a tower task, Stroop-like task, categorization task, and BRIEF-Parent) predicted math achievement at age 6 years (as measured by math fluency and teacher ratings of math achievement) after controlling for general cognitive and reading abilities.[27] Similarly, another study found that performance on measures of inhibition, WM, planning, and monitoring at age 4 years predicted math proficiency at age 7 years.[28] These studies imply that early detection of EdF may be useful in identifying children at risk for later math disorder and implementing early preventative intervention. Given that early EF performance is predictive of later math achievement, it is not surprising that lower EF performance has been found to correlate with math disorder. As compared with typically developing peers, children with math disorder are substantially weaker on average in planning, organizing, and strategizing skills ($g = -1.049$) as well as verbal WM ($g = -.909$).[3] As seen with RD, the effect size for visual WM ($g = -.441$) is lower than verbal WM. Other studies have shown that children with math disorder underperform relative to typical controls in set shifting (WCST perseverative errors),[29] inhibition (Stroop task),[29] task switching (verbal and visual TMT),[30] and verbal WM.[29,30]

Some studies have focused on mathematical word problem solving. Fourth graders who struggle with arithmetic word problem solving also have difficulty selecting relevant information, updating information, and suppressing irrelevant information relative to children without problem solving difficulties.[31] In a study of first-grade children, Concept Formation (WJ-III) and a composite central executive score (comprised of three dual-task subtests from the Working Memory Test Battery for Children or WMTB: Listening Recall, Counting Recall, and Backward Digit Recall) significantly explained variation in math word-problem performance after controlling for numerosity (i.e., numerical ability) measures, language, attention, visuospatial performance, concept formation, nonverbal reasoning, and processing speed.[32] This relationship did not predict math fact fluency in the same sample, suggesting that EF contributes differentially to word-problem performance and fact fluency within the larger construct of math ability. A similar relationship emerged in another sample of first-grade children, some of whom were at risk for math difficulty and received intervention. After controlling for risk status, treatment group, attention, language, nonverbal problem solving, phonological processing, processing speed, and concept formation, WM (WMTB Listening Recall) explained a significant amount of variation in end-of-first-grade performance on an experimental story problems measure and on curriculum-based measures of computation and concepts/applications.[33,34] Again, WM did not explain unique variance in calculation nor fact fluency outcomes.[34] Concept Formation (WJ-III) emerged as a unique predictor of arithmetic word-problem performance in a sample of third-grade children when controlling for language, nonverbal problem solving, WM, LTM, attention, and sight word efficiency.[35] Concept Formation (WJ-III) and WM (WJ-III Numbers Reversed and WMTB Listening Recall) explained significant variation in Double-Digit Addition and Subtraction Estimation[36] after partialling out the influence of language, nonverbal reasoning, processing speed, LTM, inattentive behavior, basic reading skill, arithmetic number combination, and double-digit computation skill.[37] In a sample of 2nd–4th graders, performance on a set-shifting task (TMT) predicted performance on an experimenter-designed mathematical word problem solving measure after controlling for age, visual and verbal STM, reading ability, and verbal fluency.[38] Such findings suggest that solving word problems likely requires the use of the higher cognitive skills that comprise EF.

Mathematical processes involve EF skills such as planning, strategizing, and WM to work toward and achieve the goal of problem solving. Practical applications of arithmetic skills, such as solving word problems, necessitate the ability to utilize relevant information while ignoring irrelevant information. Students who are less proficient at these skills are at a clear disadvantage and may fall behind in math achievement. In sum, there appears to be solid evidence of involvement of EdF in math disorder; some authors have suggested that EdF, among other variables, should be used in the identification of math disorder.[3] Nevertheless, further exploration is needed to determine the exact area(s) of EdF that are linked to specific aspects of math disorder (i.e., calculation vs. word problem solving).

Disorder of written expression

A small number of studies have addressed the relation of direct EF measures and writing. In typical development, switching and inhibition (Stroop, rapid automated switching) are significant predictors of children's written expression during the late elementary grades.[39–41] Fourth and fifth grade students who have difficulties in written expression, as evidenced by developing a cohesive narrative containing necessary story elements, exhibit significantly lower performance on measures of initiation (the Sentence Formulation subtest total score from the *CELF-R*, the *Visual Search and Attention Test or VSAT*, and the *COWAT* total score) and set shifting (WCST categories correct, WCST perseverations, and *Tower of Hanoi*) in comparison to students with typical levels of written expression.[42] Deficits in WM have been associated with written expression deficits in children aged 6 to 7 years, including vocabulary, sentence length, and coherence.[43] Particularly, complex span ability was predictive of vocabulary usage and coherence in text. In accordance, a longitudinal study showed measures of WM (as assessed by backwards digit recall, naming recall, nonword repetition, word list recall, and word list matching) at age 4 accurately predicted spelling and writing skills at age 7 (as assessed by the reading comprehension test, writing task, and spelling test of the National Curriculum assessments at Key Stage 1 developed by the Qualifications and Curriculum Authority in the UK).[44] These studies indicate that successful writing requires the higher-order skills that comprise EF, whether at the level of spelling or that of producing a cohesive narrative.

The neurological basis of executive dysfunction in LD

Behavioral studies provide tremendous insight into EdF and LD, and neuroimaging may further distinguish these phenotypes. It is not yet clear whether EdF and LD are overlapping but separable in terms of brain activation, and relatively few neuroimaging studies have explored EdF and LD in conjunction. Brain regions known to be involved in EF in children and adolescents (including bilateral dorsolateral, prefrontal, and inferior prefrontal cortices and insula[45–47] may also be affected in LD.

RD has been more extensively studied with neuroimaging than have other LD. During fMRI reading tasks, images of readers with RD are characterized by under-activation in left hemisphere regions including inferior parietal, superior temporal, middle and inferior temporal, precuneus, thalamus, and fusiform areas, as well as overactivation in right fusiform, postcentral, and superior temporal gyri relative to typically developing controls.[48] These areas affected during reading tasks do not show substantial overlap with EF areas. However, in a recent fMRI study using a verbal WM task, adolescents and young adults with RD showed decreased functional connectivity in the bilateral DLPFC, left cuneus, left insula, right inferior parietal lobule, and right precuneus while exhibiting increased connectivity in the left angular gyrus, right super-ior parietal cortex, left inferior frontal gyrus, left hippocampal gyrus, and right thalamus relative to the comparison group of typical readers.[49] This offers evidence that, when performing WM tasks, children and adolescents with RD exhibit a neurobiological profile of impaired WM. The decreased functional connectivity, particuarly in the bilateral DLPFC and left insula, may represent areas of weakness common to RD and WM deficits.

The complex brain differences between groups of individuals with LD and typical achievement are not limited to RD. An fMRI study of children during a visuospatial WM task showed greater activation in the left intraparietal sulcus was predictive of poor math performance 2 years later.[50] Another study examined nonverbal WM in middle school students with good vs. poor spelling performance and found good spellers activated two clusters of brain regions while the poor spellers activated five clusters; the poor spellers overactivated frontal and cingulate areas (bilateral medial superior frontal gyrus, orbital middle frontal gyrus, and ACC) relative to the comparison group.[51]

As these and other studies indicate, interpreting relative amounts of brain activation, either in intensity or extensiveness, is not a straightforward process. That is, increased activation is not necessarily correlated with increased skill, experience, or proficiency. Rather, less activation may be reflective of knowledge consolidation and hence indicate more efficient, less effortful cognitive processing. After receiving training, non-LD novice performers can exhibit increased activation, while consolidation or automaticity gained through more extensive practice, experience, and development leads to decreased acti-vation.[52,53] However, participants with LD are by definition resistant to treatment (i.e. training) to varying degrees. Their low responsiveness to treatment may result in decreased activation relative to non-LD novice controls. Conversely, upon gaining consoli-dation and automaticity, non-LD controls may exhibit less activation than children with LD who must exert effort and neurological resources in performing the task.[54] A challenge lies in interpreting data that is influenced by the interplay of LD, development, and training.

Generalization of EF intervention to academic skill

Several studies have examined the effects of WM training on cognition, including changes in brain activation following WM training.[55] Yet, few studies have measured transfer to academic performance and fewer still have explored a causal relationship between EF remediation and LD remediation. Further research on the strength of this correlation and possible causal relationship is crucial to our understanding of better ways to provide effective remediation for LD. Of the studies that have explored transfer to academic performance, results have been mixed. For example, after a 4-week verbal and spatial WM span intervention, a group of non-LD college undergraduates significantly outperformed no-treatment controls on a standardized measure of reading comprehension, with growth in spatial complex WM correlating significantly with growth in reading comprehension.[56]

A recent study comparing groups of children with dyslexia, language difficulties, and typical achievement found that 6–8 weeks of verbal and visuo-spatial WM training significantly improved WM and basic reading scores for the group with dyslexia.[57] In another study, adolescents with mild disabilities who received 5 weeks of computerized visuo-spatial WM training showed greater growth in academic skills (reading and math) tests at follow-up than did a control group.[58] However, other WM intervention studies in children failed to find similar transfer effects on standardized tests of reading or math.[59,60] Differences may be due to type of training, amount of training, or time elapsed between training and testing. Additional research may further elucidate the relationship between EF training and LD remediation, leading to changes in types of intervention for LD and educational practice.

Teaching executive control routings for the planning process in writing has resulted in positive effects on writing (effect size of 0.80).[61] More specifically, the self-regulated strategy development (SRSD) model is specifically designed to support aspects of EF: analysis, decision making and planning, execution and coordination of mental and affective resources, attention control, and flexible adaptation.[61] Skilled writing requires self-regulation, a strong memory, and attention control, skills that students with writing difficulties lack.[62] SRSD helped mitigate EF difficulties through writing strategies such as goal setting, self-monitoring, self-instruction, and self-reinforcement, resulting in an average weighted effect size of 1.14.[61]

Summary and future directions

The higher cognitive skills that comprise EF are needed throughout childhood and adolescence, and adulthood to accomplish goal-oriented behavior. Because students lacking in these skills may experience academic difficulty, educational researchers are accruing evidence on EF and its connection to learning and LD. EdF is associated with low performance in reading, math, and writing, and deficits in these are likely to result in low achievement in other academic areas. While research has somewhat connected different EF skills to specific academic domains, it is also arguable that WM, shifting attention, inhibition, goal planning, and monitoring underlie all learning, not just one specific academic area.[28] To add further complexity, the relations among EF skills shift over the course of typical childhood development, especially as these skills are applied to increasingly complex tasks.[63,39] Relative to LD, this shift may cause EF deficits to present as late-emerging LD or, conversely, as early-emerging LD that later is resolved. EdF is clearly associated with LD, and more research is needed to determine which of its contributions are domain-general and which are domain-specific, to explore the causal direction(s) of the relationship between EdF and LD.

The interface and overlap of LD and EdF remain somewhat unclear. However, evidence points toward a common involvement of prefrontal areas, possibly insulae, and perhaps some parietal areas. Like the construct of EF, the roles of EF neural circuitry and neural activity in LD appear to be complex and with nebulous boundaries. The central questions revolve around how the brains of individuals with LD and EdF differ from those with typical academic achievement. Perhaps the most exciting question is whether neural plasticity allows for the amelioration of deficits in EF and/or academic skill after intervention. Furthermore, the relative amount of functional activation for EF may change with development or training such that lower, rather than higher, activation is observed over time. Refining our understanding of brain activation patterns across the continua of skill and development could potentially lead to the use of neuroimaging techniques in diagnostic and prescriptive capacities for EdF and LD.

In the educational field, remediation is the paramount goal. Though no consensus has been reached, the suggestion that gains from EF training could transfer to academic achievement is enticing. Early EF intervention could potentially curtail the later confounding effects of LD or completely prevent LD from emerging. For example, measuring EF in preschool has the potential to identify children at-risk for later math difficulties and allows for embedding EF intervention into early math instruction.[27,28,30] Additionally, if differences in EF affect responsiveness to intervention,[19] identification of EdF in specific domains could tailor instruction to corresponding academic areas. Future research could explore coupling EF training with academic intervention to address underlying EdF alongside academic difficulties.

References

1. Fuchs D, Compton DL, Fuchs LS, Bryant J, Davis GN. Making "secondary intervention" work in a three-tier responsiveness-to-intervention model: findings from the first-grade longitudinal reading study of the National Research Center on Learning Disabilities. *Read Writ* 2008; **21**: 413–36.

2. McMaster KL, Fuchs D, Fuchs LS, Compton DL. Responding to nonresponders: an experimental field trial of identification and intervention methods. *Except Child* 2005; **4**: 445–63.

3. Johnson ES, Humphrey M, Mellard DF, Woods K, Swanson HL. Cognitive processing deficits and students with specific learning disabilities: A selective meta-analysis of the literature. *Learn Disab Quart* 2010; **33**: 3–18.

4. Kavale KA. Identifying specific learning disability: Is responsiveness to intervention the answer? *J Learn Disab* 2005; **38**: 553–62.

5. Fuchs LS, Fuchs D. Mathematical problem-solving profiles of students with mathematics disabilities with and without comorbid reading disabilities. *J Learn Disab* 2002; **35**: 564–74.

6. Katusic SK, Colligan RC, Weaver AL, Barbaresi WJ. The forgotten learning disability: Epidemiology of written-language disorder in a population-based birth cohort (1976–1982), Rochester, Minnesota. *Pediatrics* 2009; **123**: 1306–13.

7. Data Accountability Center. "Part B Child Count, 2008." http://www.ideadata.org/PartBChildCount.asp 23 June 2010.

8. Identification of specific learning disabilities. US Department of Education, Office of Special Education Programs. 2006 Oct 4. Available from: http://idea.ed.gov/object/fileDownload/model/TopicalBrief/field/PdfFile/primary_key/23.

9. American Psychiatric Association. *Diagnostic and Statistical Manual of Mental Disorders*, 4th edn., Text Revision. Washington, DC: American Psychiatric Publ; 2000.

10. Fletcher JM, Francis DJ, Rourke BP, Shaywitz SE, Shaywitz BA. The validity of discrepancy-based definitions of reading disabilities. *J Learn Disab* 1992; **25**: 555–61.

11. Vellutino FR, Scanlon DM, Lyon GR. Differentiating between difficult-to-remediate and readily remediated poor readers: More evidence against the IQ-achievement discrepancy definition of reading disability. *J Learn Disab* 2000; **33**: 223–38.

12. Siegel LS. IQ is irrelevant to the definition of learning disabilities. *J Learn Disab* 1989; **22**: 469–79.

13. Stuebing K, Fletcher JM, LeDoux JM, Lyon GR, Shaywitz SE, Shaywitz BA. Validity of IQ-discrepancy classification of reading difficulties: a meta-analysis. *Am Educ Res J* 2002; **39**: 469–518.

14. Reschly DJ, Hosp JL. State SLD identification policies and practices. *Learn Disabi Quart* 2004; **27**: 197–213.

15. Booth JN, Boyle JME, Kelly SW. Do tasks make a difference? Accounting for heterogeneity of performance of children with reading difficulties on tasks of executive function: Findings from a meta-analysis. *Br J Dev Psychol* 2010; **28**: 133–76.

16. Li JJ, Cutting LE, Ryan M, Zilioli M, Denckla M, Mahone EM. Response variability in rapid automatized naming predicts reading comprehension. *J Clin Exp Neuropsychol* 2009; **7**: 877–88.

17. Locascio G, Mahone EM, Eason SH, Cutting LE. Executive dysfunction among children with reading comprehension deficits. *J Learn Disabil* 2010; **43**: 441–54.

18. Cutting LE, Materek A, Cole CAS, Levine TM, Mahone EM. Effects of fluency, oral language, and executive function on reading comprehension performance. *Ann Dyslexia* 2009; **59**: 34–54.

19. Sesma HW, Mahone EM, Levine T, Eason SH, Cutting LE. The contribution of executive skills to reading comprehension. *Child Neuropsychol* 2009; **15**: 232–46.

20. Swanson HL. Age-related differences in learning disabled and skilled readers' working memory. *J Exp Child Psychol* 2003; **85**: 1–31.

21. Swanson HL, Sachse-Lee C. Mathematical problem solving and working memory in children with learning disabilities: Both executive and phonological processes are important. *J Exp Child Psychol* 2001; **79**: 294–321.

22. St. Clair-Thompson HL, Gathercole SE. Executive functions and achievements in school: shifting, updating, inhibition, and working memory. *Quart J Exp Psychol* 2006; **59**: 745–59.

23. Vellutino FR, Fletcher JM, Snowling MJ, Scanlon DM. Specific reading disability (dyslexia): What have we learned in the past four decades? *J Child Psychol Psychiatry* 2004; **45**: 2–40.

24. Gathercole SE, Alloway TP, Willis C, Adams A-M. Working memory in children with reading disabilities. *J Exp Child Psychol* 2006; **93**: 265–81.

25. Menghini D, Finzi A, Benassi R, *et al.* Different underlying neurocognitive deficits in developmental dyslexia: a comparative study. *Neuropsychologia* 2010; **48**: 863–72.

26. Borella E, Carretti B, Pelegrina S. The specific role of inhibition in reading comprehension in good and poor comprehenders. *J Learn Disab* 2010; **43**: 541–51.

27. Clark CAC, Pritchard VE, Woodward LJ. Preschool executive functioning abilities predict early mathematics achievement. *Dev Psychol* 2010; **46**: 1176–91.

28. Bull R, Espy KA, Wiebe SA. Short-term memory, working memory, and executive functioning in preschoolers: longitudinal predictors of mathematical achievement at age 7 years. *Dev Neuropsychol* 2008; **33**: 205–28.

29. Bull R, Scerif G. Executive functioning as a predictor of children's mathematics ability: Inhibition, switching, and

working memory. *Dev Neuropsychol* 2001; 19: 273–93.

30. D'Amico AD, Guarnera M. Exploring working memory in children with low arithmetical achievement. *Learn Individ Differ* 2005; 15: 189–202.

31. Passolunghi MC, Pazzaglia F. A comparison of updating processes in children good or poor in arithmetic word problem-solving. *Learn Individ Differ* 2005; 15: 257–69.

32. Fuchs LS, Geary DC, Compton DL, Fuchs D, Hamlett CL, Bryant JD. The contributions of numerosity and domain-general abilities to school readiness. *Child Dev* 2010; 81: 1520–33.

33. Fuchs LS, Hamlett CL, Fuchs D. *Curriculum-based math computation and concepts/applications.* Available from Author, 328 Peabody, Vanderbilt University, Nashville, TN 37203; 1990.

34. Fuchs LS, Compton DL, Fuchs D, Paulsen K, Bryant JD, Hamlett CL. The prevention, identification, and cognitive determinants of math difficulty. *J Ed Psychol* 2005; 97: 493–513.

35. Fuchs LS, Fuchs D. Mathematical problem-solving profiles of students with mathematics disabilities with and without comorbid reading disabilities. *J Learn Disab* 2002; 35: 564–74.

36. Fuchs LS, Hamlett CL, Powell SR. *Grade 3 Math Battery.* Available from Author, 328 Peabody, Vanderbilt University, Nashville, TN 37203; 2003.

37. Seethaler PM, Fuchs LS. The cognitive correlates of computational estimation skill among third-grade students. *Learn Disab Res Pract* 2006; 21: 233–43.

38. Andersson U. The contribution of working memory to children's mathematical word problem solving. *Appl Cogn Psychol* 2007; 21: 1201–16.

39. Altemeier L, Jones J, Abbott RD, Berninger VW. Executive functions in becoming writing readers and reading writers: note taking and report writing in third and fifth graders. *Dev Neuropsychol* 2006; 29: 161–73.

40. Berninger VW, Abbott RD, Jones J, *et al.* Early development of language by hand: Composing, reading, listening, and speaking connections; three-letter writing modes; and fast mapping in spelling. *Dev Neuropsychol* 2006; 29: 61–92.

41. Altemeier LE, Abbott RD, Berninger VW. Executive functions for reading and writing in typical literacy development and dyslexia. *J Clin Exp Neuropsychol* 2008; 30: 588–606.

42. Hooper SR, Swartz CW, Wakely MB, de Kruif REL, Montgomery JW. Executive functions in elementary school children with and without problems in written expression. *J Learn Disabil* 2002; 35: 57–68.

43. Bourke L, Adams AM. The relationship between working memory and early writing assessed at the word, sentence and text level. *Educ Child Psychol* 2003; 20: 19–36.

44. Gathercole SE, Brown L, Pickering SJ. Working memory assessments at school entry as longitudinal predictors of national curriculum attainment levels. *Educ and Child Psychol* 2003; 20: 109–22.

45. Houdé O, Rossi S, Lubin A, Joliot M. Mapping numerical processing, reading, and executive functions in the brain: an fMRI meta-analysis of 52 studies including 842 children. *Dev Sci* 2010; 13: 876–85.

46. Dove A, Pollmann S, Schubert T, Wiggnes CJ, von Cramon DY. Prefrontal cortex activation in task switching: an event-related fMRI study. *Cogn Brain Res* 2000; 9: 103–9.

47. Menon V, Uddin LQ. Saliency, switching, attention and control: a network model of insula function. *Brain Struct Funct* 2010; 214: 655–67.

48. Maisog JM, Einbinder ER, Flowers DL, Turkeltaub PE, Eden GF. A meta-analysis of functional neuroimaging studies of dyslexia. *Ann NY Acad Sci* 2008; 1145: 237–59.

49. Wolf RC, Sambataro F, Lohr C, Steinbrink C, Martin C, Vasic N. Functional brain network abnormalities during verbal working memory performance in adolescents and young

adults with dyslexia. *Neuropsychologia* 2010; **48**: 309–18.

50. Dumontheil I, Klingberg T. Brain activity during a visuospatial working memory task predicts arithmetical performance 2 years later. *Cereb Cortex*. 2011; in press.

51. Richards T, Berninger V, Winn W, *et al.* Differences in fMRI activation between children with and without spelling disability on 2-back/0-back working memory contrast. *J Writing Res* **1**: 93–123.

52. Meyler A, Keller TA, Cherkassky VL, Gabrieli JDE, Just MA. Modifying the brain activation of poor readers during sentence comprehension with extended remedial instruction: A longitudinal study of neuroplasticity. *Neuropsychologia* 2008; **46**: 2580–92.

53. Chein JM, Schneider W. Neuroimaging studies of practice-related change: fMRI and meta-analytic evidence of a domain-general control network for learning. *Cogn Brain Res* 2005; **25**: 607–23.

54. Pugh KR, Frost SJ, Sandak R, *et al.* Effects of stimulus activity and repetition on printed work identification: An fMRI comparison of nonimpaired and reading-disabled adolescent cohorts. *J Cog Neurosci* 2008; **20**: 1146–60.

55. Morrison AB, Chein JM. Does working memory training work? The promise and challenges of enhancing cognition by working memory. *Psychoneurol Bull Rev* 2011; **18**: 46–60.

56. Chein JM, Morrison AB. Expanding the mind's workspace: Training and transfer effects with a complex working memory span task. *Psychoneurol Bull Rev* 2010; **17**: 193–9.

57. Holmes J, Dunning D, Gathercole SE. Can working memory training improve children's reading skills? Paper presented at: Eighteenth Annual Conference of the Society for the Scientific Study of Reading; 2011 July 15; St. Pete Beach, Florida.

58. Van der Molen MJ, Van Luit JEH, Van der Molen MW, Klugkist I, Jongmans MJ. Effectiveness of a computerised working memory training in adolescents with mild to borderline intellectual disabilities. *J Intell Disab Res* 2010; **54**: 433–47.

59. Holmes J, Gathercole SE, Dunning DL. Adaptive training leads to sustained enhancement of poor working memory in children. *Dev Science* 2009; **12**: F9–15.

60. St. Clair-Thompson HL, Stevens R, Hunt A, Bolder E. Improving children's working memory and classroom performance. *Educ Psychol* 2010; **30**: 203–19.

61. Graham, S, Harris KR, Olinghouse N. Addressing executive function problems in writing: an example from the self-regulated strategy development model. In Lynn Meltzer, ed. *Executive Function in Education from Theory to Practice*. NY: The Guilford Press; 2007.

62. Harris KR, Graham S, Mason LH, Friedlander B. *Powerful Writing Strategies for All Students*. Baltimore: Paul H Brookes Publishing Co; 2008.

63. Best JR, Miller PH, Jones LL. Executive functions after age 5: changes and correlates. *Dev Rev* 2009; **29**: 180–200.

Chapter 10

Executive functions in mood and anxiety disorders

Jennifer P. Edidin and Scott J. Hunter

Mood and anxiety disorders in children and adolescents have been widely examined empirically, yet relatively few studies have focused on the effects of these disorders on developing EF skills. This lack of knowledge regarding a core cognitive capacity has hampered efforts at understanding and addressing potential disruptions in problem solving, memory, and engagement that often co-occur with mood and anxiety disorders.

Mood disorders

Mood disorders include diagnoses for which the primary symptoms are a change in emotional state. This category of psychopathology includes significantly elevated or depressed mood, inappropriate affect, or a limited range of feelings,[1] and is diagnostically composed of major depressive disorder (MDD), bipolar disorder (BD), cyclothymic disorder, and dysthymic disorder in the DSM-IV-TR. In the upcoming DSM-5, this group of disorders will likely be divided further into two categories, bipolar and related disorders and depressive disorders.[2] While few changes to the diagnosis of MDD are anticipated, the criteria for BD will likely be developmentally based, and include increased specificity in order to capture the presentation of manic symptoms observed in children. The DSM-5 may include a new disorder, temper dysregulation disorder with dysphoria (TDD), characterized by temper outbursts that begin before 10 years of age,[2] although its inclusion remains both controversial and uncertain.

Current diagnostic criteria for the affective disorders suggest disruption in EF. For example, individuals with MDD or dysthymic disorder often present with impaired thinking, decision-making, and concentration.[1] Individuals with BD are often distractible, impulsive, and emotionally dysregulated.[1]

Because children and adolescents are more likely to present with subsyndromal levels of affective disorders, cognitive symptoms are often overlooked. However, studies indicate that mild mood disorder symptoms experienced during childhood can disrupt typical development (as well as being predictive of later depression).[3-5] This is particularly true when symptoms are experienced during adolescence, which is a critical period of development for the frontal lobes and associated executive circuits.[3]

Executive Function and Dysfunction, ed. Scott J. Hunter and Elizabeth P. Sparrow. Published by Cambridge University Press. © Cambridge University Press 2012.

Executive dysfunction in major depressive disorder

Studies of EF in children and adolescents with MDD have produced variable results; however, it appears that MDD can affect multiple aspects of EF. Deficits are observed on tests of WM, cognitive flexibility and set shifting (often studied in pediatric MDD with the WISC Digit Span, WCST, TMT, and Stroop). Relative to age-matched controls, youth with MDD tend to have lower scores on the WCST.[6] Another study found high levels of perseverative errors on the TMT and low scores on the WJ-R-Cog Concept Formation subtest in boys with comorbid anxious and depressive symptoms.[7] These results are consistent with studies of adults[8] that have argued for likely EdF in depression.

In contrast, other studies have found intact EF in youth with MDD, across results from the WCST, COWAT, and TMT.[9] Differences in patient populations with regard to gender, comorbidity, and age may account for these discrepant findings. Depressive symptoms are typically less severe and may be of shorter duration in pediatric MDD, leading to less consistent evidence of EdF. Some researchers suggest that severe EdF is seen during more severe depressive episodes only.[9] While some adult studies indicate EF deficits are only present during a depressive episode, others suggest EF may be impaired for a protracted period of time following a depressive episode.

Executive dysfunction in pediatric bipolar disorder

Studies of pediatric bipolar disorder (PBD) consistently find evidence of EdF, including deficits in WM, fluency, inhibition, attention, organization, and cognitive flexibility. Several studies have found poorer WM in adolescents with BD, based on results from the WISC-IV or WAIS-III Digit Span and Letter-Number Sequencing subtests.[10,11] These deficits have been attributed to alterations in the ventral PFC, which some researchers believe to play an important role in the deficits observed in PBD.[10] Two meta-analyses have shown that youth with BD have impaired category and first letter verbal fluency, with effect sizes ranging from small to large.[12,13] This finding for youth with BD is different from studies of adults with BD, for whom semantic fluency is impaired and phonemic fluency is relatively spared.[14-16] This difference may reflect differences in deficits in memory retrieval, as the frontal and temporal regions of the brain appear to be recruited differently across age cohorts.[14]

In a recent study of children with BD, inhibitory control, as measured by the Stroop and WCST nonperseverative errors, was impaired[10] relative to non-affected peers; this is consistent with adult studies.[14] Difficulty with inhibition has also been attributed to dysfunction in the ventral PFC proposed to be characteristic of PBD, and is believed to represent one of the core deficits of the disorder.[10] Sustained attention is also problematic in pediatric and adult BD, based on data from the TMT, CPT, Wechsler Digit Span and Letter-Number Sequencing, and the Digit Symbol Substitution Test.[10,11,13,17]

A number of PBD studies have found deficits in attention across both manic and depressive episodes, as well as in euthymic phases.[11,18-22] A 23-year prospective study found increased rates of attentional problems in children who were later diagnosed with BD as young adults compared with those who were later diagnosed with MDD, or no mood disorder.[21] These youth who were later diagnosed with BD completed fewer WCST categories than those later diagnosed with MDD or no affective disorder, even after controlling for premorbid attentional dysfunction; this suggests that the relationship between PBD and EdF extends beyond just attentional deficits.[21]

Children with BD also exhibit deficits in organization, including poor performance on the RCFT.[10] PBD is also associated with deficits in set shifting and cognitive flexibility, assessed with the WCST, Category Test, Stroop, and the Penn Conditional Exclusion Test (a task conceptually similar to the WCST) relative to children with unipolar depression and healthy controls.[21]

Despite individual study findings of EdF in mood disorders, meta-analyses have not shown a consistent pattern of impairment across areas of cognitive functioning in pediatric mood disorders.[17] For example, a meta-analysis of neurocognitive functioning in PBD found attentional deficits when PBD groups were compared to healthy control groups; however, findings were inconsistent in a qualitative review of studies that examined differences in attention in a range of other psychiatric diagnoses. This suggests that attentional problems and other types of EdF may be representative of cognitive difficulties seen within a broader pediatric psychopathology phenotype rather than unique to the mood disorders.[17]

The neurological basis of executive dysfunction in mood disorders

Neuroimaging studies of youth with affective disorders have identified differences in the PFC and limbic system, with significant variability across studies. Although one MRI study showed a significantly larger bilateral amygdala to hippocampus ratio in children and adolescents with MDD relative to controls, the positive correlation between this same ratio and severity of comorbid anxiety suggests that alterations in structural symmetry may not be associated with MDD alone.[23] An early fMRI study showed hypoactivation of the amygdala in pediatric MDD when the participants examined fearful faces,[24] but a more recent study found that adolescents with MDD presented with significantly greater left amygdala activation relative to healthy controls during a facial emotion-matching task.[25] The discrepancy between these results may reflect task differences.

Studies of cerebral blood flow and metabolism in pediatric MDD have found hypoactivation of the right dorsal PFC and the dorsal ACC, areas thought to be involved with planning, organization, regulation, inhibition, motivation, and pleasure.[26] As these are among the last areas to myelinate, alterations in these areas during brain development may cause delayed effects on the development of EF.

MRI studies in PBD have found reduced gray matter volume in the DLPFC, an area thought to be involved in emotion regulation.[20,27] Smaller hippocampal volumes relative to healthy controls have been noted in children and adolescents with BD. Further, there is a significant positive correlation between hippocampal volume and age, the reverse of what occurs in healthy controls.[5] Localized alterations in the volume of the subiculum (part of the hippocampus that projects into the PFC) also have been observed in PBD; alterations in this structure may disrupt the frontotemporal neural pathway,[5] contributing to broader EdF.

PBD has been associated with alterations in activation of the left putamen, thalamus, ACC gyrus, left DLPFC, VLPFC, right inferior frontal gyrus, right insula, left frontal gyrus, and mesial temporal lobes.[28] These areas are involved in affect regulation, verbal memory, attention, and inhibition.[28–30] A recent magnetoencephalography (MEG) study examined the theta band associated with the ACC in youth with BD. Compared with healthy controls, greater power was observed in the right ACC and parietal lobes of youth with BD in response to negative feedback. In contrast, lower power was noted in the left ACC in response to positive feedback.[31] In another study that examined the relation between the emotional valence of stimuli and limbic system activation, higher levels of bilateral activation were found in the pregenual ACC and in the left amygdala, and lower levels of activation were found in the right rostral VLPFC and DLPFC when words with a negative valence were presented.[30] Words with a positive valence did not precipitate activation in the PFC or amygdala.[30]

These findings are consistent with other studies of youth with BD that suggest that alterations or disruptions observed in the PFC and the limbic system, and their neural circuitry, are associated with impairments in cognitive, affective, and behavior regulation. Although maturational changes that occur in these areas during childhood and adolescence are typically associated with improvements in EF, this does not appear to be the case in youth with BD.[32-34] In contrast to typically developing children, youth with BD appear to process negative responses more diffusely in the brain.[31] They also exhibit disinhibition in the limbic system and reduced function in PFC systems that regulate emotion regulation.[30] Further, the DLPFC appears to be adversely affected by high levels of emotional responsivity to negative affect.[30] Relative to studies of adults, these neuroimaging findings with PBD are consistent across studies; this may reflect the relatively greater severity of early-onset BD.[3]

Anxiety disorders

The hallmarks of the anxiety disorders are worry and fear. In addition to the cognitive experience of worry, many individuals also experience a strong fight-or-flight response, which may include sweating, heart palpitations, shaking or trembling, feeling faint, and gastrointestinal upset.[1] Although worry, fear, and anxiety are normal reactions to a range of experiences, they become problematic when they are unprovoked, excessive in relation to the stimulus encountered, associated with avoidance, and cause disruptions in daily functioning and interpersonal relationships.[1] The anxiety disorders include: acute stress disorder, agoraphobia, generalized anxiety disorder (GAD), obsessive-compulsive disorder (OCD), panic disorder, phobias, post-traumatic stress disorder (PTSD), and separation anxiety disorder (SAD; listed in the DSM-IV-TR under "Disorders first diagnosed in childhood").[1]

Several changes have been proposed for the anxiety disorders in the DSM-5. OCD will likely be reclassified under "Obsessive-compulsive and related disorders," while PTSD and acute stress disorder may be placed in a new category, "Trauma and stressor-related disorders." Developmentally sensitive criteria have also been proposed for diagnosing PTSD in preschool-age children.[2]

Executive dysfunction in obsessive-compulsive disorder

Studies of EF in the anxiety disorders tend to focus on OCD, particularly the specific vulnerability of frontal regulatory networks in OCD. Studies of verbal fluency (COWAT) in pediatric OCD have varied in findings, including deficits, typical performance,[35,36] and even strengths relative to controls.[37] It is possible that differences in population characteristics, such as severity, age of onset, or duration of illness, contribute to the discrepancy in findings. Inconsistencies in findings may reflect differences in participant characteristics, including age, test and subtest selection, and exclusion criteria, as well as onset and duration of OCD symptoms.[37]

Across tests of cognitive flexibility, such as the WCST, Stroop, and Object Alternation Test, deficits have been observed in pediatric OCD.[36,38,39] On the WCST, children with OCD had more errors and completed fewer sorts in comparison to controls.[39] This pattern of performance suggests orbitofrontal and frontal-striatal deficits in youth with OCD.[38,39]

Perceptual–organizational abilities and planning also seem to be impacted in pediatric OCD. Children with OCD performed in the low average range on the copy trial of the ROCF[40] and required more moves to solve items on the D-KEFS Tower Test, particularly as difficulty level increased.[36] This suggests that in addition to planning, inhibition and rule learning may also be negatively impacted by OCD.[36] In contrast, studies with the traditional Tower of Hanoi did not find significant differences for children with OCD vs. controls;[37] this may reflect differences in the two Tower versions. In particular, tower tests that require fewer moves to correctly complete the item may be less sensitive than those that require a greater number of moves.[36]

Executive dysfunction in other anxiety disorders

There are fewer studies of EdF in panic disorder, agoraphobia, social phobia, and GAD. What has been published has suggested primary impairments in memory and attention.[6] Some studies also have found increased response inhibition.[41] It is of note that similar to the studies of mood disorders, EdF are noted even during symptom remission[42] in studies of anxiety disorders, suggesting an extended impact of the disorder on problem solving.

The neurological basis of executive dysfunction in anxiety disorders

Most neuroimaging research in the anxiety disorders has focused on OCD. Although fear is primarily processed in the amygdala, research has determined that it is also influenced and mediated by the PFC.[43] It has been hypothesized that the PFC is responsible for "'cognitive' control of conditioned fear".[44] The PFC also has been implicated in the overinhibition of repetitive cognitions and behaviors characteristic of OCD.[45] This highlights that the areas of the brain specifically involved in problem solving and behavioral regulation are also involved in the processing and management of anxiety. As such, elevated levels of fear and worry can influence and interfere with executive processing.

When youth with pediatric OCD were presented with alternating blocks of symptom provocation, neutral stimuli, and imagined scenarios, lower levels of brain activation relative to healthy controls were observed in the right insula, putamen, thalamus, DLPFC, left OFC, right thalamus, and right insula during the provocation condition. The lower levels of activation in the right DLPFC were associated with elevated symptom severity.[46] This suggests that youth with OCD have lower levels of neural activation in areas of the brain responsible for emotional and cognitive processing.[46]

Recent studies have provided support for the frontal-striatal-thalamic model of OCD.[47] When youth were presented with a task of cognitive flexibility (requiring set-shifting), the OCD group had a significantly slower response time relative to healthy controls when the target alternated and exhibited less activation in the left inferior frontal gyrus when required to shift sets.[48]

In an fMRI study, children with GAD displayed an exaggerated amygdala response when shown fearful faces when compared to controls, and the magnitude of the difference between the signal change for neutral and fearful stimuli was positively correlated with symptom severity.[24] These results support an amplified response of the limbic system in response to fear in pediatric anxiety disorders. This disruption, in turn, may be associated with impaired EF, particularly with emotion and behavioral regulation and cognitive flexibility.

Summary and future directions

While there is growing evidence for specific impairments in EF across neuropsychological and neuroimaging studies in pediatric mood and anxiety disorders, relative to studies of adults, there is still a great deal of research to be done. Cumulatively, the current body of research suggests that early adolescence may be a uniquely critical period for brain development, and as such, a particularly vulnerable time for the impact of mood or excessive anxiety. Affective disorders that occur during this time may interrupt or even alter development in regions of the brain involved in EF. The frontotemporal and prefrontal cortices, the limbic system, as well as the connections among these areas appear to be particularly vulnerable during adolescence. Alterations in these areas have been implicated in many of the EF deficits observed in pediatric affective disorders.[3] However, the overlap in deficits observed among the affective disorders suggests that they are not unique to any one disorder, but rather to affective psychopathology more broadly.[36] This is consistent with the findings of studies with adults.[49]

Future research needs to address discrepancies in pediatric and adult findings, with a focus on the development and continuity of these disorders across the lifespan. With a more comprehensive understanding of the neurocognitive development associated with these disorders, research can begin to develop more targeted and effective prevention and intervention programs. These programs may be able to significantly impact the development and progression of mood and anxiety disorders if implemented during childhood and adolescence.[3]

References

1. American Psychiatric Association. *Diagnostic Statistical Manual of Mental Disorders*, 4th edn., Text Revision. Washington, DC: APA; 2000.

2. American Psychiatric Association. *Issues pertinent to a developmental approach to bipolar disorder in DSM-5 [Internet].* 2010 [cited 2011 June 13]. Available from: http://www.dsm5.org/Proposed%20Revision%20Attachments/APA%20Developmental%20Approaches%20to%20Bipolar%20Disorder.pdf.

3. Blumberg HP. The next wave in neuroimaging research in pediatric bipolar disorder. *J Am Acad Child Psychol* 2008; **47**(5): 483–5.

4. Frazier JA, Chiu S, Breeze JL, *et al.* Structural brain magnetic resonance imaging of limbic and thalamic volumes in pediatric bipolar disorder. *Am J Psychiatry* 2005; **162**(7): 1256–65.

5. Bearden CE, Soares JC, Klunder AD, *et al.* Three-dimensional mapping of hippocampal anatomy in adolescents with bipolar disorder. *J Am Acad Child Psychol* 2008; **47**(5): 515–25.

6. Micco J, Henin A, Biederman J, *et al.* Executive functioning in offspring at risk for depression and anxiety. *Depress Anxiety* 2009; **26**(9): 780–90.

7. Emerson CS, Mollet GA, Harrison DW. Anxious-depression in boys: an evaluation of executive functioning. *Arch Clin Neuropsychol* 2005; **20**(4): 539–46.

8. Taconnat L, Baudouin A, Fay S, *et al.* Episodic memory and organizational strategy in free recall in unipolar depression: the role of cognitive support and executive functions. *J Clin Exp Neuropsychol* 2010; **32**(7): 719–27.

9. Favre T, Hughes C, Emslie G, Stavinoha P, Kennard B, Carmody T. Executive functioning in children and adolescents

with Major Depressive Disorder. *Child Neuropsychol* 2009; **15**(1): 85–98.

10. Lera-Miguel S, Andrés-Perpiñá S, Calvo R, Fatjó-Vilas M, Lourdes F, Lázaro L. Early-onset bipolar disorder: how about visual-spatial skills and executive functions? *Eur Arch Psychol Clin Neurol* 2011; **261**(3): 195–203.

11. Pavuluri MN, West A, Hill SK, Jindal K, Sweeney JA. Neurocognitive function in pediatric bipolar disorder: 3-year follow-up shows cognitive development lagging behind healthy youths. *J Am Acad Child Psychol* 2009; **48**(3): 299–307.

12. Arts B, Jabben N, Krabbendam L, Os JV. Meta-analyses of cognitive functioning in euthymic bipolar patients and their first-degree relatives. *Psychol Med* 2008; **38**(6): 771–85.

13. Robinson LJ, Thompson JM, Gallagher P, et al. A meta-analysis of cognitive deficits in euthymic patients with bipolar disorder. *J Affect Disord* 2006; **93**(1–3): 105–15.

14. Juselius S, Kieseppä T, Kaprio J, Lönnqvist J, Tuulio-Henriksson A. Executive functioning in twins with bipolar I disorder and healthy co-twins. *Arch Clin Neuropsychol* 2009; **24**(6): 599–606.

15. Martínez-Arán A, Vieta E, Torrent C, et al. Functional outcome in bipolar disorder: The role of clinical and cognitive factors. *Bipolar Disord* 2007; **9**(1–2): 103–13.

16. Olley AL, Malhi GS, Bachelor J, Cahill CM, Mitchell PB, Berk M. Executive functioning and theory of mind in euthymic bipolar disorder. *Bipolar Disord* 2005; **7**(Suppl. 5): 43–52.

17. Joseph MF, Frazier TW, Youngstrom EA, Soares JC. A quantitative and qualitative review of neurocognitive performance in pediatric bipolar disorder. *J Child Adol Psychophamacol* 2008; **18**(6): 595–605.

18. Dickstein DP, Treland JE, Snow J, et al. Neuropsychological performance in pediatric bipolar disorder. *Biol Psychiatry* 2004; **55**(1): 32–9.

19. Doyle AE, Wilens TE, Kwon A, et al. Neuropsychological functioning in youth with bipolar disorder. *Biol Psychiatry* 2005; **58**(7): 540–8.

20. Luby JL, Navsaria N. Pediatric bipolar disorder: evidence for prodromal states and early markers. *J Child Psychol Psychiatry* 2010; **51**(4): 459–71.

21. Meyer SE, Carlson GA, Wiggs EA, et al. A prospective study of the association among impaired executive functioning, childhood attentional problems, and the development of bipolar disorder. *Dev Psychopathol* 2004; **16**(2): 461–76.

22. Pavuluri MN, Schenkel LS, Aryal S, et al. Neurocognitive function in unmedicated manic and medicated euthymic pediatric bipolar patients. *Am J Psychiatry* 2006; **163**(2): 286–93.

23. MacMillan S, Szeszko PR, Moore GJ, et al. Increased amygdala: hippocampal volume ratios major depression. *J Child Adol Psychopharmacol* 2003; **13**(1): 65–73.

24. Thomas KM, Drevets WC, Dahl RE, et al. Amygdala Response to Fearful Faces in Anxious And Depressed Children. *Arch Gen Psychiatry* 2001; **58**(11): 1057–63.

25. Yang TT, Simmons AN, Matthews SC, et al. Adolescents with major depression demonstrate increased amygdala activation. *J Am Acad Child Psychol* 2010; **49**(1): 42–51.

26. Liotti M, Mayberg HS. The role of functional neuroimaging in the neuropsychology of depression. *J Clin Exp Neuropsychol* 2001; **23**(1): 121–36.

27. Dickstein DP, Milham MP, Nugent AC, et al. Frontotemporal alterations in pediatric bipolar disorder: results of a voxel-based morphometry study. *Arch Gen Psychiatry* 2005; **62**(7): 734–41.

28. Frazier JA, Ahn MS, DeJong S, Bent EK, Breeze JL, Giuliano AJ. Magnetic resonance imaging studies in early-onset bipolar disorder: *a critical review. Harvard Rev Psychiatry* 2005; **13**(7): 125–40.

29. Leibenluft E, Rich BA, Vinton DT, et al. Neural circuitry engaged during unsuccessful motor inhibition in pediatric bipolar disorder. *Am J Psychiatry* 2007; **164**(1): 52–60.

30. Pavuluri MN, O'Connor MM, Harral EM, Sweeney JA. An fMRI study of the interface between affective and cognitive neural circuitry in pediatric bipolar disorder. *Psychiatry Res* 2008; **162**(3): 244–55.

31. Rich BA, Holroyd T, Carver FW, *et al.* A preliminary study of the neural mechanisms of frustration in pediatric bipolar disorder using magnetoencephalography. *Depress Anxiety* 2010; **27**(3): 276–86.

32. Crone EA. Executive functions in adolescence: inferences from brain and behavior. *Dev Sci* 2009; **12**(6): 825–30.

33. Romer D, Betancourt L, Giannetta JM, Brodsky ML, Farah M, Hurt H. Executive cognitive functions and impulsivity as correlates of risk taking behavior and problem behavior in preadolescents. *Neuropsychologia* 2009; **47**(13): 2916–26.

34. Steinberg L. Cognitive and affective development in adolescence. *Trends Cogn Sci* 2005; **9**(2): 69–74.

35. Andres S, Boget T, Lazaro L, *et al.* Neurosychological performance in children and adolescents with obsessive–compulsive disorder and influence of clinical variables. *Biol Psychiatry* 2007; **61**(8): 946–51.

36. Ornstein TJ, Arnold P, Manassis K, Mendlowitz S, Schachar R. Neuropsychological performance in childhood OCD: a preliminary study. *Depress Anxiety* 2010; **27**(4): 372–80.

37. Beers SR, Rosenberg DR, Dick EL, *et al.* Neuropsychological study of frontal lobe function in psychotropic-naive children with obsessive–compulsive disorder. *Am J Psychiatry* 1999; **156**(5): 777–9.

38. Freedman M. Object alternation and orbitofrontal system dysfunction in Alzheimer's and Parkinson's disease. *Brain Cogn* 1990; **14**(2): 134–43.

39. Shin MS, Choi H, Kim H, Hwang JW, Kim BN, Cho SC. A study of neuropsychological deficit in children with obsessive-compulsive disorder. *Eur Psychiatry* 2008; **23**(4): 512–20.

40. Flessner CA, Allgair A, Garcia A, *et al.* The impact of neuropsychological functioning on treatment outcome in pediatric obsessive-compulsive disorder. *Depress Anxiety* 2010; **27**(4): 365–71.

41. Oosterlaan J, Sergeant JA. Response inhibition and response re-engagement in attention-deficit/hyperactivity disorder, disruptive, anxious and normal children. *Behav Brain Res* 1998; **94**(1): 33–43.

42. Gualtieri CT, Johnson LG, Benedict KB. Neurocognition in depression: Patients on and off medication versus healthy comparison subjects. *J Neuropsychiatry Clin Neurosci* 2006; **18**(2): 217–25.

43. Barkley RA. Behavioral inhibition, sustained attention and executive functions, constructing a unifying theory of ADHD. *Psychol Bull* 1997; **121**(1): 65–94.

44. Ninan PT. The functional anatomy, neurochemistry, and pharmacology of anxiety. *J Clin Psychiatry* 1999; **60**(Suppl. 2): 12–17.

45. Cummins TK, Ninan PT. The neurobiology of anxiety in children and adolescents. *Growth* 2002; **1**(2): 114–28.

46. Gilbert AR, Akkal D, Almeida JRC, *et al.* Neural correlates of symptom dimensions in pediatric obsessive-compulsive disorder: a functional magnetic resonance imaging study. *J Am Acad Child Psychol* 2009; **48**(9): 936–44.

47. MacMaster FP, O'Neill J, Rosenberg DR. Brain imaging in pediatric obsessive-compulsive disorder. *J Am Acad Child Psychol* 2008; **47**(11): 1262–72.

48. Britton JC, Rauch SL, Rosso IM, *et al.* Cognitive inflexibility and frontal-cortical activation in pediatric obsessive-compulsive disorder. *J Am Acad Child Psychol* 2010; **49**(9): 944–53.

49. Bédard M, Joyal CC, Godbout L, Chantal S. Executive Functions and the Obsessive-Compulsive Disorder: On the Importance of Subclinical Symptoms and Other Concomitant Factors. *Arch Clin Neuropsychol* 2009; **24**(6): 585–98.

Chapter

11

Executive functions in childhood epilepsy

Frank A. Zelko and Lev Gottlieb

Epilepsy, which is defined by a pattern of recurring seizures, comprises an array of diseases and syndromes within an evolving classification framework.[1] The cardinal feature of epilepsy is the electroclinical event, an anomalous behavior or sensory alteration that correlates with abnormal electrophysiological activity in the brain. Clinical manifestations of childhood epilepsy are broad, ranging from fleeting reductions of consciousness, to simple sensory and motor events, to complex behaviors and disruptions of higher-level cognition. Electrophysiological events associated with seizures also vary in form and localization.[2]

Cognition in childhood epilepsy is influenced by several factors, including: (1) underlying genetic, metabolic, and neuropathologic processes that give rise to epileptic events, (2) transient event-related neurophysiological disruptions, (3) neuronal injury caused by epileptic events leading to progressive neurologic and cognitive deterioration, and (4) adverse effects of antiepileptic drugs (AEDs). Environmental and disease factors such as age of onset, seizure frequency, and epilepsy type or syndrome have also been associated with cognitive outcome in childhood epilepsy.[3–6] In light of this heterogeneity, the failure to identify a "signature profile" of neuropsychological impairment in childhood epilepsy is not surprising.[7,8] However, many forms of childhood epilepsy are associated with disruptions of behavior or cognition that are potentially indicative of EdF.

Executive dysfunction in childhood epilepsy
General findings

Consistent with findings in the adult literature,[9] deficits of attention have long been a concern in childhood epilepsy.[10] Early studies of parent and teacher ratings indicated greater attention difficulties in children with epilepsy compared to controls.[11,12] However, the phenomenology of ADHD in childhood epilepsy appears to differ from that of ADHD in the general population, in that the inattentive subtype is more prevalent, and a gender difference may not exist.[13–15] A recent review estimated the prevalence of ADHD in childhood epilepsy to fall between 12% and 17%, though rates approaching 30% have been reported in epilepsy clinic samples.[16] Conversely, children

Executive Function and Dysfunction, ed. Scott J. Hunter and Elizabeth P. Sparrow. Published by Cambridge University Press. © Cambridge University Press 2012.

with ADHD were found to be 2.7 times more likely than non-ADHD controls to have epilepsy.[17] Epilepsy with comorbid ADHD is associated with earlier epilepsy diagnosis, greater seizure frequency, and poorer AED treatment response.[17] A history of ADHD prior to seizure onset is not uncommon.[14,15] ADHD may be considered a risk factor for childhood epilepsy[14] and an indicator of neurodevelopmental vulnerability, which predisposes to both conditions.[15]

Children with epilepsy have often been found to do poorly on CPTs and subtests of intelligence and memory scales sensitive to attention problems.[8,11,18–20] However, some studies have failed to show differences between children with epilepsy and controls on such tasks,[21,22] suggesting that the relationship between attention deficits and childhood epilepsy is not straightforward. It has been proposed that the poor performance of children with epilepsy on attention tasks may be largely attributable to other factors such as slow processing speed[23] or even contextual variables such as disruptions of the home environment or parenting strategies.[24]

Two recent investigations have considered executive aspects of spatial attention in childhood epilepsy.[25,26,31] In one, methodology developed by Posner and colleagues[27] to study neuroanatomic networks underlying alerting, orienting, and executive components of visual attention was applied to the investigation of children with newly diagnosed idiopathic generalized epilepsy.[30] Children with idiopathic generalized epilepsy were found to respond more slowly than controls on an executive control task but not on alerting and orienting tasks lacking an executive component. Oculomotor response and control mechanisms were examined in a very recent study of saccadic task performance in childhood epilepsy.[31] Regardless of task conditions, children with epilepsy were found to have generally slower response times than normal controls, but they performed especially poorly on an antisaccadic response inhibition task, suggesting disruption of top-down modulation processes necessary for executive attention control. Together, these studies implicate executive components of attention in childhood epilepsy and suggest that further analysis of executive attention systems may be fruitful.

EdF has been reported in children with epilepsy on a variety of clinical measures involving inhibition, problem-solving, set-shifting, and fluency.[19,25,28–30] EdF frequently manifests early in the disease process and, in fact, predates seizure onset in many children.[25] EdF has been associated with early onset of epilepsy, high seizure frequency, and use of multiple AEDs.[28] Multiple AEDs may have a direct impact upon EF secondary to side effects such as depressed processing speed, or they may reflect the severity and intractability of a child's epilepsy. In light of conceptualizations linking EF to information processing speed,[31–33] it is also important to note that processing speed deficits have been consistently demonstrated in studies of childhood epilepsy.[25,26,34,35]

Parent ratings on the BRIEF were more often elevated in a clinic-referred sample of children with epilepsy than in the BRIEF standardization sample, with particular elevations on scales sampling planning/organization skills and WM.[36] Comparisons of children with epilepsy to healthy controls have found mean BRIEF parent ratings to be significantly higher for children with epilepsy.[26,29] BRIEF ratings in childhood epilepsy have correlated significantly with psychometric measures of sorting, verbal fluency, color-word interference,[29] and health-related quality of life.[37] These findings are consistent with the general view that children with epilepsy are at substantial risk for EdF affecting everyday life, and they also support the use of parent rating scales in assessment of children with epilepsy.

Localization-related epilepsies: frontal-lobe epilepsy and temporal-lobe epilepsy

Frontal-lobe epilepsy (FLE) represents the prototypical seizure disorder for associated EdF, including impaired attention, inhibition, self-monitoring, cognitive flexibility, problem-solving, fluency, and planning.[38-40] These deficits have been documented in children with both symptomatic and nonsymptomatic FLE.[41-47] Importantly, these EF deficits often occur in the context of intact overall intelligence,[38,45,46] making them a defining neurocognitive feature of the disorder.

Although memory dysfunction constitutes the most prominent neurocognitive deficit in temporal-lobe epilepsy (TLE),[48] EdF has been identified as well. Individuals with TLE and EdF experience greater cognitive decline over time than those with memory impairment alone.[49] A variety of EF deficits involving attention, inhibition, cognitive flexibility, and fluency have been documented in children with symptomatic and nonsymptomatic TLE,[50-55] suggesting that temporal lobe epileptogenic activity also affects extratemporal regions including the frontal lobes.[51-53,56] Nevertheless, direct comparisons between TLE and FLE suggest that FLE is associated with greater overall EdF.[42-44,47]

Age-related idiopathic epilepsies: benign childhood epilepsy with centrotemporal spikes, childhood absence epilepsy, and juvenile myoclonic epilepsy

Benign childhood epilepsy with centrotemporal spikes (BCECTS, a.k.a. Rolandic epilepsy) constitutes the most common genetically determined epilepsy syndrome in childhood.[2] Evidence suggests that BCECTS is not associated with lasting EdF once seizures remit,[28,57-60] with the exception of minor deficits of attentional control[61] and verbal fluency.[62] Rolandic seizures, however, may exacerbate EF deficits when comorbid with ADHD.[63]

Childhood absence epilepsy is commonly associated with deficits of attention, inhibition, cognitive flexibility, problem solving, and fluency,[64,65] though these symptoms frequently improve with remission of absence seizures in adolescence.[2]

Of all the age-related idiopathic epilepsies, juvenile myoclonic epilepsy has been most directly associated with EdF as manifested in difficulties with attention, inhibition, cognitive flexibility, problem solving, fluency, planning, and prospective memory.[66-71] Similar but less severe deficits have also been observed in siblings of patients with juvenile myoclonic epilepsy, suggesting that a component of EdF in juvenile myoclonic epilepsy may be genetically determined and independent of the epileptogenic process.[64,68,71]

The neurological basis of executive dysfunction in childhood epilepsy

Several studies by Hermann and colleagues have considered the neural substrate of pediatric epilepsy in relation to patients' cognitive status. Their findings suggest the presence of subclinical anomalies of gray and white matter as early as the time of a child's initial diagnosis.[35] Significant reductions of temporal and extratemporal white matter including the corpus callosum have been reported in adults with childhood-onset TLE compared to both late-onset TLE and normal controls, with volumetric reductions that correlate with performance on executive and other neuropsychological tasks.[72–74] Volumetric analyses of thalamic and frontal lobe structures have revealed children with juvenile myoclonic epilepsy to have larger frontal cerebrospinal fluid (CSF) volumes and smaller right thalami than healthy controls, and larger CSF volumes than a BCECTS comparison group.[69] In the same study, frontal white matter, gray matter, and thalamic volumes correlated significantly with executive task indices in patients with juvenile myoclonic epilepsy but not in patients with BCECTS or healthy controls. This research group has recently described an anomalous pattern of brain development in childhood epilepsy characterized by subnormal white matter development over time, particularly in the frontal lobes, and has proposed that reduced brain connectivity in childhood epilepsy may be a major contributor to EdF in this population.[75]

Summary and future directions

Deficits of attention and EF occur early in childhood epilepsy, often predating formal epilepsy diagnosis. Current conceptualizations of childhood epilepsy are increasingly linking disruptions of EF and attention to anomalies of brain development which it is now possible to detail with current imaging technologies, with an emphasis on reduced white matter connectivity between frontal cortex and extrafrontal structures. These anomalies may comprise the substrate of both early neurocognitive dysfunction and epileptic events.

Though our ability to identify the discrete processes underlying poor individual performance on clinical measures of attention and EF is limited, such tasks are clearly useful in monitoring and managing childhood epilepsy. They reflect disease-intrinsic neurocognitive risk and serve as markers of disease progression and AED side effects. Observer ratings of "real world" EdF hold the promise of efficient and ecologically valid assessment of this important functional domain. An alternate approach to monitoring the neurocognitive impact of childhood epilepsy is also suggested by the development of brief and easily repeatable EF screening batteries sensitive to CNS-related changes in mental status.[76] Recent applications of chronometric methods[26,30] demonstrate the potential for fine-grained analysis of attention and EF to advance our understanding of neurocognitive dysfunction in childhood epilepsy. Future integration of this approach with structural and functional imaging methodology is a particularly exciting prospect.

The effectiveness of stimulant medication therapy as a treatment for attention deficits in childhood epilepsy has been addressed in several studies. The consensus of these investigations is that stimulant medications have beneficial effects upon parent and teacher ratings of attentional difficulties, improve patient performance on tasks of attention, and do not potentiate seizures in most children with epilepsy.[12,77–79] A study of surgical outcomes in childhood TLE and FLE showed pre- to post-surgery improvement on a cancellation task but no improvement on measures of response inhibition, verbal fluency, or a visual maze task.[80] Aside from research on stimulant medications and this isolated study of surgical outcomes, the topic of interventions for deficits of attention and executive skills in childhood epilepsy remains largely unexplored.

Unfortunately, this is also the case for other childhood neurologic disorders such as brain tumors and hydrocephalus, in part due to the difficulty involved in designing and conducting such studies. The emergence of computerized cognitive intervention methods targeting functions such as WM[81] may facilitate such research, though it will be important to incorporate metacognitive and other approaches as well.[82]

Future research of EF in childhood epilepsy will be enhanced by a developmental perspective and consideration of the existing literature on the emergence of EF in childhood and adolescence. Among other findings, this literature indicates that the primary executive components of inhibition, WM, and shifting have different developmental trajectories, with particularly dramatic gains of inhibitory capacity during the preschool years.[83] Functional imaging research suggests that as development proceeds, inhibitory task performance is associated with a transition from broad engagement of brain structures in early childhood to activation patterns in adulthood that are more circumscribed, efficient, and task specific.[83,84] It is not yet clear how this transition is accomplished. Do broad early activation patterns reflect plasticity of EF, or do they represent a network that must be intact in order for normal EF to emerge? The association of early onset childhood epilepsy with greater EdF[28] suggests that the latter may be the case, and is consistent with the general impression that epilepsy in early childhood exerts a particularly disruptive effect upon cognition.[6] Similar findings in other populations[85] reinforce the view that EF skills are especially vulnerable in a child's early years. These findings highlight the importance of early identification of EdF, to facilitate interventions that will hopefully ameliorate its impact upon academic attainment and overall quality of life in children with epilepsy.

References

1. Berg AT, Berkovic SF, Brodie MJ, et al. Revised terminology and concepts for organization of seizures and epilepsies: report of the ILAE Commission on Classification and Terminology, 2005–2009. *Epilepsia* 2010; **51**: 676–85.

2. Panayiotopoulos CP. *The Epilepsies: Seizures, Syndromes and Management. Chipping Norton*, Oxfordshire, UK, Bladon Medical Publishing; 2005.

3. Fastenau PS, Shen J, Dunn DW, et al. Neuropsychological predictors of academic underachievement in pediatric epilepsy: moderating roles of demographic, seizure, and psychosocial variables. *Epilepsia* 2004; **45**: 1261–72.

4. Dunn DW, Johnson CS, Perkins SM, et al. Academic problems in children with seizures: relationships with neuropsychological functioning and family variables during the 3 years after onset. *Epilepsy Behav* 2010; **19**: 455–61.

5. Nolan MA, Redoblado MA, Lah S, et al. Intelligence in childhood epilepsy syndromes. *Epilepsy Res* 2003; **53**: 139–50.

6. Berg AT. Epilepsy, cognition, and behavior: The clinical picture. *Epilepsia* 2011; **52** Suppl 1: 7–12.

7. Vermeulen J, Kortstee SW, Alpherts WC, et al. Cognitive performance in learning disabled children with and without epilepsy. *Seizure* 1994; **3**: 13–21.

8. Williams J, Griebel ML, Dykman RA. Neuropsychological patterns in pediatric epilepsy. *Seizure* 1998; **7**: 223–8.

9. Mirsky AF, Primac DW, Marsan CA, et al. A comparison of the psychological test performance of patients with focal and nonfocal epilepsy. *Exp Neurol* 1960; **2**: 75–89.

10. Ounsted C. The hyperkinetic syndrome in epileptic children. *Lancet* 1955; **269**: 303–11.

11. Stores G, Hart J, Piran N. Inattentiveness in schoolchildren with epilepsy. *Epilepsia* 1978; **19**: 169–75.

12. Semrud-Clikeman M, Wical B. Components of attention in children with complex partial seizures with and without ADHD. *Epilepsia* 1999; **40**: 211–15.

13. Dunn DW, Austin JK, Harezlak J, *et al.* ADHD and epilepsy in childhood. *Dev Med Child Neurol* 2003; **45**: 50–4.

14. Hesdorffer DC, Ludvigsson P, Olafsson E, *et al.* ADHD as a risk factor for incident unprovoked seizures and epilepsy in children. *Arch Gen Psychiatry* 2004; **61**: 731–6.

15. Hermann B, Jones J, Dabbs K, *et al.* The frequency, complications and aetiology of ADHD in new onset paediatric epilepsy. *Brain* 2007; **130**: 3135–48.

16. Reilly CJ. Attention deficit hyperactivity disorder (ADHD) in childhood epilepsy. *Res Dev Disabil* 2011; **32**: 883–93.

17. Davis SM, Katusic SK, Barbaresi WJ, *et al.* Epilepsy in children with attention-deficit/hyperactivity disorder. *Pediatr Neurol* 2010; **42**: 325–30.

18. Henkin Y, Sadeh M, Kivity S, *et al.* Cognitive function in idiopathic generalized epilepsy of childhood. *Dev Med Child Neurol* 2005; **47**: 126–32.

19. Hermann BP, Jones JE, Sheth R, *et al.* Growing up with epilepsy: a two-year investigation of cognitive development in children with new onset epilepsy. *Epilepsia* 2008; **49**: 1847–58.

20. Fastenau PS, Johnson CS, Perkins SM, *et al.* Neuropsychological status at seizure onset in children: risk factors for early cognitive deficits. *Neurology* 2009; **73**: 526–34.

21. Berg AT, Langfitt JT, Testa FM, *et al.* Residual cognitive effects of uncomplicated idiopathic and cryptogenic epilepsy. *Epilepsy Behav* 2008; **13**: 614–19.

22. Sogawa Y, Masur D, O'Dell C, *et al.* Cognitive outcomes in children who present with a first unprovoked seizure. *Epilepsia* 2010; **51**: 2432–9.

23. Aldenkamp A, Braken BK, van M, *et al.* A clinical comparative study evaluating the effect of epilepsy versus ADHD on timed cognitive tasks in children. *Child Neuropsychol* 2000; **6**: 209–17.

24. Oostrom KJ, Smeets-Schouten TH, van A, *et al.* Three to four years after diagnosis: cognition and behavior in children with

25. 'epilepsy only'. A prospective, controlled study. *Brain* 2005; **128**: 1546–55.

25. Tian Y, Dong B, Ma J, *et al.* Attention networks in children with idiopathic generalized epilepsy. *Epilepsy Behav* 2010; **19**: 513–17.

26. Asato MR, Nawarawong N, Hermann B, *et al.* Deficits in oculomotor performance in pediatric epilepsy. *Epilepsia* 2011; **52**: 377–85.

27. Fan J, McCandliss BD, Sommer T, *et al.* Testing the efficiency and independence of attentional networks. *J Cogn Neurosci* 2002; **14**: 340–7.

28. Hoie B, Mykletun A, Waaler PE, *et al.* Executive functions and seizure-related factors in children with epilepsy in Western Norway. *Dev Med Child Neurol* 2006; **48**: 519–25.

29. Parrish J, Geary E, Jones J, *et al.* Executive functioning in childhood epilepsy: parent-report and cognitive assessment. *Dev Med Child Neurol* 2007; **49**: 412–16.

30. Hermann BP, Lin JJ, Jones JE, *et al.* The emerging architecture of neuropsychological impairment in epilepsy. *Neurol Clin* 2009; **27**: 881–907.

31. Fry A, Hale S. Processing speed, working memory, and fluid intelligence: Evidence for a developmental cascade. *Psychol Sci* 2011; **7**: 237–41.

32. Span MM, Ridderinkhof KR, van der Molen MW. Age-related changes in the efficiency of cognitive processing across the life span. *Acta Psychol (Amst)* 2004; **117**: 155–83.

33. McAuley T, White DA. A latent variables examination of processing speed, response inhibition, and working memory during typical development. *J Exp Child Psychol* 2011; **108**: 453–68.

34. O'Leary SD, Burns TG, Borden KA. Performance of children with epilepsy and normal age-matched controls on the WISC-III. *Child Neuropsychol* 2006; **12**: 173–80.

35. Hermann BP, Jones J, Sheth R, *et al.* Cognitive and magnetic resonance

volumetric abnormalities in new-onset pediatric epilepsy. *Semin Pediatr Neurol* 2007; **14**: 173–80.

36. Slick DJ, Lautzenhiser A, Sherman EM, *et al.* Frequency of scale elevations and factor structure of the Behavior Rating Inventory of Executive Function (BRIEF) in children and adolescents with intractable epilepsy. *Child Neuropsychol* 2006; **12**: 181–9.

37. Sherman EM, Slick DJ, Eyrl KL. Executive dysfunction is a significant predictor of poor quality of life in children with epilepsy. *Epilepsia* 2006; **47**: 1936–42.

38. Luton LM, Burns TG, DeFilippis N. Frontal lobe epilepsy in children and adolescents: a preliminary neuropsychological assessment of executive function. *Arch Clin Neuropsychol* 2010; **25**: 762–70.

39. Risse GL. Cognitive outcomes in patients with frontal lobe epilepsy. *Epilepsia* 2006; **47** Suppl 2: 87–9.

40. Braakman HM, Vaessen MJ, Hofman PA, *et al.* Cognitive and behavioral complications of frontal lobe epilepsy in children: a review of the literature. *Epilepsia* 2011; **52**: 849–56.

41. Upton D, Thompson PJ. Age at onset and neuropsychological function in frontal lobe epilepsy. *Epilepsia* 1997; **38**: 1103–13.

42. Hernandez MT, Sauerwein HC, Jambaque I, *et al.* Deficits in executive functions and motor coordination in children with frontal lobe epilepsy. *Neuropsychologia* 2002; **40**: 384–400.

43. Hernandez MT, Sauerwein HC, Jambaque I, *et al.* Attention, memory, and behavioral adjustment in children with frontal lobe epilepsy. *Epilepsy Behav* 2003; **4**: 522–36.

44. Culhane-Shelburne K, Chapieski L, Hiscock M, *et al.* Executive functions in children with frontal and temporal lobe epilepsy. *J Int Neuropsychol Soc* 2002; **8**: 623–32.

45. Riva D, Saletti V, Nichelli F, *et al.* Neuropsychologic effects of frontal lobe epilepsy in children. *J Child Neurol* 2002; **17**: 661–7.

46. Riva D, Avanzini G, Franceschetti S, *et al.* Unilateral frontal lobe epilepsy affects executive functions in children. *Neurol Sci* 2005; **26**: 263–70.

47. McDonald CR, Delis DC, Norman MA, *et al.* Is impairment in set-shifting specific to frontal-lobe dysfunction? Evidence from patients with frontal-lobe or temporal-lobe epilepsy. *J Int Neuropsychol Soc* 2005; **11**: 477–81.

48. MacAllister WS, Schaffer SG. Neuropsychological deficits in childhood epilepsy syndromes. *Neuropsychol Rev* 2007; **17**: 427–44.

49. Hermann B, Seidenberg M, Lee EJ, *et al.* Cognitive phenotypes in temporal lobe epilepsy. *J Int Neuropsychol Soc* 2007; **13**: 12–20.

50. Bigel MG, Smith ML. Single and dual pathologies of the temporal lobe: effects on cognitive function in children with epilepsy. *Epilepsy Behav* 2001; **2**: 37–45.

51. Guimaraes CA, Li LM, Rzezak P, *et al.* Temporal lobe epilepsy in childhood: comprehensive neuropsychological assessment. *J Child Neurol* 2007; **22**: 836–40.

52. Rzezak P, Fuentes D, Guimaraes CA, *et al.* Frontal lobe dysfunction in children with temporal lobe epilepsy. *Pediatr Neurol* 2007; **37**: 176–85.

53. Rzezak P, Fuentes D, Guimaraes CA, *et al.* Executive dysfunction in children and adolescents with temporal lobe epilepsy: is the Wisconsin Card Sorting Test enough? *Epilepsy Behav* 2009; **15**: 376–81.

54. Black LC, Schefft BK, Howe SR, *et al.* The effect of seizures on working memory and executive functioning performance. *Epilepsy Behav* 2010; **17**: 412–19.

55. Tuchscherer V, Seidenberg M, Pulsipher D, *et al.* Extrahippocampal integrity in temporal lobe epilepsy and cognition: thalamus and executive functioning. *Epilepsy Behav* 2010; **17**: 478–82.

56. Oyegbile TO, Dow C, Jones J, *et al.* The nature and course of neuropsychological morbidity in chronic temporal lobe epilepsy. *Neurology* 2004; **62**: 1736–42.

57. Hommet C, Billard C, Motte J, et al. Cognitive function in adolescents and young adults in complete remission from benign childhood epilepsy with centro-temporal spikes. Epileptic Disord 2001; 3: 207–16.

58. Lindgren S, Kihlgren M, Melin L, et al. Development of cognitive functions in children with rolandic epilepsy. Epilepsy Behav 2004; 5: 903–10.

59. Hoie B, Sommerfelt K, Waaler PE, et al. The combined burden of cognitive, executive function, and psychosocial problems in children with epilepsy: a population-based study. Dev Med Child Neurol 2008; 50: 530–6.

60. Danielsson J, Petermann F. Cognitive deficits in children with benign rolandic epilepsy of childhood or rolandic discharges: a study of children between 4 and 7 years of age with and without seizures compared with healthy controls. Epilepsy Behav 2009; 16: 646–51.

61. Deltour L, Quaglino V, Barathon M, et al. Clinical evaluation of attentional processes in children with benign childhood epilepsy with centrotemporal spikes (BCECTS). Epileptic Disord 2007; 9: 424–31.

62. Goldberg-Stern H, Gonen OM, Sadeh M, et al. Neuropsychological aspects of benign childhood epilepsy with centrotemporal spikes. Seizure 2010; 19: 12–16.

63. Holtmann M, Matei A, Hellmann U, et al. Rolandic spikes increase impulsivity in A. Brain Dev 2006; 28: 633–40.

64. Levav M, Mirsky AF, Herault J, et al. Familial association of neuropsychological traits in patients with generalized and partial seizure disorders. J Clin Exp Neuropsychol 2002; 24: 311–26.

65. Conant LL, Wilfong A, Inglese C, et al. Dysfunction of executive and related processes in childhood absence epilepsy. Epilepsy Behav 2010; 18: 414–23.

66. Sonmez F, Atakli D, Sari H, et al. Cognitive function in juvenile myoclonic epilepsy. Epilepsy Behav 2004; 5: 329–36.

67. Pascalicchio TF, de Araujo Filho GM, da Silva Noffs MH, et al. Neuropsychological profile of patients with juvenile myoclonic epilepsy: a controlled study of 50 patients. Epilepsy Behav 2007; 10: 263–7.

68. Iqbal N, Caswell HL, Hare DJ, et al. Neuropsychological profiles of patients with juvenile myoclonic epilepsy and their siblings: a preliminary controlled experimental video-EEG case series. Epilepsy Behav 2009; 14: 516–21.

69. Pulsipher DT, Seidenberg M, Guidotti L, et al. Thalamofrontal circuitry and executive dysfunction in recent-onset juvenile myoclonic epilepsy. Epilepsia 2009; 50: 1210–19.

70. Ciumas C, Wahlin TB, Espino C, et al. The dopamine system in idiopathic generalized epilepsies: identification of syndrome-related changes. Neuroimage 2010; 51: 606–15.

71. Wandschneider B, Kopp UA, Kliegel M, et al. Prospective memory in patients with juvenile myoclonic epilepsy and their healthy siblings. Neurology 2010; 75: 2161–7.

72. Hermann B, Seidenberg M, Bell B, et al. The neurodevelopmental impact of childhood-onset temporal lobe epilepsy on brain structure and function. Epilepsia 2002; 43: 1062–71.

73. Hermann BP, Seidenberg M, Bell B. The neurodevelopmental impact of childhood onset temporal lobe epilepsy on brain structure and function and the risk of progressive cognitive effects. Prog Brain Res 2002; 135: 429–38.

74. Hermann B, Hansen R, Seidenberg M, et al. Neurodevelopmental vulnerability of the corpus callosum to childhood onset localization-related epilepsy. Neuroimage 2003; 18: 284–92.

75. Hermann BP, Dabbs K, Becker T, et al. Brain development in children with new onset epilepsy: a prospective controlled cohort investigation. Epilepsia 2010; 51: 2038–46.

76. Krull KR, Okcu MF, Potter B, et al. Screening for neurocognitive impairment in pediatric cancer long-term survivors. J Clin Oncol 2008; 26: 4138–43.

77. Feldman H, Crumrine P, Handen BL, et al. Methylphenidate in children with seizures

and attention-deficit disorder. *Am J Dis Child* 1989; **143**: 1081–6.

78. Gross-Tsur V, Manor O, van der MJ, *et al.* Epilepsy and attention deficit hyperactivity disorder: is methylphenidate safe and effective? *J Pediatr* 1997; **130**: 670–4.

79. Kaufmann R, Goldberg-Stern H, Shuper A. Attention-deficit disorders and epilepsy in childhood: incidence, causative relations and treatment possibilities. *J Child Neurol* 2009; **24**: 727–33.

80. Lendt M, Gleissner U, Helmstaedter C, *et al.* Neuropsychological outcome in children after frontal lobe epilepsy surgery. *Epilepsy Behav* 2002; **3**: 51–9.

81. Klingberg T. Training and plasticity of working memory. *Trends Cogn Sci* 2010; **14**: 317–24.

82. Butler RW, Copeland DR, Fairclough DL, *et al.* A multicenter, randomized clinical trial of a cognitive remediation program for childhood survivors of a pediatric malignancy. *J Consult Clin Psychol* 2008; **76**: 367–78.

83. Best JR, Miller PH. A developmental perspective on executive function. *Child Dev* 2010; **81**: 1641–60.

84. Casey BJ, Trainor RJ, Orendi JL, *et al.* A developmental functional MRI study of prefrontal activation during performance of a Go-No-Go task. *J Cogn Neurosci* 1997; **9**: 835–47.

85. Anderson V, Anderson P, Grimwood K, *et al.* Cognitive and executive function 12 years after childhood bacterial meningitis: effect of acute neurologic complications and age of onset. *J Pediatr Psychol* 2004; **29**: 67–81.

Chapter

12

Executive functions in pediatric cancer

Marsha Nortz Gragert and Lisa S. Kahalley

Cancer is the leading cause of death by disease in children under the age of 15 years.[1] Brain tumors and acute lymphoblastic leukemia (ALL) are the two most common forms of pediatric cancer, collectively accounting for more than half of all newly diagnosed cases annually.[2,3] Most research into the neuropsychological sequelae of pediatric cancer and its associated treatment has involved the study of ALL and brain tumors because of their high prevalence as well as their greater associated neuropsychological morbidity. This morbidity has become increasingly prevalent as survival rates for ALL and brain tumors have improved over the last several decades.

The neuropsychological sequelae of pediatric cancer extend into adolescence and adulthood and are not only associated with the cancer itself but the treatments employed, including surgical intervention, chemotherapy, cranial/craniospinal radiation therapy (CRT), or a combination of these treatments. Other disease- and treatment-related outcome moderators include neurologic complications (e.g., intracranial bleeding, hydrocephalus, leukoencephalopathy) and sensorimotor deficits related to the primary disease and/or to iatrogenic effects.[4] CRT, in particular, has been one of the greatest contributors to improved survival in the treatment of brain tumors and higher risk forms of ALL, but it has also been associated with numerous neurologic and neurocognitive effects that vary according to the extent and location of CNS involvement, size of area irradiated, and total dose administered.[5–9] Intrathecal and high-dose intravenous chemotherapies, particularly methotrexate, are now routinely employed without adjuvant radiation in the treatment of standard-risk ALL. While evidence regarding the neuropsychological risk associated with such isolated chemotherapy is mixed,[10–14] it is generally acknowledged that both intrathecal chemotherapy and the chemotherapy agents administered in the treatment of various brain tumors have a less significant effect on neuropsychological outcome than does CRT.[15]

Although CRT is among the strongest predictors of post-treatment neuropsychological outcome, there is significant variability in outcome that is not accounted for by disease and treatment factors. Until recently,[16] the available literature has been characterized by rather crude methods for measuring biological insults such as the "radiation lesion." This as well as our relatively imprecise clinical instrumentation for measuring neuropsychological functions has limited our ability to more accurately predict neuropsychological outcome, particularly for heterogeneous cognitive functions like EF. Furthermore, consistent with a developmental model of neurobehavioral outcome in at-risk medical populations proposed by Dennis (17; see Fig. 12.1 part A), factors beyond those related to cancer, its treatment,

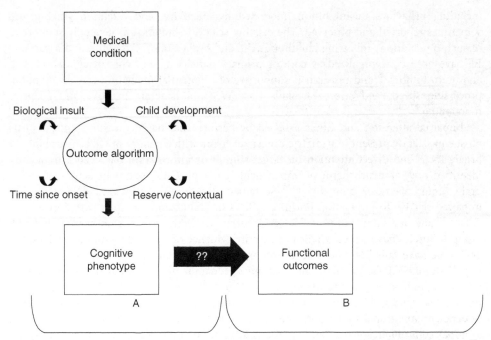

Fig. 12.1. Model of the relationship between medical condition (cancer) and outcome, adapted from Dennis.[17]

and related medical complications have been found to be important moderators of neuro-cognitive outcome. Studies have strongly indicated that neurocognitive status declines with increasing time since CRT and chemotherapy.[9,18,19] Child factors, such as younger age at time of treatment,[6,7,9,20] female gender,[6,20,21] and higher baseline neurocognitive function-ing[6,9,22] are also documented moderators of outcome associated with greater neurocogni-tive decline. Well-established abilities associated with early brain development, such as basic language and gross motor functioning, are typically only minimally affected in the absence of focal neurologic insult (e.g., cerebellar lesion impacting gross motor skills), whereas skills that develop later or that have a more prolonged course of development (e.g., processing speed, EF) are more consistently impaired.[23,24] Our understanding of the complex, predict-ive relationships among such moderators of neurocognitive outcome remains limited and in need of ongoing study.

Executive dysfunction in pediatric cancer

Comprehensive reviews of the neuropsychological sequelae of pediatric cancers and associ-ated treatments that impact the CNS are available in the recent literature.[4,7,10,25,26] Attention, processing speed, new learning, visuospatial/visuomotor functioning, WM and other EF skills, and areas of academic achievement have been found to be at particular risk, consistent with our knowledge of the timing and developmental course of such functions. Clinically, common presenting concerns observed and reported by parents of childhood cancer survivors include inattention, distractibility, forgetfulness, poor "short-term memory," inconsistent learning, slowed processing and task completion, organizational difficulties, and specific areas of academic deficit. Other attention and EF symptoms, including behavioral disinhibition, increased hyperactivity, and attention seeking, are sometimes reported and observed. The existing scientific literature is generally supportive of such observations following childhood ALL and brain tumor. Attention and associated EF have been conceptualized as core or primary deficits in survivors of childhood ALL and brain tumors,[25] and research is supportive of a potential mediating role of attention, processing speed, and select EF skills (i.e., WM) in general cognitive and adaptive functioning.[27-30]

Impaired attention and EF as assessed by performance-based measures appear to be most consistently present in pediatric cancer survivors with a history of CRT. The ability to briefly focus and direct attention on target stimuli or information has been a frequently identified area of neurocognitive impairment following CRT treatment across ALL and brain tumor diagnosis groups.[15,31-34] Sustained attention has also been documented as impaired relative to population norms on CPTs in brain tumor samples with a history of CRT[30,35] and in a sample of post-CRT ALL survivors relative to a chemotherapy only ALL group.[32] Studies have typically failed to identify evidence of impulsivity on these CPTs,[33,35] and some have failed to find evidence of impairment on any component of such measures.[33] Beyond CPTs, Vaquero and colleagues[36] documented impaired inhibitory control and set maintenance on the Stroop Color Word Test and the WCST in a sample of medulloblastoma survivors previously treated with CRT. These authors also found evidence of deficient attentional shifting and cognitive flexibility on verbal fluency measures as well as impaired problem solving and hypothesis formation on the WCST and Raven's Progressive Matrices. This is consistent with findings on verbal fluency measures, TMT, and measures of problem solving and hypothesis formation in a separate sample of patients with malignant posterior fossa tumors.[23] The areas of EF assessed by Spiegler and colleagues evidenced delayed but progressive decline in the early post-treatment years, consistent with studies documenting this pattern in global IQ.[6,19] Evidence of impaired metacognitive skills is also documented following CRT in samples of ALL survivors.[37,38]

Though the findings are less robust, attention and EF risks are seen in nonirradiated samples of childhood cancer survivors as well. Following intrathecal chemotherapy alone, findings of deficient sustained attention, attentional shifting, and set-maintenance have been reported.[14,39,40] A recent meta-analysis of studies involving ALL survivors treated with chemotherapy alone found evidence of weak WM, processing speed, and attentional shifting (TMT-B), but verbal fluency effect sizes were not significant.[10] In samples of posterior fossa brain tumor survivors following surgical resection without chemotherapy or CRT, processing speed, attentional shifting, and inhibitory control have been identified as at risk,[36,41,42] which has been related to neural circuitry connecting the cerebellum and the PFC. Perhaps the most common area of EF documented to be at risk among childhood cancer survivors is WM, or the storage and online manipulation of information necessary to perform a task. This has been documented in ALL and brain tumor survivors following CRT,[29,31,36,43] ALL patients treated with intrathecal chemotherapy alone,[10,39] and patients with focal posterior fossa brain tumors that required only surgical resection.[36] WM is a potential mediator of global IQ in childhood cancer survivors,[29] consistent with similar findings in typically developing children.[44]

Deficits in attention and EF have also been documented on behavior rating scales completed by parents and/or teachers of ALL and brain tumor survivors. A recent abstract reported that child and adolescent brain tumor survivors with a history of CRT performed significantly worse than controls (both untreated healthy siblings and solid tumor cancer patients who received treatments other than CRT) on the Working Memory scale of the BRIEF, and modest but significant correlations were found between this measure and performance-based measures of WM (digit span, self-ordered search).[45] In a sample of adolescent ALL and brain tumor survivors, many experienced clinically significant post-treatment inattention based on Conners 3 parent and teacher reports, although the rate of patients meeting full diagnostic criteria for DSM-IV ADHD or criteria for secondary ADHD (i.e., meeting all criteria for ADHD except the age of onset) was broadly consistent with population base rates.[46] EdF are also reported on self-report measures completed by adult survivors of pediatric cancers. Data from the Childhood Cancer Survivor Study (CCSS), a multi-institutional collaborative examining long-term outcomes in survivors treated between 1970 and 1986,[47] include results from a 19-item, self-report Neurocognitive Questionnaire (CCSS-NCQ), which was derived from the BRIEF and found to possess four reliable and valid factors: Task Efficiency, Organization, Emotional Regulation, and Memory. Relative to the other CCSS-NCQ factors, survivors of brain tumors and other CNS-malignancies were most likely to report dysfunction on the Task Efficiency (speed of performance, self-initiation, multitasking) and Memory factors (LTM and WM), with risk for such deficits significantly associated with CRT history or other neurologic complication.[48] Similar findings were reported in ALL and acute myeloid leukemia survivors who received CRT, but emotional regulation was also significant.[49] Adult, long-term follow-up studies of EF are largely limited to self-report data, but Maddrey and colleagues[50] documented EdF in adult survivors (mean age at testing = 22.2 years) of childhood medulloblastoma treated with CRT relative to population norms on performance-based measures of focused and sustained attention, processing speed, attentional shifting and inhibitory control. Performance on these measures was weaker than the participants' self-report on a questionnaire assessing neuropsychological impairment.[50]

Clearly, survivors of childhood cancer are at risk for lasting impairment in EF and attention, as evidenced by a wealth of neurocognitive outcome studies with this population.[10,15,32,33,50-52] Less is known about the functional impact of EdF post-treatment, although emerging findings regarding health-related quality of life, social functioning, and health-related decision-making are concerning.

Limitations in EF have been associated with worse overall health-related quality of life in cancer survivors.[53] Much of what we know about more specific functional outcomes associated with EF following treatment for pediatric cancer comes from the CCSS. Reports from the CCSS have identified significant financial burden associated with post-treatment EdF once survivors reach adulthood. Specifically, childhood cancer survivors with EdF were less likely to graduate from high school, had lower household income, and had higher rates of unemployment compared to survivors without EdF.[48,53] For survivors with EdF, these areas of functional vulnerability are understandable given the EF demands (planning, organization, self-monitoring, behavioral regulation, and WM) of most academic and occupational environments.

CNS-directed therapies (e.g., CRT, intrathecal chemotherapy) used to treat many pediatric cancers are associated with post-treatment social difficulties.[54] These treatments also place children at risk for cognitive late effects (i.e., lasting cognitive changes resulting from disease and treatment), including deficits in EF and attention.[10,15,32,33,51,52,55] Treatment-related EdF may make it more difficult for childhood cancer survivors to process and respond appropriately to new social situations, although there is little published research to date that examines such relations. In a sample of adolescent and young adult survivors of childhood ALL, survivors with EdF were less likely to use adaptive coping strategies (e.g., distraction, cognitive restructuring, acceptance, and positive thinking) to regulate emotions and respond appropriately to social stressors, leading to increases in emotional and behavioral problems.[39] Without adequate EF, survivors may be unable to engage necessary skills to adapt to novel events and complex situations successfully, resulting in distress or problematic adjustment. The influence of EdF on social maladjustment may persist into adulthood for survivors of pediatric cancer, as recent CCSS studies reported that adult survivors were less likely to be married if they experienced EdF.[48,53] Further study is needed to better understand the emerging associations between EdF and social difficulties among childhood cancer survivors as well as the mechanisms underlying these associations.

Post-treatment EdF may have important health implications as well. Adult survivors with EdF in the CCSS cohort exhibited increased smoking risk.[56] This finding is consistent with a growing literature documenting increased risk for smoking among adolescents and adults with ADHD, another clinical population vulnerable to EdF.[57-60] The mechanism underlying the association between smoking and EdF in childhood cancer survivors is unknown. Survivors with post-treatment WM deficits may be unable to adequately retain and apply important information about their medical risks when faced with health behavior decisions. It is also possible that these childhood cancer survivors may spontaneously experiment with smoking due to behavioral disinhibition, with the smoking behavior maintained by certain benefits of nicotine. For example, other clinical groups and general population samples have shown nicotine can improve performance on cognitive and behavioral measures of attention[61-66] as well as help regulate emotion.[67]

Childhood cancer survivors who have EdF post-treatment may be at risk for making other dangerous health decisions beyond the decision to smoke, but associations between EF and other health behaviors remain unexplored at this time. In other pediatric populations (e.g., Human immunodeficiency virus or HIV, Type I diabetes), EdF has been associated with medication non-adherence.[68,69] As childhood cancer survivors age and assume more individual responsibility for their own health management, their ability to maintain post-treatment medication regimens, adhere to follow-up clinical appointments, and engage in other healthy behaviors may be related to their EF abilities, and such associations require further study.

The neurological basis of executive dysfunction in pediatric cancer

Although the pathophysiology of EdF and the other documented neurocognitive effects in childhood cancer survivors is not fully understood, it is now generally accepted that CRT is associated with reductions in normal appearing white matter.[35,70] Furthermore, some studies have documented a direct correlation between normal appearing white matter and neurocognitive outcome,[70] and normal appearing white matter explains a significant amount of the variance in the relationships between age at time of CRT and IQ.[71] Intrathecal chemotherapies (e.g., methotrexate) that are now routinely employed in the treatment of standard risk ALL have also been inconsistently associated with similar pathophysiological changes in a subset of survivors.[12,13,40,72] Carey and colleagues[12] employed voxel-based morphometry to document reduced right frontal white matter volumes in a small sample of childhood ALL survivors without a history of CRT, and there was a trend toward a significant relationship between these white matter findings and performance on measures of focused attention and attentional switching/set shifting. More recently, DTI technology has demonstrated reduced functional anisotropy suggestive of radiosensitivity of the frontal lobe relative to the parietal lobe in medulloblastoma survivors,[73] and functional anisotropy in a mixed ALL and brain tumor sample was significantly correlated with IQ. The functional implication of white matter changes is significant, as overall white matter volume and specific regional volumes of white matter in the prefrontal area, larger frontal lobe, and cingulate gyrus are associated with EF (e.g., attention, WM) as well as processing speed and visual-spatial processing.[29,35,74] Also particularly relevant to EF outcome are focal effects of tumor location and the surgical site when the frontal lobe, frontal-subcortical circuitry, and cerebellar lesions impinging on cerebellar-frontal neural pathways are involved.[36,41,42]

Summary and future directions

In summary, pediatric cancer research has come far in delineating the range of neurocognitive risks among survivors of pediatric cancer, particularly those who have experienced CNS insult as a result of their primary disease, the treatments required, or other secondary complications. EF deficits are well-documented as one such neurocognitive risk, but further scientific study is needed to explicate what is likely a complex relationship between disease factors and their associated neurocognitive phenotype (see Fig. 12.1, part A). Although the moderating role of the nature and timing of the biological insult incurred as a result of cancer- and treatment-related factors has and continues to be the focus of scientific inquiry, there is a less extensive literature documenting the role of other potential moderators, such as child development factors (e.g., stage of ongoing neurocognitive development) and other contextual factors (e.g., cognitive reserve, family factors, access to educational resources). Furthermore, the functional impact of post-treatment EdF is only starting to be explored in survivors of childhood cancer (see Fig. 12.1, part B). Further study of these associations is an important future direction in childhood cancer research, and the findings will serve as a needed foundation for the development of targeted interventions that are effective in promoting improved functioning in affected survivors.

References

1. National Cancer Institute. *CANCER FACTS. National Cancer Institute at the National Institutes of Health*; 2008 [cited 2011 July 17]; Available from: http://www.cancer.gov/cancertopics/factsheet/Sites-Types/childhood.

2. Sklar CA. Childhood brain tumors. *J Pediatr Endocrinol Metab* 2002; 15 Suppl **2**: 669–73.

3. Ries LAG, Melbert D, Krapcho M, et al. *SEER Cancer Statistics Review, 1975–2005*. Bethesda, MD: National Cancer Institute; 2008. Available from: http://seer.cancer.gov/csr/1975_2005/.

4. Nortz MJ, Hemme-Phillips JM, Ris MD. Neuropsychological sequelae in children treated for cancer. In Hunter SJ, Donders J, editors. *Pediatric Neuropsychological Intervention*. Cambridge: Cambridge University Press; 2007.

5. Ris MD, Noll RB. Long-term neurobehavioral outcome in pediatric brain-tumor patients: review and methodological critique. *J Clin Exp Neuropsychol* 1994;**16**(1): 21–42.

6. Ris MD, Packer R, Goldwein J, Jones-Wallace D, Boyett JM. Intellectual outcome after reduced-dose radiation therapy plus adjuvant chemotherapy for medulloblastoma: a Children's Cancer Group study. *J Clin Oncol* 2001; **19**(15): 3470–6.

7. Mulhern RK, Merchant TE, Gajjar A, Reddick WE, Kun LE. Late neurocognitive sequelae in survivors of brain tumours in childhood. *Lancet Oncol* 2004; **5**(7): 399–408.

8. Reddick WE, Russell JM, Glass JO, *et al.* Subtle white matter volume differences in children treated for medulloblastoma with conventional or reduced dose craniospinal irradiation[star, open]. *Magne Reson Imagi.* [doi: DOI: 10.1016/S0730-725X(00)00182-X]. 2000; **18**(7): 787–93.

9. Silber JH, Radcliffe J, Peckham V, *et al.* Whole-brain irradiation and decline in intelligence: the influence of dose and age on IQ score. *J Clin Oncol* 1992; **10**(9): 1390–6.

10. Peterson CC, Johnson CE, Ramirez LY, *et al.* A meta-analysis of the neuropsychological sequelae of chemotherapy-only treatment for pediatric acute lymphoblastic leukemia. *Pediatr Blood Cancer* 2008; **51**(1): 99–104.

11. Spiegler BJ, Kennedy K, Maze R, *et al.* Comparison of long-term neurocognitive outcomes in young children with acute lymphoblastic leukemia treated with cranial radiation or high-dose or very high-dose intravenous methotrexate. *J Clin Oncol* 2006; **24**(24): 3858–64.

12. Carey ME, Haut MW, Reminger SL, Hutter JJ, Theilmann R, Kaemingk KL. Reduced frontal white matter volume in long-term childhood leukemia survivors: a voxel-based morphometry study. *Am J Neuroradiol* 2008; **29**(4): 792–7.

13. Carey ME, Hockenberry MJ, Moore IM, *et al.* Brief report: effect of intravenous methotrexate dose and infusion rate on neuropsychological function one year after diagnosis of acute lymphoblastic leukemia. *J Pediatr Psychol* 2007; **32**(2): 189–93.

14. Buizer AI, de Sonneville LM, van den Heuvel-Eibrink MM, Veerman AJ. Chemotherapy and attentional dysfunction in survivors of childhood acute lymphoblastic leukemia: effect of treatment intensity. *Pediatr Blood Cancer* 2005; **45**(3): 281–90.

15. Langer T, Martus P, Ottensmeier H, Hertzberg H, Beck JD, Meier W. CNS late-effects after ALL therapy in childhood. Part III: neuropsychological performance in long-term survivors of childhood ALL: impairments of concentration, attention, and memory. *Med Pediatr Oncol* 2002; **38**(5): 320–8.

16. Ris MD, Ryan PM, Lamba M, *et al.* An improved methodology for modeling neurobehavioral late-effects of radiotherapy in pediatric brain tumors. *Pediatr Blood Cancer* 2005; **44**(5): 487–93.

17. Dennis M. Childhood medical disorders and cognitive impairment: biological risk, time, development, and reserve. In Yeates KO, Ris MD, Taylor HG, eds. *Pediatric Neuropsychology: Research, Theory, and Practice.* 1st edn. New York, NY: The Guilford Press; 2000, 3–22.

18. Radcliffe J, Packer RJ, Atkins TE, *et al.* Three- and four-year cognitive outcome in children with noncortical brain tumors treated with whole-brain radiotherapy. *Ann Neurol* 1992; **32**(4): 551–4.

19. Palmer SL, Goloubeva O, Reddick WE, *et al.* Patterns of intellectual development among survivors of pediatric medulloblastoma: a longitudinal analysis. *J Clin Oncol* 2001; **19**(8): 2302–8.

20. Buizer AI, de Sonneville LM, Veerman AJ. Effects of chemotherapy on neurocognitive function in children with acute lymphoblastic leukemia: a critical review of the literature. *Pediatr Blood Cancer* 2009; **52**(4): 447–54.

21. Temming P, Jenney M. The neurodevelopmental sequelae of childhood leukaemia and its treatment. *Arch Dis Child* 2010; **95**: 936–40.

22. Palmer SL, Gajjar A, Reddick WE, *et al.* Predicting intellectual outcome among children treated with 35–40 Gy craniospinal irradiation for medulloblastoma. *Neuropsychology* 2003; **17**(4): 548–55.

23. Spiegler BJ, Bouffet E, Greenberg ML, Rutka JT, Mabbott DJ. Change in neurocognitive functioning after treatment with cranial radiation in childhood. *J Clin Oncol* 2004 15; **22**(4): 706–13.

24. Armstrong FD, Blumberg MJ, Toledano SR. Neurobehavioral issues in childhood cancer. *School Psychol Rev* 1999; **28**(2): 194–205.

25. Butler RW, Mulhern RK. Neurocognitive interventions for children and adolescents surviving cancer. *J Pediatr Psychol* 2005; **30**(1): 65–78.

26. Moore BD. Neurocognitive outcomes in survivors of childhood cancer. *J Pediatr Psychol* 2005; **30**(1): 51–63.

27. Papazoglou A, King TZ, Morris RD, Morris MK, Krawiecki NS. Attention mediates radiation's impact on daily living skills in children treated for brain tumors. *Pediatr Blood Cancer* 2008; **50**(6): 1253–7.

28. Papazoglou A, King TZ, Morris RD, Krawiecki NS. Cognitive predictors of adaptive functioning vary according to pediatric brain tumor location. *Dev Neuropsychol* 2008; **33**(4): 505–20.

29. Schatz J, Kramer JH, Ablin A, Matthay KK. Processing speed, working memory, and IQ: A developmental model of cognitive deficits following cranial radiation therapy. *Neuropsychology* 2000; **14**(2): 189–200.

30. Reeves CB, Palmer SL, Reddick WE, *et al.* Attention and memory functioning among pediatric patients with medulloblastoma. *J Pediatr Psychol* 2006; **31**(3): 272–80.

31. Patel SK, Lai-Yates JJ, Anderson JW, Katz ER. Attention dysfunction and parent reporting in children with brain tumors. *Pediatr Blood Cancer* 2007; **49**(7): 970–4.

32. Lockwood KA, Bell TS, Colegrove RW. Long-term effects of cranial radiation therapy on attention functioning in survivors of childhood leukemia. *J Pediatr Psychol* 1999; **24**: 55–66.

33. Rodgers J, Horrocks J, Britton PG, Kernahan J. Attentional ability among survivors of leukaemia. *Arch Dis Child* 1999; **80**(4): 318–23.

34. Merchant TE, Kiehna EN, Miles MA, Zhu J, Xiong X, Mulhern RK. Acute effects of irradiation on cognition: changes in attention on a computerized continuous performance test during radiotherapy in pediatric patients with localized primary brain tumors. *Inte J Radiati Oncol*Biol*Physi*. [doi: DOI: 10.1016/S0360-3016(02)02828-6]. 2002; **53**(5): 1271–8.

35. Mulhern RK, White HA, Glass JO, *et al.* Attentional functioning and white matter integrity among survivors of malignant brain tumors of childhood. *J Int Neuropsychol Soc* 2004; **10**(2): 180–9.

36. Vaquero E, Gomez CM, Quintero EA, Gonzalez-Rosa JJ, Marquez J. Differential prefrontal-like deficit in children after cerebellar astrocytoma and medulloblastoma tumor. *Behav Brain Funct* 2008; **4**: 18.

37. Waber DP, Isquith PK, Kahn CM, Romero I. Metacognitive factors in the visuospatial skills of long-term survivors of acute lymphoblastic leukemia: an experimental approach to the Rey-Osterrieth complex figure test. *Dev Neuropsychol* 1994; **10**: 349–67.

38. Kleinman SN, Waber DP. Prose memory strategies of children treated for leukemia: a story grammar analysis of the Anna Thompson passage. *Neuropsychology* 1994; **8**: 464–70.

39. Campbell LK, Scaduto M, Van Slyke D, Niarhos F, Whitlock JA, Compas BE. Executive function, coping, and behavior in survivors of childhood acute lymphocytic leukemia. *J Pediatr Psychol* 2009; **34**(3): 317–27.

40. Reddick WE, Shan ZY, Glass JO, *et al.* Smaller white-matter volumes are associated with larger deficits in attention and learning among long-term survivors of acute lymphoblastic leukemia. *Cancer* 2006; **106**(4): 941–9.

41. Stargatt R, Rosenfeld JV, Maixner W, Ashley D. Multiple factors contribute to neuropsychological outcome in children with posterior fossa tumors. *Dev Neuropsychol* 2007; **32**(2): 729–48.

42. Steinlin M, Imfeld S, Zulauf P, *et al.* Neuropsychological long-term sequelae after posterior fossa tumour resection during childhood. *Brain* 2003; **126**(9): 1998–2008.

43. Dennis M, Hetherington CR, Spiegler BJ. Memory and attention after childhood brain tumors. *Med Pediatr Oncol Suppl* 1998; **1**: 25–33.

44. Fry AF, Hale S. Processing speed, working memory, and fluid intelligence: Evidence for a developmental cascade. *Psychol Sci* 1996; **7**: 237–41.

45. Howarth RA, Conklin HM, Ashford JM, *et al.* Performance- and rater-based

measures of working memory among childhood brain tumor survivors. Clin Neuropsychol. *[published abstract]* 2011; **25**(4): 587.

46. Kahalley LS, Conklin HM, Tyc VL, *et al.* ADHD and secondary ADHD criteria fail to identify many at-risk survivors of pediatric ALL and brain tumor. *Pediatr Blood Cancer* 2011; **57**(1): 110–18.

47. Robison LL, Armstrong GT, Boice JD, *et al.* The Childhood Cancer Survivor Study: a National Cancer Institute-supported resource for outcome and intervention research. *J Clin Oncol* 2009; **27**(14): 2308–18.

48. Ellenberg L, Liu Q, Gioia G, *et al.* Neurocognitive status in long-term survivors of childhood CNS malignancies: a report from the Childhood Cancer Survivor Study. *Neuropsychology* 2009; **23**(6): 705–17.

49. Kadan-Lottick NS, Zeltzer LK, Liu Q, *et al.* Neurocognitive functioning in adult survivors of childhood non-central nervous system cancers. *J Natl Cancer Inst* 2010; **102**(12): 881–93.

50. Maddrey AM, Bergeron JA, Lombardo ER, *et al.* Neuropsychological performance and quality of life of 10 year survivors of childhood medulloblastoma. *J Neurooncol* 2005; **72**(3): 245–53.

51. Anderson V, Godber T, Smibert E, Ekert H. Neurobehavioural sequelae following cranial irradiation and chemotherapy in children: an analysis of risk factors. *Pediatr Rehabil* 1997; **1**(2): 63–76.

52. Holmquist LA, Scott J. Treatment, age, and time-related predictors of behavioral outcome in pediatric brain tumor survivors. *J Clin Psychol Med Settings* 2002; **9**: 315–21.

53. Ness KK, Gurney JG, Zeltzer LK, *et al.* The impact of limitations in physical, executive, and emotional function on health-related quality of life among adult survivors of childhood cancer: a report from the Childhood Cancer Survivor Study. *Arch Phys Med Rehabil* 2008; **89**(1): 128–36.

54. Vannatta K, Gerhardt CA, Wells RJ, Noll RB. Intensity of CNS treatment for pediatric cancer: prediction of social outcomes in survivors. *Pediatr Blood Cancer* 2007; **49**(5): 716–22.

55. Fossen A, Abrahamsen TG, Storm-Mathisen I. Psychological outcome in children treated for brain tumor. *Pediatr Hematol Oncol* 1998; **15**(6): 479–88.

56. Kahalley LS, Robinson LA, Tyc VL, *et al.* Attentional and executive dysfunction as predictors of smoking within the Childhood Cancer Survivor Study cohort. *Nicotine Tob Res* 2010; **12**(4): 344–54.

57. Kollins SH, McClernon FJ, Fuemmeler BF. Association between smoking and attention-deficit/hyperactivity disorder symptoms in a population-based sample of young adults. *Arch Gen Psychiatry* 2005; **62**(10): 1142–7.

58. Lambert NM, Hartsough CS. Prospective study of tobacco smoking and substance dependencies among samples of ADHD and non-ADHD participants. *J Learn Disabil* 1998; **31**(6): 533–44.

59. Milberger S, Biederman J, Faraone SV, Chen L, Jones J. ADHD is associated with early initiation of cigarette smoking in children and adolescents. *J Am Acad Child Adolesc Psychiatry* 1997; **36**(1): 37–44.

60. Pomerleau OF, Downey KK, Stelson FW, Pomerleau CS. Cigarette smoking in adult patients diagnosed with attention deficit hyperactivity disorder. *J Subst Abuse* 1995; **7**(3): 373–8.

61. Ernst M, Heishman SJ, Spurgeon L, London ED. Smoking history and nicotine effects on cognitive performance. *Neuropsychopharmacology* 2001; **25**(3): 313–19.

62. Levin ED, Conners CK, Silva D, Canu W, March J. Effects of chronic nicotine and methylphenidate in adults with attention deficit/hyperactivity disorder. *Exp Clin Psychopharmacol* 2001; **9**(1): 83–90.

63. Levin ED, Conners CK, Silva D, *et al.* Transdermal nicotine effects on attention. *Psychopharmacology (Berl).* 1998; **140**(2): 135–41.

64. Levin ED, Conners CK, Sparrow E, *et al.* Nicotine effects on adults with attention-

deficit/hyperactivity disorder. *Psychopharmacology (Berl)* 1996; **123**(1): 55–63.

65. Levin ED, Rezvani AH. Development of nicotinic drug therapy for cognitive disorders. *Eur J Pharmacol* 2000; **393**(1–3): 141–6.

66. Potter AS, Newhouse PA. Effects of acute nicotine administration on behavioral inhibition in adolescents with attention-deficit/hyperactivity disorder. *Psychopharmacology (Berl)* 2004; **176**(2): 182–94.

67. Kassel JD, Stroud LR, Paronis CA. Smoking, stress, and negative affect: correlation, causation, and context across stages of smoking. *Psychol Bull* 2003; **129**(2): 270–304.

68. Ettenhofer ML, Foley J, Castellon SA, Hinkin CH. Reciprocal prediction of medication adherence and neurocognition in HIV/AIDS. *Neurology* 2010; **74**(15): 1217–22.

69. McNally K, Rohan J, Pendley JS, Delamater A, Drotar D. Executive functioning, treatment adherence, and glycemic control in children with type 1 diabetes. *Diabetes Care* 2010; **33**(6): 1159–62.

70. Fouladi M, Chintagumpala M, Laningham FH, *et al.* White matter lesions detected by magnetic resonance imaging after radiotherapy and high-dose chemotherapy in children with medulloblastoma or primitive neuroectodermal tumor. *J Clin Oncol* 2004; **22**(22): 4551–60.

71. Mulhern RK, Palmer SL, Reddick WE, *et al.* Risks of Young Age for Selected Neurocognitive Deficits in Medulloblastoma Are Associated With White Matter Loss. *J Clin Oncol* 2001; **19**(2): 472–9.

72. Paakko E, Harila-Saari A, Vanionpaa L, Himanen S, Pyhtinen J, Lanning M. White matter changes on MRI during treatment in children with acute lymphoblastic leukemia: correlation with neuropsychological findings. *Med Pediatr Oncol* 2000; **35**(5): 456–61.

73. Qiu D, Kwong DL, Chan GC, Leung LH, Khong PL. Diffusion tensor magnetic resonance imaging finding of discrepant fractional anisotropy between the frontal and parietal lobes after whole-brain irradiation in childhood medulloblastoma survivors: reflection of regional white matter radiosensitivity? *Int J Radiat Oncol Biol Phys* 2007; **69**(3): 846–51.

74. Reddick WE, White HA, Glass JO, *et al.* Developmental model relating white matter volume to neurocognitive deficits in pediatric brain tumor survivors. *Cancer* 2003; **97**(10): 2512–19.

Chapter

13

Executive functions in HIV

Sharon Nichols

Most of the literature on infectious disease and the CNS has focused on broader aspects of cognitive and behavioral functioning with less emphasis on EF. However, the role of EF in mediating some behavioral and functional outcomes, as well as recognition of the potential for infectious diseases to strike at various points during the protracted development of brain regions subserving EF, has increased interest in this area.

Infectious diseases vary in their actions on the CNS, including direct attacks and secondary effects such as encephalitis (irritation and inflammation of the brain), meningitis (inflammation of the protective membranes covering the brain and spinal cord), or encephalomyelitis (a.k.a. myeloencephalitis; inflammation of the brain and meninges). Acute disseminated encephalomyelitis (ADEM) can occur following infection, and is associated with damage to white matter.

Infectious disease impacting the CNS can be bacterial in nature, including *Bartonella henselae* (a.k.a. "cat scratch disease"), the *Borrelia* family (causing Lyme disease), and *Mycobacterium tuberculosis* (TB). Viral causes of CNS inflammation in pediatric populations include the herpes viruses (including herpes simplex, Epstein–Barr, and varicella-zoster), cytomegalovirus (CMV), mosquito- and tick-borne viruses, and enteroviruses (e.g., poliovirus, echovirus, coxsackievirus). Although measles, mumps, rabies, rubella, streptococcus pneumonia, and haemophilus influenza type B were cause for concern in the past, they are less prevalent now in the United States given the effectiveness of immunizations.

One viral infection that has been well studied in conjunction with EF is human immunodeficiency virus (HIV). Not only has HIV been linked to EdF and to brain networks involved in EF, but, importantly, EdF has potential impact on both the management and spread of HIV. Thus, EdF in youth with HIV can have public health as well as clinical implications. HIV can directly attack the neurologic system; the weakened immune system associated with later stages of HIV disease also causes vulnerability to other infectious diseases that can cause encephalitis or meningitis, although this is less common in children than in adults. This chapter focuses on HIV as the best-studied example of EdF secondary to infectious disease in children.

Human immunodeficiency virus

HIV is a retrovirus that affects children primarily through pre- and perinatal mother-to-child transmission since effective screening of blood products has reduced the risk of infection in children with bleeding disorders such as hemophilia, a group affected by

Executive Function and Dysfunction, ed. Scott J. Hunter and Elizabeth P. Sparrow. Published by Cambridge University Press. © Cambridge University Press 2012.

HIV early in the epidemic. Since studies demonstrated that antiretroviral medications given during pregnancy and perinatally could dramatically reduce mother to child transmission of HIV, the incidence of pediatric HIV has decreased in countries where these medications are most available. Worldwide, however, HIV in children continues to be a significant issue, with 2.5 million children under 15 living with HIV infection in 2009 and an estimated 370 000 new infections occurring that year alone.[1] The 260 000 deaths of children from acquired immune deficiency syndrome (AIDS) in 2009 demonstrate that effective treatments are unavailable for many children. Furthermore, youth age 15–24 years continue to represent more than 40% of new HIV infections each year, with an estimated 1.2 billion young people in this age group living with HIV as of 2007.[2] These HIV-infected adolescents and young adults present special concerns since they have a virus with the potential to affect development of frontostriatal regulatory circuits, in addition to the typical adolescent lag between emergence of the propensity to engage in risk behaviors and development of self-regulation skills.

Treatment approaches for HIV have evolved from single antiretroviral agents to combinations of antiretroviral therapies from multiple drug classes. Used correctly, these therapies have proven effective in controlling systemic viral replication, although the medications vary in their ability to penetrate into the brain and treat virus sequestered there. The phrase "used correctly" is an important one since a high level of adherence to medication doses and schedules is required in order to achieve viral control; furthermore, HIV can rapidly mutate into a drug-resistant form if sufficient drug levels are not maintained. For this reason, cognitive impairments that could interfere with medication adherence have been a focus of research in adults and are beginning to receive increased attention in children and adolescents, particularly those at an age where they are typically expected to assume responsibility for taking medications.

Executive dysfunction in HIV

Prior to the development of antiretroviral therapy, neurocognitive and motor dysfunction were commonly seen in both children and adults with HIV.[3] This dysfunction, in some cases, took the form of a progressive dementia with a loss of skills and knowledge or, in the case of infants and children, a failure to achieve expected motor and cognitive milestones. In other children, cognitive development would diverge from the typical developmental trajectory or would plateau.

With treatment advances, HIV has evolved from a progressive illness to a chronic condition. Severe HIV-associated neurocognitive and neurodevelopmental impairments occur much less frequently in both adults[4] and children.[5,6] However, milder cognitive impairment continues to be seen, potentially at an even higher level as people live with HIV for many years.[4] In adults with HIV, these impairments tend to appear in functional domains subserved by frontostriatal and hippocampal areas of the brain, including EF, memory (particularly prospective memory), and processing speed.[7,8]

Children and adolescents with HIV typically encountered by clinicians face many additional developmental risks that may at least in part account for functioning lower than population norms. These risks include prematurity, prenatal drug and alcohol exposure, environmental and educational disadvantage, disrupted caregiving and family stress, and possibly genetic predispositions to psychiatric or learning disorders. In addition, prenatal exposure to antiretroviral medications may have as yet unknown effects on long-term development. Studies that compare children with HIV with uninfected children born to HIV-infected mothers, and thus exposed perinatally to HIV and to antiretroviral therapy as well as sharing other risk factors, find that they, in general, perform comparably on tests of general intellectual functioning, falling in the average to low average range.[9–11] However, a subset of children and youth who experienced periods of significant immunocompromise and illness early in development continue to show significant impairment long term.[9,10,12] There is also concern that persisting subtle deficits may have a disproportionate impact on functional outcomes in this population already facing other significant environmental, educational and economic hurdles.

It is likely that problems with EF would be among the subtle deficits seen in children and youth with HIV for two reasons. First, as noted above, EF is an area in which deficits are well documented in adults with HIV infection, even in the combination antiretroviral therapy era.[13] In adults, EdF may emerge even in the early stages of HIV disease and include deficits on measures of control of inhibitory interference and cognitive flexibility, supporting the frontostriatal nature of HIV's impact on the brain.[14,15] When present, deficits in EF appear to increase the risk of poor functional outcomes[16] such as risky automobile driving[17] and medication management impairment.[18,19] Second, in both children and adults, the areas of the brain primarily affected by HIV (see below) overlap significantly with those that subserve EF.

Thus far, only a few small studies of children with HIV have been published that included measures of EF, although larger studies are ongoing. Bisiacchi, Suppiej, and Laverda[20] compared the performance of 29 perinatally infected, but neurologically asymptomatic, children and 13 control children perinatally exposed to HIV. All children were age 6–15. The investigators used a wide-ranging neuropsychological battery that contained several tests of EF. Only performance on tests of EF distinguished all infected children from controls, while the 9 children with AIDS diagnoses showed deficits in memory and visuo-praxis as well. Koekkoek and colleagues[21] studied 22 children (median age = 9.46 years) with HIV infection using a measure of global functioning and tests from the Amsterdam Neuropsychological Tasks (ANT) program. Children with HIV infection performed more poorly than predicted by age norms, with EF (attentional control, and visuospatial WM) and processing speed showing the strongest association with indicators of HIV disease severity. The authors also found significantly impaired verbal fluency relative to age norms. In a study of 41 infected children treated with combination antiretroviral therapy, Martin and colleagues[10] found that children with computed tomography (CT) brain scan abnormalities had lower scores on subtests of a measure of cognitive functioning that were likely to involve EF, and a measure of WM was related to CD4+ counts and percent. Related findings using tests of memory include research by Klaas and colleagues showing that infected children with CNS disease performed worse than those without CNS disease on recall but not recognition of verbal information,[22] a pattern seen with subcortical impairment.

Unfortunately, the literature on neurocognitive impacts of HIV in youth with behaviorally acquired HIV is even leaner than that regarding perinatal acquisition of HIV. A small study by Hosek and colleagues[23] looked at the development of formal reasoning in 42 youth age 16–25 with HIV infection and found that 69% of youth had not begun the transition from concrete to formal or abstract reasoning. No studies of this population specifically incorporate measures of EF. Because of the ongoing maturation of EF occurring in late adolescence, it is possible that individuals who acquire HIV before or during that period may face even greater risks to EF, and the functional consequences of EF impairments, than has been clearly demonstrated in adults with HIV.

The neurological basis of executive dysfunction in HIV

In adults with HIV, cognitive impairments tend to appear in functional domains subserved by frontostriatal and hippocampal areas of the brain.[8] The few neuroimaging studies performed with children indicate that the impact of HIV during development parallels the adult pattern in falling primarily in subcortical areas and white matter. Imaging and autopsy studies have shown that in children, as in adults, significant HIV-related neuropathology is seen most often in the subcortical white matter and frontostriatal systems.[24] Imaging studies using magnetic resonance spectroscopy have shown metabolic abnormalities in frontal areas[25] that correlate with cognitive performance.[26] Furthermore, these are brain areas that undergo active development during childhood and through adolescence.[27] Thus, it is reasonable to hypothesize that HIV would interfere with the development of complex executive skills, as well as other functions, that rely on the integrity of white matter and of frontostriatal circuits.

Summary and future directions

Small studies of children with perinatal HIV infection suggest that EF deficits are likely in that population. The adult HIV literature, as well as our knowledge of EF development, suggests that individuals who acquire HIV during adolescence are also at risk for EdF. Updated, longitudinal studies incorporating neuroimaging and using larger samples of children and youth are needed to clarify what, if any, EF deficits are currently seen, their neuropathological underpinnings, and what treatment regimens may be associated with better EF outcomes. For HIV, and for other childhood infectious diseases where likelihood of survival into adulthood has increased, understanding the association of EdF with functional outcomes such as adult employment and social functioning is important.

It is recommended that future research be designed to facilitate the development and targeting of EF-related interventions to maximize successful adult outcome. This might be done by incorporating measures of functional outcomes as well as by using tasks that have clear links to those outcomes (for example, measures of prospective memory might be linked with medication adherence tasks) and to remediation, as well as by examining the availability of environmental and other supports that could be enlisted to improve transition to adulthood. With the greater survival of children and adolescents with HIV and other infectious diseases, research that can increase their chances of successful adult outcome should receive particular focus.

References

1. World Health Organization. *Global Report: UNAIDS report on the global AIDS epidemic, 2010.* Geneva, Switzerland: World Health Organization; 2010.

2. Wilson CM, Wright PF, Safrit JT, Rudy B. Epidemiology of HIV infection and risk in adolescents and youth. *J Acquir Immune Defic Synd.* 2010; **54**: S5–6. 10.1097/QAI.0b013e3181e243a1.

3. Van Rie A, Harrington PR, Dow A, Robertson K. Neurologic and neurodevelopmental manifestations of pediatric HIV/AIDS: a global perspective. *Eur J Paediatr Neurol* 2007; **11**(1): 1–9.

4. Heaton RK, Franklin DR, Ellis RJ, *et al.* HIV-associated neurocognitive disorders before and during the era of combination antiretroviral therapy: differences in rates, nature, and predictors. *J Neurovirol* 2011; **17**(1): 3–16.

5. Shanbhag MC, Rutstein RM, Zaoutis T, Zhao H, Chao D, Radcliffe J. Neurocognitive functioning in pediatric human immunodeficiency virus infection: effects of combined therapy. *Arch Pediatr Adolesc Med* 2005; **159**(7): 651–6.

6. Chiriboga CA, Fleishman S, Champion S, Gaye-Robinson L, Abrams EJ. Incidence and prevalence of HIV encephalopathy in children with HIV infection receiving highly active anti-retroviral therapy (HAART). *J Pediatr* 2005; **146**(3): 402–7.

7. Moore DJ, Masliah E, Rippeth JD, *et al.* Cortical and subcortical neurodegeneration is associated with HIV neurocognitive impairment. *AIDS* 2006; **20**(6): 879–87.

8. Woods SP, Moore DJ, Weber E, Grant I. Cognitive neuropsychology of HIV-associated neurocognitive disorders. *Neuropsychol Rev* 2009; **19**(2): 152–68.

9. Smith R, Malee K, Leighty R, *et al.* Effects of perinatal HIV infection and associated risk factors on cognitive development among young children. *Pediatrics* 2006; **117**(3): 851–62.

10. Martin SC, Wolters PL, Toledo-Tamula MA, Zeichner SL, Hazra R, Civitello L. Cognitive functioning in school-aged children with vertically acquired HIV infection being treated with highly active antiretroviral therapy (HAART). *Dev Neuropsychol* 2006; **30**(2): 633–57.

11. Malee K, Williams PL, Montepiedra G, *et al.* The role of cognitive functioning in medication adherence of children and adolescents with HIV infection. *J Pediatr Psychol* 2009; **34**(2): 164–75.

12. Wood SM, Shah SS, Steenhoff AP, Rutstein RM. The impact of AIDS diagnosis on long-term neurocognitive and psychiatric outcomes of surviving adolescents with perinatally acquired HIV. *AIDS* 2009; **23**: 1859–65.

13. Hardy DJ, Hinkin CH. Reaction time performance in adults with HIV/AIDS. *J Clin Exp Neuropsychol* 2002; **24**(7): 912–29.

14. Baldewicz TT, Leserman J, Silva SG, *et al.* Changes in neuropsychological functioning with progression of HIV-1 infection: Results of an 8-year longitudinal investigation. *AIDS Behav* 2004; **8**(3): 345–55.

15. Stern Y, McDermott MP, Albert S, *et al.* Factors associated with incident human immunodeficiency virus-dementia. *Arch Neurol* 2001; **58**(3): 473–9.

16. Heaton RK, Marcotte TD, Mindt MR, *et al.* The impact of HIV-associated neuropsychological impairment on everyday functioning. *J Int Neuropsychol Soc* 2004; **10**(3): 317–31.

17. Marcotte TD, Heaton RK, Albert S. Everyday impact of HIV-associated neurocognitive disorders. In Gendelman HE, Grant I, Everall IP, Lipton SA, Swindells S, eds. *The Neurology of AIDS*: 2nd edn. Oxford: Oxford University Press; 2005.

18. Ettenhofer ML, Foley J, Castellon SA, Hinkin CH. Reciprocal prediction of medication adherence and neurocognition in HIV/AIDS. *Neurology* 2010 13; **74**(15): 1217–22.

19. Waldrop-Valverde D, Jones DL, Weiss S, Kumar M, Metsch L. The effects of low literacy and cognitive impairment on medication adherence in HIV-positive injecting drug users. *AIDS Care* 2008; **20**(10): 1202–10.

20. Bisiacchi PS, Suppiej A, Laverda A. Neuropsychological evaluation of neurologically asymptomatic HIV-infected children. *Brain Cogn* 2000; **43**(1–3): 49–52.

21. Koekkoek S, de Sonneville LM, Wolfs TF, Licht R, Geelen SP. Neurocognitive function profile in HIV-infected school-age children. *Eur J Paediatr Neurol* 2008; **12**(4): 290–7.

22. Wolters PL, Brouwers P. Evaluation of neurodevelopmental deficits in children with HIV-1 infection. In Gendelman HE, Grant I, Everall IP, Lipton SA, Swindells S,

editors. *The Neurology of AIDS*: 2nd edn. Oxford: Oxford University Press; 2005.

23. Hosek SG, Zimet GD. Behavioral considerations for engaging youth in HIV clinical research. *J Acquir Immune Defic Syndr* 2010; 54 Suppl 1: S25–30.

24. Sharer LR. Neuropathological aspects of HIV-1 infection in children. In Gendelman HE, Grant I, Everall IP, Lipton SA, Swindells S, editors. *The neurology of AIDS*: 2nd edn. Oxford: Oxford University Press; 2005.

25. Banakar S, Thomas MA, Deveikis A, Watzl JQ, Hayes J, Keller MA. Two-dimensional 1H MR spectroscopy of the brain in human immunodeficiency virus (HIV)-infected children. *J Magn Reson Imaging* 2008; 27(4): 710–17.

26. Keller MA, Venkatraman TN, Thomas A, *et al.* Altered neurometabolite development in HIV-infected children: correlation with neuropsychological tests. *Neurology* 2004; 62(10): 1810–17.

27. Sowell ER, Peterson BS, Thompson PM, Welcome SE, Henkenius AL, Toga AW. Mapping cortical change across the human life span. *Nat Neurosci* 2003; 6(3): 309–15.

Chapter

14

Executive functions and neurotoxic exposure

Jill Kelderman

Neurotoxicity refers to adverse alteration of CNS functioning due to exposure to either a natural or manmade substance. The impact of neurotoxic exposures on development can be quite significant, given both the underlying vulnerabilities of the maturing brain and the potential for early neurotoxic exposures to alter a child's developmental trajectory. This chapter reviews the relationship between the most commonly encountered neurotoxins and EF in children and adolescents. We will begin with a review of environmental neurotoxins (lead, PCBs, manganese, and pesticides), followed by a discussion of substances of abuse. This will include prenatal exposures to teratogens, and the impact of voluntary consumption of alcohol, marijuana, and cocaine during adolescence.

Environmental neurotoxins

The effects of environmental neurotoxins are undoubtedly multifaceted and bidirectional, with numerous variables contributing to ultimate outcomes. From a methodological perspective, this has resulted in an increasing appreciation of variables including maternal education, nutrition, and other high risk environmental variables which are more likely to co-exist in an environment with neurotoxins. A full summary of the literature, particularly in regards to lead and related SES variables, is extensive and beyond the scope of this chapter. The review below is intended to be succinct and focused on EdF associated with environmental neurotoxins in childhood.

Lead

Lead is the most studied environmental neurotoxin, with a large research base outlining its negative effects on cognition and behavior. The United States phased out the use of lead in gasoline and paints used in homes and toys in the 1970s, and it is now highly regulated. This has led to a decline in the amount of environmental lead; however, it continues to be found in soil, household dust, drinking water, and lead smelters (metal processing facilities), as lead does not degrade and is easily absorbed into soil. Leaded paint can still be found in homes built prior to 1950; this is currently the most common source of lead exposure for children in the United States.[1,2]

The Centers for Disease Control and Prevention (CDC) guidelines have gradually lowered the blood lead level (BLL) considered adverse.[3] In screening guidelines published in 1991, the CDC reduced acceptable exposure levels from 25 mcg/dl to <10 mcg/dl, following the accumulation of evidence associating lower BLLs with poorer performance on tests assessing cognition. Numerous studies have reported a relationship between BLLs <10 mcg/ml and significant disruptions in intellectual abilities, academic skills, and behavior problems.[4-7] BLLs as low as 7 mcg/dl have been inversely associated with intellectual ability in children exposed to lead, even after controlling for a variety of SES variables.[3,8]

Dose-dependent relationships between lead and cognitive dysfunction are consistently reported in the literature, and no BLL threshold has been identified as harmless.[9-12] The impact of a BLL increase of 1 mcg/dl at lower BLLs (<10 mcg/dl) appears relatively greater than at higher BLLs (>10 mcg/dl), suggesting a non-linear relationship between lead and cognitive functioning in children.[7] In light of this increasing evidence of adverse effects even at low levels of exposure, arguments have been made to lower the threshold for acceptable exposure to 2 mcg/dl.[13]

EdF has been identified to varying degrees in children with BLLs below 10 mcg/dl. A prospective study of 5-year-old children with a mean lifetime BLL of 7.2 mcg/dl demonstrated impairment in spatial WM, spatial memory span, set-shifting, and planning as assessed using the CANTAB, after controlling for both protective and risk factors.[14] Decreased attention and WM were reported by Surkan and colleagues in their study of 534 children aged 6–10 with BLLs between 5–10 mcg/dl.[15] Weaknesses with EF (WCST number of errors, WCST conceptual level responses, WISC-III Digit Span, Seashore Rhythm Task) have been identified in children with mean BLLs as low as 3 mcg/dl.[6] Additionally, cognitive flexibility has been implicated in lead exposure studies. Specifically, several studies have identified a significant relationship between increased BLL and increases in WCST perseverative errors[6,15,16] as well as poorer performance on the CANTAB Intradimensional-Extradimensional Shift Test.[14] Reduced vigilance/alertness has been linked to BLL. Vigilance deficits reported in association with BLLs include decreased total correct, increased omission errors, and slower processing speeds/alertness on CPTs.[6,17,18] Other aspects of EF have been inconsistently related to BLLs, including response inhibition[6,17,19] and planning.[6,15,17] In sum, the emerging literature suggests sustained attention, WM, and cognitive flexibility may be particularly vulnerable to the effects of lead exposure, even at low BLLs, while other aspects of EF including inhibitory control and planning may be relatively resistant to low BLLs.

Socio-economic variables have been shown to be strong moderating variables in regard to neurocognitive effects of lead exposure in childhood. Lower SES is usually associated with higher lead exposure.[19] Children from a lower SES are more likely to live in older housing, where the presence of leaded paint is higher. Furthermore, in high-density urban areas, higher lead levels in soil result from proximity to dense traffic areas in the era of leaded gasoline. Children from a lower SES may also be more vulnerable to the effects of lead due to poor diet; iron deficiency has been linked to higher lead levels, which may reflect the role iron plays in blocking lead absorption in the digestive tract.[20] Additionally, the protective impact of enriched environments may play an important role, as children from high SES show fewer neurocognitive deficits following lead exposure.[21] Hubbs-Tait et al.[22] proposed a multilevel model of development outlining the impacts of social environments, micronutrients, and neurotoxicants on child cognition and behavior, whereby the three domains influence one another in a multidirectional manner. This complex model may explain the sometimes divergent findings reported in the literature, as these variables are not consistently measured or controlled.

The literature base on the biomechanics of lead neurotoxicity is extensive.[23,24] Animal and human research have both indicated that lead causes damage to the CNS by inducing apoptosis and neurotransmitter excitotoxicity, and altering neurotransmitter receptors, mitochondria, second messengers, cerebrovascular endothelial cells, astroglia, and oligo-dendroglia. Lead crosses the blood–brain barrier rapidly, primarily due to its ability to substitute for calcium ions. Lead disrupts neurotransmitter functioning, and glutamatergic, dopaminergic, and cholinergic systems have been implicated. The glutamatergic system plays a key role in long-term potentiation, and thereby learning and memory. Lead may lead to decreased dopamine synthesis and release in nigrostriatal and mesolimbic systems, which has been associated with failure to inhibit in animals. In addition, lead blocks release of acetylcholine and diminishes cholinergic function.

The effects of lead on the CNS may be permanent. Lower brain volume in PFC and ACC has been reported in adults with a history of lead exposure in childhood.[25] Childhood BLLs have also been associated with atypical metabolic functioning in adults, including decreases in gray matter metabolites in basal ganglia and cerebellum, and decreases in white matter metabolites in frontal and parietal lobes.[26]

PCBs

Polychlorinated biphenyls (PCBs) are a constellation of synthetic organic compounds that were widely used as coolants and lubricants in transformers and capacitors. After discovering a buildup of PCBs in the environment, they were phased out of electrical equipment in the 1970s and eventually banned. Like lead, PCBs do not break down easily and remain in air, water, and soil for extended periods of time. Currently, PCB exposure primarily occurs through exposure to contaminated food, especially seafood, and also through air containing PCBs released from disposal and incineration sites.[27]

Deleterious effects of prenatal PCB exposure on neurodevelopment have been reported in several studies.[28–33] Prenatal PCB exposure has been correlated with lower scores on tests assessing verbal WM including WISC-III Freedom from Distractibility, WISC-R Digit Span, and Sternberg Memory Test.[34,35] Increased rates of commission errors on CPT tests have been associated with prenatal PCB exposures.[36,37] There is limited investigation into cognitive flexibility and planning among children exposed to PCBs prenatally. One study reported difficulties with cognitive flexibility on the WCST, but not the Stroop.[35] As PCBs have been associated with reductions in prefrontal and striatal dopamine,[38–39] additional work delineating the impact of prenatal PCB exposure on EdF is warranted. Notably, comparison of studies examining the effects of PCBs is particularly difficult given the wide variability in methodologies and PCB congeners that are considered.

Manganese

Although an essential nutrient, manganese is neurotoxic at high levels. Decreased levels of dopamine and lesions of the basal ganglia are considered characteristic of chronic manganese exposure.[40] Several studies have reported an inverse relationship between manganese exposure and children's intellectual abilities.[41–43] Studies specifically exploring the relationship between manganese exposure and EdF, however, are limited. Children with ADHD have been found to have higher hair manganese as compared to controls.[44] Among a Canadian sample, higher hair manganese concentration was associated with hyperactivity and oppositional behaviors as assessed via teacher reports.[45] Impaired manual dexterity and speed and decreased digit span were reported in a sample of Chinese children exposed to high-level manganese sewage irrigation in comparison to controls.[46] Children with higher hair manganese and arsenic levels had impaired verbal memory (CVLT-C, WRAML Stories Recall), but no deficits on the WRAVMA, CELF-3, or CCT Level II.[42] No significant findings were reported between hair metals and behavior questionnaires, including the CDI, BASC, Conners' ADHD/DSM Scales (CADS-IV),[47,48] or BRIEF. Certainly, further investigation is warranted to more fully evaluate the relationship between manganese neurotoxicity and EdF.

Pesticides

Pesticides represent another family of environmental neurotoxins. There are many different classes of pesticides, each of which includes numerous specific exemplars. Despite their variety, accumulating research suggests that exposure to many types of pesticides in utero and during early childhood is associated with attention problems and EdF. Prenatal exposure to organophosphates pesticides has been associated with attention problems. For example, children who were highly exposed to chlorpyrifos prenatally were significantly more likely than those with lower exposure levels to experience attention problems according to parent ratings.[49]

Marks et al.[50] reported prenatal levels of organophosphate metabolites were not associated with the ADHD Confidence Index on the K-CPT at 3.5 years of age, but were associated with maternal report of attention problems and ADHD on the CBCL at 5 years of age. Concurrently, organophosphates pesticides exposure was not negatively associated with performance on the NEPSY-II Visual Attention subtest at age 3, but was at age 5. These findings suggest delayed manifestation of EdF secondary to prenatal exposure to organophosphates pesticides.

Comparable results have been documented in response to organophosphates pesticides exposure during childhood, with several studies demonstrating problems with attention and EF (parent ratings,[51] verbal cancellation test,[52] or WCST[53]) either concurrent with or following organophosphates pesticides exposure. In general, results typically indicate more severe and pervasive neurocognitive deficits when exposed to pesticides prenatally as compared to exposure during childhood.

Drugs of abuse

While the above mentioned neurotoxins are often ingested unintentionally and, unknowingly, other neurotoxins are volitionally consumed. The following section focuses on the effects of alcohol, marijuana, cocaine, and nicotine on EF, differentiating between prenatal exposure and voluntary use during adolescence. When considering the following results, it is essential to bear in mind the inherent methodological challenges and shortcomings within this area. The confounding effect of polysubstance use during pregnancy lends significant obstacles for those attempting to delineate the impact of prenatal exposure. Furthermore, is it virtually impossible to accurately quantify precise levels of substance exposure within a natural population. Methods of ingestion, differing levels of neurotoxic substances, poly-substance use, and willingness to disclose substance use during pregnancy represent significant impediments to researchers' efforts to determine actual levels of exposure. Additionally, the effects of early environments and SES undoubtedly contribute additional variance to neurocognitive outcomes.

Prenatal alcohol exposure

The effects of prenatal alcohol exposure on later cognitive development may be the most widely appreciated example of prenatal neurotoxic sequelae. Fetal alcohol spectrum disorder (FASD) affects approximately 97 in 1000 births worldwide.[56] FASD captures a continuum of impairment ranging from the more affected, traditional fetal alcohol syndrome (FAS) presentation to the more mild, partial FAS or alcohol-related neurodevelopmental disorder (ARND), which includes individuals who do not have all of the traditional characteristics (e.g., facial dysmorphology), but nevertheless experience CNS dysfunction.

In utero exposure to alcohol commonly results in specific deficits to the executive system, with the most persistent and commonly reported limitations in the domain of WM, including visual and spatial WM.[57–59] Children and adults with prenatal exposure to alcohol perform more poorly on digit span than their unexposed peers, even when controlling for intelligence.[60–63] Children with prenatal exposure to alcohol also display variability in attention.[64]

Children and adolescents with FASD have limitations in cognitive planning on the Tower of London,[65] with FAS and ARND performing similarly.[66] This suggests that specific deficits in EF exist even when characteristic features, such as facial dysmorphology, are not present. Conceptual set shifting, inhibition, and integration of feedback (WCST) are also impaired in children and adolescents with FASD.[60,65,67–69] Impairments have been observed in affective set-shifting,[69] response inhibition,[70] concept formation,[71] and verbal and nonverbal fluency.[67,72] Aspects of inhibition and concrete rule learning appear relatively intact in FASD.[69] History of exposure to alcohol predicted performance on a tapping inhibition task among 4-year-olds, even when controlling for intelligence and environmental factors such as SES.[70] No relationship was found between alcohol exposure and tasks of category fluency and motor planning, suggesting that limitations in these domains may be more subtle and emerge over time.

In infancy and toddlerhood, history of prenatal exposure is related to decreased frontal cortex size.[73] Adolescents with FASD have smaller, abnormally shaped brains, with the frontal lobes and left hemisphere particularly affected.[74] These anatomical differences persist into adulthood, with lower total brain volume, particularly in the hippocampus.[75] In addition, for adults with FASD and dysmorphic features, hippocampal size predicts WM ability. Taken together, prenatal exposure to alcohol appears to have a unique and negative effect on the development of the frontal cortex and hippocampus.

Alcohol abuse in adolescence

The neuropsychological effects of chronic alcohol exposure in adulthood are well researched. Chronic alcoholism in adults is associated with neuropsychological deficits in visual-spatial processing, memory, cognitive speed, and EF.[76–78] Adolescence is a period of development and refinement of systems involved in EF, including those that mediate reward and possibly sensitize networks related to addiction. These systems, therefore, may be particularly vulnerable to the neurotoxic effects of alcohol.[79,80]

It is essential to consider premorbid EF when exploring the impact of alcohol use on neurocognition. EdF has been postulated as contributing to problem drug use, possibly moderating the relationship between family history of substance abuse and use in adolescence.[81] Poor response inhibition, but not set shifting or WM, is a moderating variable in the relationship between adolescents at high-risk for substance abuse and whether they develop alcohol-use related problems and illicit drug use.[82]

Heavy alcohol exposure has been linked to poor attention among adolescents diagnosed with alcohol dependence, even after three weeks of abstinence.[83] Deficits were identified on WAIS-R Arithmetic, Coding, Digits Forward, and Digits Backward, as well as on TMT-B. Female, but not male, adolescent alcohol users exhibited poorer performance on the WCST.[84] Lesser amounts of alcohol consistent with alcohol abuse among adolescents have not been linked with EdF,[85] suggesting a dose-dependent relationship.

Adolescents who drink heavily show subtle differences upon imaging. Adolescent heavy drinkers show reduced PFC volumes relative to nondrinking controls; this finding is more pronounced among females.[86] Tapert and colleagues[87] reported poorer performance on a test of spatial WM among adolescents who drank heavily for one to two years. The heavy drinkers showed increased activation in parietal cortex and decreased activation in occipital and cerebellar regions when compared to light drinkers, supporting the hypothesis that high levels of alcohol use may lead to cortical reorganization and compensation.[88]

Prenatal marijuana exposure

Two major longitudinal studies have examined the long-term effect of prenatal marijuana exposure (PME); although they differ in demographics (Ottawa Prenatal Prospective Study, mostly low risk, middle class, white mothers, and Maternal Health Practices in Child Development study, mostly high-risk, low SES, black families), findings are generally consistent across samples and at various time points. In general, PME is associated with EdF throughout childhood, despite the finding that children with PME could not be distinguished from non-exposed children on global measures such as IQ.

Studies have found EdF in children with PME including state regulation in infants,[89,90] STM, visual reasoning, and verbal reasoning in preschoolers,[91,92] visual problem-solving tasks in older children,[93,94] and commissions on CPTs.[95] A dose-dependent relationship has been reported between PME and CPT performance, including increased omission errors and decreased correct hits.[96] Young adolescents with PME show higher response time variability and increased omission errors.[97] Parent and teacher ratings indicate higher levels of inattention, hyperactivity, and impulsivity.[96,98]

There are several possible mechanisms of neurotoxicity in PME.[99] Multiple neurotransmitters are likely affected including dopamine, GABA, glutamate, and acetylcholine. Marijuana causes CB1 cannabinoid receptors to release endogenous opioids which act on opioid receptors in the ventral tegmental area, causing release of dopamine in the nucleus accumbens.[100] PME thereby increases activity in dopaminergic pathways of the nucleus accumbens.[101]

PME likely plays a large role in prenatal CNS development by altering typical neuronal proliferation, migration, differentiation, survival, and synaptogenesis. Indeed, MRI studies show decreased levels of cortical gray matter in PME children aged 10–14 relative to controls.[102] Functional neuroimaging studies identify atypical activation patterns suggestive of compensatory responses to altered or delayed development of PFC,[103] and altered lateralization and functional connectivity.[104]

Marijuana abuse in adolescence

Marijuana is a commonly used illicit substance with neurotoxic effects. In addition to differences in learning and memory, attention, visual-spatial skills, and processing speed, adult chronic marijuana use (CMU) is associated with EdF. Imaging studies have identified activation differences in PFC areas among adult CMU, including DLPFC, OFC, ACC, and basal ganglia.[105,106]

Deficits in attention and spatial WM have been demonstrated in adolescent CMU who had abstained for a month.[107] Evidence for a gradual recovery of cognitive abilities following a week of abstinence, with normalization after a month of abstinence has been shown in some studies, while ongoing weaknesses have been shown in other CMU 28 days after abstinence.[107,108] Adolescent marijuana use, regardless of gender, was associated with poorer EF, represented by a construct score based on scores from the D-KEFS (Verbal Fluency Total Correct, Tower Total Achievement, and Tower Error Score) and larger PFC volume.[109] Although adolescent CMU scored similarly to controls on a spatial WM task, activation differences relative to controls suggest CMU may exert alternative strategies to complete these tasks, leading to increased activation in compensatory brain areas even after a period of abstinence.[110] Adolescent marijuana users presenting for a neuropsychological evaluation may perform within expected limits on testing of WM and inhibitory control, however they may do so only with increased processing effort and by recruiting compensatory neural networks.

Several studies have identified differences in brain activation during spatial WM tasks for CMU relative to controls.[110,111] Structural brain differences have also been identified among adolescent CMU, including smaller cerebellar volumes (even after abstinence).[112] Female adolescent marijuana users show larger PFC volume as compared to their male counterparts,[109] which may reflect interruption of the normal pruning process.

Prenatal cocaine exposure

Extensive research efforts have been aimed at evaluating the degree of impairment in attention and EF in children with a history of prenatal cocaine exposure (PCE). Results typically indicate deficits in sustained attention,[113–117] deficits in selective attention,[116,118] slowed motor and processing speed,[119] and deficits in inhibitory control and impulsivity.[95,113,117,120] School-aged children with a history of PCE show poorer performance on Stroop Interference, but no differences on the ROCF.[121] Additional work is needed to determine the effect of PCE on other aspects of EF.

Exposure to cocaine in utero inhibits reuptake of monoamines that are present early in corticogenesis, which in turn may interfere with neuronal growth mechanisms.[122–124] Neuroimaging of children with PCE generally finds abnormalities in structure and function in areas reliant on dopamine. For example, decreased caudate and putamen volumes have been described in a PCE population,[125,126] as has increased diffusion in bifrontal projection fibers.[127] PCE has also been associated with decreased global cerebral blood flow during Stroop[128] and N-back[129] tasks, as well as greater BOLD signal activation in frontal and striatal regions[130] compared to nonexposed controls.

Cocaine abuse in adolescence

There is some evidence that PCE may increase the risk for later substance abuse during adolescence. This heightened risk could be related to alterations in fetal brain development or exposure to unhealthy environments, or both. For example, Bennett and colleagues[131] found that males (but not females) who were exposed to cocaine prenatally demonstrated increased risk behaviors such as aggression, substance abuse, and disregard for safety precautions, and these risk behaviors, in turn, were associated with problems with inhibitory control, emotional regulation, and antisocial behaviors. Moreover, while some researchers have found that PCE has no direct relationship with experimentation with cocaine in early adolescence, proximal risk and protective factors may play a crucial role in adolescent cocaine use.[132] That is, teens who tested positive for current cocaine use (both +/− PCE) had greater availability of drugs in the home, caregivers who abused alcohol and presented with more depressive symptoms, less nurturing home environments, less positive attachments to caregivers and peers, more externalizing and social problems, and more experimentation with drugs relative to teens who tested negative to current cocaine use (both +/− PCE). Availability of drugs in the home had the greatest predictive value for current cocaine use irrespective of PCE status; higher IQ, more nurturing home environments, and positive attachment to caregivers and peers provided some protective effect.

Prenatal nicotine exposure

The effects of prenatal nicotine exposure (PNE) are apparent in the neonate. PNE infants age 10 to 27 days showed lower scores on measures of self-regulation.[134] The amount of nicotine exposure has been correlated with poorer attention and decreased response to auditory stimuli as assessed using the Brazelton Neonatal Behavioral Assessment Scale.[135] PNE 6-month-olds had less focused attention, lowered reactivity to basic sensory stimulation, and more distractibility compared to nonexposed infants.[136] As early as 24 months, children with PNE exhibit higher rates of internalizing, externalizing and total problem per parent report to the CBCL, as compared to nonexposed children.[137] PNE predicted increased activity, inattention, and behavioral problems per parent CBCL among 6-year-olds.[138] PNE predicted more activity, impulsivity, and deficits in selective attention and response on the Stroop test among 10-year-olds.[139] These effects were observable with PNE levels as low as ten cigarettes per day. Among a sample of children with ADHD, hyperactive-impulsive symptoms and CD symptoms were significantly higher among children with PNE compared to non-PNE children.[140]

Nicotine binds to nicotinic acetylcholine receptors, and acetylcholine is crucial to brain development, including cell division and differentiation. Derauf et al.[99] outlined numerous mechanisms of neurotoxicty including maternal and fetal undernutrition secondary to smoking-induced anoxia, hypoxia due to increased carboxyhemoglobin and vasoconstriction, placental hypertrophy, reduced transplacental transport of nutrients, and interference with norepinephrine and acetylcholine.

Structurally, PNE has been linked to reduced cranial volume,[141,142] reduced cortical gray matter in total parenchymal volumes,[102] and cortical thinning in orbitofrontal, middle frontal, and parahippocampal cortices of PNE females, but not males.[143] PNE combined with current adolescent smoking was associated with increased white matter diffusion in a larger number of areas (e.g., genu of the corpus callosum, left frontal white matter, right superior longitudinal fasciculus, and anterior limb of the right internal capsule).[144]

Genetics may serve as a moderating variable between PNE and EdF. Current research suggests genetic polymorphisms can act in concert with PNE to offer either protective or risk factors for developing later problems with executive functioning and behavior. Males with PNE who were homozygous for DAT1 had higher rates of hyperactivity and impulsivity than all other groups on the K-SADS.[145] In children with PNE, the odds of a DSM-IV ADHD diagnosis were 2.9 times greater in twins with the DAT1 allele, 2.6 times greater in those with the DRD4 allele, and 9.0 times greater with both alleles.[146] PNE males (but not females) with low activity MAOA 5' have an increased risk of CD symptoms as measured by a phase processing task.[147]

Summary and future directions

In summary, a variety of neurotoxins are associated to varying degrees with aspects of EdF. Attention and WM appear to be some of the most commonly cited areas affected, however this may reflect a bias to explore these particular areas. Importantly, the effects of environmental contaminants are also inextricably linked with other risk factors, including premature birth, low birth weight, congenital abnormalities, endocrine and immune dysfunction, and psychosocial adversity, which may also lead to EdF in isolation, and may alter the risks associated with environmental exposures.[54,55] Along those lines, research is beginning to investigate genetic protective and/or risk factors that may mediate the effects of pesticide exposure.

Considering the numerous methodological obstacles outlined above, the need for replication is particularly important in order to make meaningful statements regarding causation. This could be achieved more efficiently if researchers were to develop research protocols allowing for cross-comparisons and summative statements. Increasing considerations of the potentially moderating roles of genetics and SES will continue to improve our understanding of the multifaceted and bidirectional roles of neurotoxins and EdF. Ongoing attempts to improve methodological weaknesses by controlling (either statistically or by experimental design) potentially confounding variables is necessary.

Recent longitudinal research has begun to show a developmental trend such that observed deficits tend to become more pronounced in mid to late childhood when academic demands increase, and these findings parallel the typical developmental progression of EF skills.[115,116,117,120,127,145,149] The observance of children growing into EdF underlies the importance of prevention. As noted by Bellinger,[5] primary prevention is the most effective manner in which to reduce the numerous negative consequences of neurotoxic exposure. Reduction and elimination of environmental neurotoxins must come from the government level and be incorporated into public policy. Public education regarding the effects of prenatal exposure to teratogens must be prioritized, as should programs supporting pregnant women's cessation efforts. Children and pre-adolescents should be informed of the consequences of heavy substance use. It will require extensive efforts at the government and community level in order to effectively eliminate prenatal and childhood exposure to neurotoxins, and thereby avoid the subsequent lifelong negative consequences.

References

1. Jones RL, Homa DM, Meyer PA, et al. Trends in blood lead levels and blood lead testing among US children aged 1 to 5 years, 1988–2004. Pediatr 2009; 123(3): e376–85.

2. Lanphear BP, Emond M, Jacobs DE, et al. A side by side comparison of dust collection methods for sampling lead-contaminated house dust. Environ Res 1995; 68: 114–23.

3. Baghurst PA, McMichael AJ, Wigg NR, et al. Environmental exposure to lead and children's intelligence at the age of seven years – The Port Pirie Cohort Study. N Engl J Med 1992; 327: 1279–84.

4. Canfield RL, Henderson CR, Cory-Slechta DA, Cox C, Jusko TA, Lanphear BP. Intellectual impairment in children with blood lead concentrations below 10 μg per deciliter. N Engl J Med 2003; 348: 1517–26.

5. Bellinger DC, Needleman HL. Intellectual impairment and blood lead levels. *N Engl J Med* 2003; **349**: 500–2.

6. Chiodo LM, Jacobson SW, Jacoson JL. Neurodevelopmental effects of postnatal lead exposure at very low levels. *Neurotoxicol Teratol* 2004; **26**: 359–71.

7. Lanphear BP, Hornung R, Khoury J, Yolton K, Baghurst P, Bellinger DC. Low-level environmental lead exposure and children's intellectual function: An international pooled analysis. *Environ Hlth Perspect* 2005; **113**(7): 894–9.

8. Jusko TA, Henderson CR, Lanphear BP, Cory-Slechta DA, Parsons PJ, Canfield RL. Blood lead concentrations <10 μ g/dL and child intelligence at 6 years of age. *Environ Health Perspect* 2008; **116**(2): 243–8.

9. Needleman H. Lead poisoning. *Annu Rev Med.* 2004; **55**: 209–22.

10. Needleman H. Low level lead exposure: history and discovery. *Ann Epidemiol* 2009; **19**(4): 235–8.

11. Lanphear BP. The conquest of lead poisoning: a pyrrhic victory. *Environ Hlth Perspect* 2007; **115**(10): A484–5.

12. Kordas K, Canfield RL, Lopez P, *et al.* Deficits in cognitive function in achievement in Mexican first-graders with low blood lead concentrations. *Environ Res* 2006; **100**: 371–86.

13. Gilbert SG, Weiss BA. A rationale for lowering the blood lead action level from 10 to 2 **μ** g/dL. *Neurotoxicology* 2006; **27**(5): 693–701.

14. Canfield RL, Gendle MH, Cory-Slechta DA. Impaired neuropsychological functioning in lead-exposed children. *Dev Neuropsychol* 2004; **26**(1): 513–40.

15. Surkan PJ, Zhang A, Trachtenberg F, Daniel DB, McKinlay S, Bellinger DC. Neuropsychological function in children with blood lead levels <10 **μ** g/dL. *Neurotoxicology* 2007; **28**(6): 1170–7.

16. Stiles K, Bellinger DC. Neueropsychological correlates of low-level lead exposure in school-age children: a prospective study. *Neurotoxicol Teratol* 1993; **15**(1): 27–35.

17. Chiodo LM, Covington C, Sokol FJ, *et al.* Blood lead levels and specific attention effects in young children. *Neurotoxicol Teratol* 2007; **29**(5): 538–46.

18. Ris MD, Dietrich KN, Succop PA, Berger OG, Bornschein RL. Early exposure to lead and neuropsychological outcome in adolescence. *J Int Neuropsychol Soc* 2004; **10**: 261–70.

19. Baghurst PA, Tong S, Sawyer MG, Burns J, McMichael AJ. Sociodemographic and behavioural determinants of blood lead concentrations in children aged 11–13 years. The Port Pirie Cohort Study. *Med J of Aust* 1999; **170**(2): 63–7.

20. Conrad ME, Umbreit JN, Moore EG, Rodning CR. Newly identified iron-binding protein in human duodenal mucosa. *Blood* 1992; **79**: 244–7.

21. Bellinger DC. Lead neurotoxicity and socioeconomic status: Conceptual and analytical issues. *Neurotoxicology* 2008; **29**(5): 828–32.

22. Hubbs-Tait L, Nation JR, Krebs NF, Bellinger DC. Neurotoxicants, micronutrients, and social environments: Individual and combined effects on children's development. *Psychol Sci Publ Interest* 2005; **6**(3): 57–121.

23. Agency for Toxic Substances and Disease Registry. *Toxicological profile for lead [paper on the internet]. US Department of Health and Human Services. 2007;* [cited 2011 June 10]. Available from: http://www.atsdr.cdc.gov/ToxProfiles/tp13.pdf.

24. Sanders T, Liu Y, Buchner V, Tchounwou PB. Neurotoxic effects and biomarkers of lead exposure: a review. *Rev of Environ Hlth* 2009; **24**(1): 15–45.

25. Cecil KM, Brubaker CH, Adler CM, *et al.* Decreased brain volume in adults with childhood lead exposure. *PLoS Med* 2008; **5**(5): 741–9.

26. Cecil KM, Dietrich KN, Altaye M, *et al.* Proton magnetic resonance spectroscopy in adults with childhood lead exposure. *Environ Hlth Perspect* 2011; **119**(3): 403–8.

27. Agency for Toxic Substances and Disease Registry (ATSDR). *Toxicological profile for PCBs. [paper on the internet]. US*

Department of Health and Human Services. 2000; [cited 2011 June 21]. Available from: http://www.atsdr.cdc.gov/ToxProfiles/tp13.pdf.

28. Schantz SL, Widholm JJ, Rice DC. Effects of PCB exposure on neuropsychological function in children. *Environ Hlth Perspect* 2003; **111**(3): 357–76.

29. Boucher O, Muckle G, Bastien CH. Prenatal exposure to polychlorinated biphenyls: A neuropsychological analysis. *Environ Hlth Perspect* 2009; **117**(1): 7–16.

30. Huisman M, Koopman-Esseboom C, Lanting CI, *et al.* Neurological conditions in 18 months-old children perinatally exposed to polychlorinated biphenyls and dioxins. *Early Hum Dev* 1995; **41**: 165–76.

31. Lonky E, Reihman J, Darvill T, Mather J Sr, Daly H. Neonatal behavioral assessment scale performance in humans influenced by maternal consumption of environmentally contaminated Lake Ontario fish. *J Great Lakes Res* 1996; **22**(2): 198–212.

32. Rogan WJ, Gladen BC, McKinney JD, *et al.* Polychlorinated biphenyls (PCBs) and dichlorodiphenyl dichloroethene (DDE) in human milk: Effects of maternal factors and previous lactation. *Am J Publ Hlth* 1986; **76**: 172–7.

33. Jacobson JL, Jacobson SW. Intellectual impairment in children exposed to polychlorinated biphenyls in utero. *N Engl J Med* 1996; **335**: 783–9.

34. Stewart PW, Lonky E, Reihman J, Pagano J, Gump BB, Darvill T. The relationship between prenatal PCB exposure and intelligence (IQ) in 9-year-old children. *Environ Hlth Perspect* 2008; **116**(10): 1416–22.

35. Jacobson JL, Jacobson SW. Prenatal exposure to polychlorinated biphenyls and attention at school age. *J Pediatr* 2003; **143**(6) 780–8.

36. Stewart P, Fitzgerald S, Reihman J, *et al.* Prenatal PCB exposure, the corpus callosum, and response inhibition. *Environ Hlth Perspect* 2003; **111**(13): 1670–7.

37. Stewart P, Reihman J, Gump B, Lonky E, Darvill T, Pagano J. Response inhibition at 8 and 9 ½ years of age

in children prenatally exposed to PCBs. *Neurotoxicol Teratol* 2005; **27**(6): 771–80.

38. Seegal FG, Bush B, Brosch KO. Comparison of effects of Aroclors 1016 and 1260 on non-human primate catecholamine function. *Toxicology* 1991; **66**(2): 145–63.

39. Seegal FG, Brosch KO, Okoniewski RJ. Effects of in utero and lactational exposure of the laboratory rat to 2,4,2',4'- and 3,4,3',4'-tetrachlorobiphenyl on dopamine function. *Toxicol Appl Pharmacol* 1997; **146**(1): 95–103

40. McMillan DE. A brief history of the neurobehavioral toxicity of manganese: Some unanswered questions. *Neurotoxicology* 1999; **20**: 499–507.

41. Wasserman GA, Liu X, Parvez F, *et al.* Water arsenic exposure and children's intellectual function in Araihazar, Bangladesh. *Environ Hlth Perspect* 2004; (**112**): 1329–33.

42. Wright RO, Amarasiriwardena C, Woolf AD, Jim R, Bellinger DC. Neuropsychological correlates of hair arsenic, manganese, and cadmium levels in school-age children residing near a hazardous waste site. *Neurotoxicology* 2006; **2**(2): 210–16.

43. Bouchard MF, Sauve S, Barbeau B, *et al.* Intellectual impairment in school-age children exposed to manganese from drinking water. *Environ Hlth Perspect* 2011; **119**(1): 138–43.

44. Crinella FM, Cordova EJ, Ericson JE. Manganese, aggression, and attention-deficit hyperactivity disorder. *Neurotoxicology* 1998; **19**(3): 468–9.

45. Bouchard M, Laforest F, Vandalac L, Bellinger D, Mergler D. Hair manganese and hyperactive behaviors: Pilot study of school-age children exposed through tap water. *Environ Hlth Perspect* 2007; **115**(1): 122–7.

46. He P, Liv DH, Zhang GG. Effects of high level manganese sewage irrigation on children's neurobehaviour. *Chung Hua Yu Fang I Hsueh Tsa Chih* 1994; **28**: 216–18.

47. Conners CK. *CADS-Parent Version*. North Tonawanda, NY: Multi-Health Systems, Inc.; 1997.

48. Conners CK. *CADS-Teacher Version*. North Tonawanda, N NY: Multi-Health Systems, Inc.; 1999.

49. Rauh VA, Garfinkel R, Perera FP, *et al.* Impact of prenatal chlorpyrifos exposure on neurodevelopment in the first 3 years of life among inner-city children. *Pediatrics* 2006; **118**(6): 1845–59.

50. Marks AR, Harley K, Bradman A, Kogut K, Barr DB, Johnson C. Organophosphate pesticide exposure and attention in young Mexican-American children: The CHAMACOS study. *Environ Hlth Perspect* 2010; **118**(2): 1768–74.

51. Bouchard MR, Chevrier J, Harley KG, *et al.* Prenatal exposure to organophosphate pesticides and IQ in 7-year-old children. *Environ Hlth Perspect* 2011; **119**(8): 1189–95.

52. Ruckart PZ, Kakolewski K, Bove FJ, Kaye WE. Long-term neurobehavioral health effects of methyl parathion exposure in children in Mississippi and Ohio. *Environ Hlth Perspect* 2004; **112**(1): 46–51.

53. Lizardi PS, O'Rourke MK, Morris RJ. The effects of organophosphate pesticide exposure on Hispanic children's cognitive and behavioral functioning. *J Pediatr Psychol* 2008; **33**(1): 91–101.

54. Banerjee TD, Middleton F, Faraone SV. Environmental risk factors for attention-deficit hyperactivity disorder. *Acta Paediatr* 2007; **96**(9): 1269–74.

55. Swanson JM, Kinsbourne M, Nigg J, *et al.* Etiologic subtypes of attention-deficit/hyperactivity disorder: brain imaging, molecular genetic and environmental factors and the dopamine hypothesis. *Neuropsychol Rev* 2007; **17**(1): 39–59.

56. Abel EL. An update on incidence of FAS: FAS is not an equal opportunity birth defect. *Neurotoxicol Teratol* 1995; **17**(4): 437–43.

57. Kodituwakku PW. Neurocognitive profile in children with fetal alcohol spectrum disorders. *Dev Disabil Res Rev* 2009; **15**(3): 218–24.

58. Green CR, Mihic AM, Nikkel SM, *et al.* Executive function deficits in children with fetal alcohol spectrum disorders (FASD) measured using the Cambridge Neuropsychological Tests Automated Battery (CANTAB). *J Child Psychol Psychiatry* 2009; **50**(6): 688–97.

59. Mattson SN, Riley EP, Auti-Ramo I. Discrimination of nondysmorphic children with prenatal alcohol exposure from nonexposed controls. *Alcohol Clin Exp Res Suppl* 2009; **33**: 7A.

60. Carmichael Olson HC, Feldman JJ, Streissguth AP, Sampson PD, Bookstein FL. Neuropsychological deficits in adolescents with fetal alcohol syndrome: clinical findings. *Alcohol Clin Exp Res* 1998; **22**(9): 1998–2012.

61. Jacobson SW, Jacobson JJ, Sokol LM, Chiodo RL, Berube S, Narang S. Preliminary evidence of working memory and attention deficits in 7-year-olds prenatally exposed to alcohol. *Alcohol Clin Exp Res* 1998; **61A**: 22.

62. Streissguth AP, Barr HM, Sampson PD. Moderate prenatal alcohol exposure: effects on child IQ and learning problems at age 7 1/2 years. *Alcohol Clin Exp Res* 1990; **14**(5): 662–9.

63. Connor PD, Sampson PD, Bookstein FL, Barr HM, Streissguth AP. Direct and indirect effects of prenatal alcohol damage on executive function. *Dev Neuropsychol* 2000; **18**(3): 331–54.

64. Kooistra L, Crawford S, Gibbard B, Ramage B, Kaplan BJ. Differentiating attention deficits in children with fetal alcohol spectrum disorder or attention-deficit-hyperactivity disorder. *Devl Med Child Neurol* 2010; **52**(2): 205–11.

65. Kodituwakku PW, Handmaker NS, Cutler SK, Weathersby EK, Handmaker SD. Specific impairments in self-regulation in children exposed to alcohol prenatally. *Alcohol Clin Exp Res* 1995; **19**(6): 1558–64.

66. Mattson SN, Goodman AM, Caine C, Delis DC, Riley EP. Executive functioning in children with heavy prenatal alcohol

exposure. *Alcohol Clin Exp Res* 1999; **23**(11): 1808–15.

67. Vaurio L, Riley EP, Mattson SN. Neuropsychological Comparison of Children with Heavy Prenatal Alcohol Exposure and an IQ-Matched Comparison Group. *J Int Neuropsychol Soc* 2011; 25;**17**: 1–11.

68. Coles CD, Platzman KA, Raskind-Hood CL, Brown RT, Falek A, Smith IE. A comparison of children affected by prenatal alcohol exposure and attention deficit, hyperactivity disorder. *Alcohol Clin Exp Res* 1997; **21**(1): 150–61.

69. Kodituwakku PW, May PA, Clericuzio CL, Weers D. Emotion-related learning in individuals prenatally exposed to alcohol: an investigation of the relation between set shifting, extinction of responses, and behavior. *Neuropsychologia* 2001; **39**(7): 699–708.

70. Noland JS, Singer LT, Arendt RE, Minnes S, Short EJ, Bearer CF. Executive functioning in preschool-age children prenatally exposed to alcohol, cocaine, and marijuana. *Alcohol Clin Exp Res* 2003; 27 (4): 647–56.

71. McGee CL, Schonfeld AM, Roebuck-Spencer TM, Riley EP, Mattson SN. Children with heavy prenatal alcohol exposure demonstrate deficits on multiple measures of concept formation. *Alcohol Clin Exp Res* 2008; **32**(8): 1388–97.

72. Schonfeld AM, Mattson SN, Lang AR, Delis DC, Riley EP. Verbal and nonverbal fluency in children with heavy prenatal alcohol exposure. *J Stud Alcohol* 2001; **62** (2): 239–46.

73. Wass TS, Persutte WH, Hobbins JC. The impact of prenatal alcohol exposure on frontal cortex development in utero. *Am J Obstet Gynecol* 2001; **185**(3): 737–42.

74. Sowell ER, Thompson PM, Mattson SN, *et al.* Regional brain shape abnormalities persist into adolescence after heavy prenatal alcohol exposure. *Cereb Cortex* 2002; **12**(8): 856–65.

75. Coles CD, Goldstein FC, Lynch ME, *et al.* Memory and brain volume in adults prenatally exposed to alcohol. *Brain Cogn* 2011; **75**(1): 67–77.

76. Knight RG, Longmore BE. *Clinical Neuropsychology of Alcoholism*. Hove, UK: Lawrence J. Erlbaum Associates; 1994.

77. Brown SA, Tapert SF, Granholm EG, Delis DC. Neurocognitive functioning of adolescents: effects of protracted alcohol use. *Alcohol Clin Exp Res* 2000; **24**(2): 164–71.

78. Glass JM, Buu A, Adams KM, *et al.* Effects of alcoholism severity and smoking on executive neurocognitive function. *Addiction* 2009; **104**(1): 38–48.

79. Gogtay N, Thompson PM. Mapping gray matter development: Implications for typical development and vulnerability to psychopathology. *Brain Cogn* 2010; **72**(1): 6–15.

80. Guerri C, Pascual M. Mechanisms involved in the neurotoxic, cognitive, and neurobehavioral effects of alcohol consumption during adolescence. *Alcohol* 2010; **44**: 15–26.

81. Giancola P, Moss H. Executive cognition functioning in alcohol use disorders. In Galanter M, ed. *Recent Developments in Alcoholism: The Consequences of Alcoholism*. New York: Plenum Press; 1998, 227–51.

82. Nigg JT, Wong MM, Martel MA, *et al.* Poor response inhibition as a predictor of problem drinking and illicit drug use in adolescents at risk for alcoholism and other substance use disorders. *J Am Acad Child Adolesc Psychiatry* 2006; **45**(4): 468–75.

83. Tapert SF, Brown SA. Substance dependence, family history of alcohol dependence and neuropsychological functioning in adolescence. *Addiction* 2000; **95**(7): 1043–53.

84. Moss HB, Kirisci L, Gordon HW, Tarter RE. A neuropsychologic profile of adolescent alcoholics. *Alcohol Clin Exp Res* 1994; **18**(1): 159–63.

85. Eckardt M, Stapleton J, Rawlings R, Davis EZ, Grodin DM. Neuropsychological functioning in detoxified alcoholics between 18 and 35 years of age. *Am J Psychiatry* 1995; **152**: 53–9.

86. Medina KL, McQueeny T, Nagel BJ, Hanson KL, Schweinsburg AD, Tapert SF. Prefrontal cortex volumes in adolescents with alcohol use disorders: Unique gender effects. *Alcohol Clin Exp Res* 2008; **32**(3): 386–94.

87. Tapert SF, Schweinsburg AD, Barlett VC, et al. BOLD response and spatial working memory in adolescents with alcohol use disorders. *Alcohol Clin Exp Res* 2004; **28**(10): 1577–86.

88. Squeglia LM, Jacobus J, Tapert SF. The influence of substance use on adolescent brain development. *Clin EEG Neurosci* 2009; **40**(1): 31–8.

89. Richardson GA, Day NL, Taylor PM. The effect of prenatal alcohol, marijuana, and tobacco exposure on neonatal behavior. *Infant Behav Dev* 1989; **12**(2): 199–209.

90. Fried PA. Prenatal exposure to marihuana and tobacco during infancy, early and middle childhood: Effects and an attempt at synthesis. *Arch Toxicol Suppl* 1995; **17**: 233–60.

91. Day NL, Richardson GA, Goldschmidt L, et al. Effect of prenatal marijuana exposure on the cognitive development of offspring at age three. *Neurotoxicol Teratol* 1994; **16**(2): 169–75.

92. Griffith DR, Azuma SD, Chasnoff IJ. Three-year outcome of children exposed prenatally to drugs. *J Am Acad Child Adolesc Psychiatry* 1994; **33**(1): 20–7.

93. Fried PA, Watkinson B, Gray R. Differential effects on cognitive functioning 9- to 12-year olds prenatally exposed to cigarettes and marijuana. *Neurotoxicol Teratol* 1998; **20**(3): 293–306.

94. Richardson GA, Day NL. A comparison of the effects of prenatal marijuana, alcohol, and cocaine use on 10-year child outcome. *Neurotoxicol Teratol* 1997; **19**(3): 257–7(1).

95. Leech SI, Richardson GA, Goldschmidt L, Day NI. Prenatal substance exposure: Effects on attention and impulsivity of 6-year-olds. *Neurotoxicol Teratol* 1999; **21**(2): 109–18.

96. Fried, PA, Watkinson B, Gray R. A follow-up study of attentional behavior in 6-year-old children exposed prenatally to marihuana, cigarettes, and alcohol. *Neurotoxicol Teratol* 1992; **14**(5): 299–311.

97. Fried PA, Watkinson B. Differential effects on facets of attention in adolescents prenatally exposed to cigarettes and marihuana. *Neurotoxicol Teratol* 2001; **23**(5): 421–30.

98. Goldschmidt L, Day NL, Richardson GA. Effects of prenatal marijuana exposure on child behavior problems at age 10. *Neurotoxicol Teratol* 2000; **22**: 325–36.

99. Derauf C, Kekatpure M, Neyzi N, Lester B, Kosofsky B. Neuroimaging of children following prenatal drug exposure. *Semin Cell Dev Biol* 2009; **20**(4): 441–54.

100. Tanda G, Goldberg SR. Cannabinoids: reward, dependence, and underlying neurochemical mechanisms – a review of recent preclinical data. *Psychopharmacology* 2003; **169**(2): 115–34.

101. Ameri A. The effects of cannabinoids on the brain. *Prog Neurobiol* 1999; **58**(4): 315–48.

102. Rivkin MJ, Davis PE, Lemaster JL, et al. Volumetric MRI study of brain in children with intrauterine exposure to cocaine, alcohol, tobacco, and marijuana. *Pediatrics* 2008; **121**(4): 741–50.

103. Smith AB, Taylor E, Brammer M, Rubia K. The neural correlates of switching set as measured in fast, event-related functional magnetic resonance imaging. *Hum Brain Mapp* 2004; **21**: 247–56.

104. Smith AB, Taylor E, Brammer M, Toone B, Rubia K. Task-specific hypoactivation in prefrontal and temporoparietal brain regions during motor inhibition and task switching in medication-naïve children and adolescents with attention deficit hyperactivity disorder. *Am J Psychiatry* 2006; **163**(6): 1044–51.

105. Loeber RT, Yurgelun-Todd DA. Human neuroimaging of acute and chronic marijuana use: Implications for frontocerebellar dysfunction. *Hum Psychopharmacol: Clin Exp* 1999; **14**: 291–304.

106. Kanayama G, Rogowska J, Pope HG, Gruber SA, Yurgelun-Todd DA. Spatial working memory in heavy cannabis users: A functional magnetic resonance imaging study. *Psychopharmacology* 2004; **16**: 16.

107. Bolla KO, Brown K, Eldreth D, Tate K, Cadet JL. Dose-related neurocognitive effects of marijuana use. *Neurology* 2002; **59**: 1337–43.

108. Pope Jr HG., Gruber AJ, Hudson JI, Huestis MA, Yurgelun-Todd DA. Neuropsychological performance in long-term cannabis users. *Arch Gen Psychiatry* 2001; **58**(10): 909–15.

109. Medina KL, McQueeny T, Nagel BJ, Hanson KL, Yang T, Tapert SF. Prefrontal cortex morphometry in abstinent adolescent marijuana users: Subtle gender effects. *Addict Biol* 2009; **14**: 457–68.

110. Padula CB, Schweinsburg AD, Tapert SF. Spatial working memory performance and fMRI activation interactions in abstinent adolescent marijuana users. *Psychol Addict Behav* 2007; **21**(4): 478–87.

111. Schweinsburg AD, Schweinsburg BC, Medina KL, McQueeny T, Brown SA, Tapert SF. The influence of recency of use on fMRI response during spatial working memory in adolescent marijuana users. *J Psychoactive Drugs* 2010; **42**(3): 401–12.

112. Medina KL, Nagel BJ, Tapert SF. Abnormal cerebellar morphometry in abstinent adolescent marijuana users. *Psychiatry Res* 2010; **182**(2): 152–9.

113. Accornero VH, Amado AJ, Morrow CE, Xue L, Anthony JC, Bandstra ES. Impact of prenatal cocaine exposure on attention and response inhibition as assessed by continuous performance tests. *J Dev Behav Pediatr* 2007; **28**(3): 195–205.

114. Ackerman JP, Llorente AM, Black MM, Ackerman CS, Mayes LA, Nair P. The effect of prenatal drug exposure and caregiving context on children's performance on a task of sustained visual attention. *J Dev Behav Pediatr* 2011; **29**(6): 467–74.

115. Bandstra ES, Morrow CE, Anthony JC, Accornero VH, Fried PA. Longitudinal investigation of task persistence and sustained attention in children with prenatal cocaine exposure. *Neurotoxicol Teratol* 2001; **23**: 545–59.

116. Noland JS, Singer LT, Short EJ, et al. Prenatal drug exposure and selective attention in preschoolers. *Neurotoxicol Teratol* 2005; **27**(3): 429–38.

117. Savage J, Brodsky N, Malmud Elsa, Giannetaa JM, Hurt H. Attentional functioning and impulse control in cocaine-exposed and control children at age ten years. *J Dev Behav Pediatr* 2005; **26**(1): 42–7.

118. Richardson GA, Conroy ML, Day NL. Prenatal cocaine exposure: Effects on the development of school-age children. *Neurotoxicol Teratol* 1996; **18**(6): 627–34.

119. Schroder MD, Snyder PJ, Sielski I, Mayes L. Impaired performance of children exposed in utero to cocaine on a novel test of visuospatial working memory. *Brain and Cogn* 2004; **55**(2): 409–12.

120. Bendersky M, Gambini G, Lastella A, Bennett DS, Lewis M. Inhibitory motor control at five years as a function of prenatal cocaine exposure. *J Dev Behav Pediatr* 2003; **24**(5): 345–51.

121. Rose-Jacobs R, Waber D, Beeghly M, et al. Intrauterine cocaine exposure and executive functioning in middle childhood. *Neurotoxicol Teratol* 2009; **31**(3): 159–68.

122. Harvey JA, Romano AG, Gabriel M, et al. Effects of prenatal exposure to cocaine on the developing brain: anatomical, chemical, physiological and behavioral consequences. *Neurotox Res* 2001; **3**(1): 117–43.

123. Malanga CJ, Kosofksy BE. Mechanisms of action of drugs of abuse on the developing fetal brain. *Clin Perinatol* 1999; **26**(1): 17–37.

124. Mayes LC. Developing brain and in utero cocaine exposure: effects of neural ontogeny. *Dev Psychopathol* 1999; **11**: 685–714.

125. Avants BB, Hurt H, Giannetta JM, et al. Effects of heavy in utero cocaine exposure on adolescent caudate morphology. *Pediatr Neurol* 2007; **37**(4): 275–9.

126. Singer LT, Nelson S, Short E, *et al*. Prenatal cocaine exposure: Drug and environmental effects at 9 years. *J Pediatr* 2008; **153**(1): 105–11.

127. Warner TD, Behnke M, Eyler FD, *et al*. Diffusion tensor imaging of frontal white matter and executive functioning in cocaine-exposed children. *Pediatrics* 2006; **118**(5): 2014–24.

128. Rao H, Wang J, Gianetta J, *et al*. Altered resting cerebral blood flow in adolescents with in utero cocaine exposure revealed by perfusion functional MRI. *Pediatrics* 2007; **120**(5): 1245–54.

129. Hurt H, Gianetta JM, Korczykowski M, *et al*. Functional magnetic resonance imaging and working memory in adolescents with gestational cocaine exposure. *J Pediatr* 2008; **152**(3): 371–7.

130. Sheinkopf SJ, Lester BM, Sanes JN, *et al*. Functional MRI and response inhibition in children exposed to cocaine in utero. *Dev Neurosci* 2009: **31**(1–2): 159–66.

131. Bennett D, Bendersky M, Lewis M. Preadolescent health risk behavior as a function of prenatal cocaine exposure and gender. *J Dev Behav Pediatr* 2007; **28**(6): 467–72.

132. Warner TD, Behnke M, Davis Eyler F, Szabo NJ. Early adolescent cocaine use as determined by hair analysis in a prenatal cocaine exposure cohort. *Neurotoxicol Teratol* 2011; **33**(1): 88–99.

133. Rose-Jacobs R, Soenksen S, Appugliese DP, *et al*. Early adolescent executive functioning, intrauterine exposures and own drug use. *Neurotoxicol Teratol* 2011; **33**(3): 379–92.

134. Stroud LR, Paster RL, Papandonatos GD, *et al*. Maternal smoking during pregnancy and newborn neurobehavior: a pilot study of effects at 10–27 days. *J Pediatr* 2009; **154**(1): 10–16.

135. Mansi G, Raimondi F, Pichini S, *et al*. Neonatal urinary cotinine correlates with behavioral alterations in newborns prenatally exposed to tobacco smoke. *Pediatr Res* 2007; **61**(2): 257–61.

136. Wiebe SA, Espy KA, Stopp C, *et al*. Gene-environment interactions across development: Exploring DRD2 genotype and prenatal smoking effects on self-regulation. *Dev Psychol* 2009; **45**(1): 31–44.

137. Carter S, Paterson J, Gao W, Iusitini L. Maternal smoking during pregnancy and behaviour problems in a birth cohort of 2-year-old Pacific children in New Zealand. *Early Hum Dev* 3008; **84**(1): 59–66.

138. Cornelius MD, Goldschmidt L, DeGenna N, Day NL. Smoking during teenage pregnancies: Effects on behavioral problems in offspring. *Nicotine Tob Res* 2007; **9**(7): 739–50.

139. Cornelius MD, De Genna NM, Leech SL, Willford AJ, Goldschmidt L, Day NL. Effects of prenatal cigarette smoke exposure on neurobehavioral outcomes in 10-year-old children of adolescent mothers. *Neurotoxicol Teratol* 2011; **33**: 137–44.

140. Langley K, Holmans PA, van den Bree M, Thaper A. Effects of low birth weight, maternal smoking in pregnancy and social class on the phenotypic manifestation of Attention Deficit Hyperactivity Disorder and associated antisocial behaviour: investigation in a clinical sample. *BMC Psychiatry [serial on the Internet]*. 2007; [cited 2011 November 27] 7(26). Available from: http://www.biomedcentral.com/1471-244X/7/26.

141. Kallen K. Maternal smoking during pregnancy and infant head circumference at birth. *Obst Gynecolo Surv* 2001; **56**(5): 262–3.

142. Shankaran S, Das A, Bauer CR, *et al*. Association between patterns of maternal substance abuse and the infant birth weight and head circumference. *Pediatrics* 2004; **114**(2): e226–34.

143. Toro R, Leonard G, Lerner JV, *et al*. Prenatal exposure to maternal cigarette smoking and the adolescent cerebral cortex. *Neuropsychopharmacology* 2008; **33**: 1019–27.

144. Jacobsen LK, Picciotto MR, Heath CJ, Frost SJ, Tsou KA, Dwan RA, *et al*. Prenatal and adolescent exposure to tobacco smoke modulates the development of white matter

microstructure. *J Neurosci* 2007; **27**(49): 13491–8.

145. Becker K, El-Faddagh M, Schmidt MH, Esser G, Launcht M. Interaction of dopamine transporter genotype with prenatal smoke exposure on ADHD symptoms. *J Pediatr* 2008; **152**(2): 263–9.

146. Neuman RJ, Lobos E, Reich W, Henderson CA, Sun LW, Todd RD. Prenatal smoking exposure and dopaminergic genotypes interact to cause a severe ADHD subtype. *Biol Psychiatry* 2007; **61**(12): 1320–8.

147. Wakschlag LS, Kistner EO, Pine DS, Biesecker G, Pickett KE, Skol A. Interaction of prenatal exposure to cigarettes and MAOA genotype in pathways to youth antisocial behavior. *Mol Psychiatry* 2010; **15**(9): 928–37.

148. Eyler FD, Warner TD, Behnke M, Hou W, Wobie K, Garvan CW. Executive functioning at ages 5 and 7 in children with prenatal cocaine exposure. *Dev Neurosci* 2009; **31**(1–2): 121–36.

149. Heffelfinger A, Craft S, Shyken J. Visual attention in children with prenatal cocaine exposure. *J Int Neuropsychol Soc* 1997; **3**(3): 237–45.

Chapter

15

Executive functions after congenital and prenatal insults

Jillian M. Schuh and Scott J. Hunter

The pre- and perinatal period of development is an especially sensitive time during which stress and insults to the brain can set in place a series of influences on the developmental trajectory of EF. Issues such as prematurity, extremely low birthweight, anoxic/hypoxic and ischemic events, spina bifida/myelomeningocele, hydrocephalus, and prenatal exposure to toxins (see Chapter 14) all provide illustrations of the impact of early insults on the developing brain. With the advancement of medical science, more children with these issues are surviving than ever before. As a result, there is a need to better understand the specific cognitive profiles associated with these complications that often occur during periods of brain development that are critical for EF, particularly when the medical concerns are ongoing.

Prematurity and low birthweight

Extreme prematurity and low birthweight are associated with variability in the development of EF, and also put an infant at greater risk for other medical conditions, such as hemorrhaging, that further implicate the ontogeny of executive processes. Better prenatal care, along with the use of exogenous surfactant in the neonatal period, has allowed many children born extremely early to survive past infancy into childhood.[1] Variations in gestational age and birthweight at the time of delivery create a spectrum of impact, resulting in effects on cognitive development that range from subtle to profound.

Long-term effects of prematurity and low birthweight on EF development vary, with more pronounced limitations for earlier births and lighter birthweights.[2–4] Birthweight between 500 to 750 grams is associated with poorer performance on EF measures than weights between 750 to 999 grams. Likewise, children born before 26 weeks gestational age perform more poorly than those born between 26 to 27 weeks.[5]

Specific EF deficits identified in this population include planning,[2,5–7] verbal conceptual reasoning,[5] inhibition and motor sequencing,[6] and WM (both spatial and verbal);[5,7,8,9–11] Spatial EF appear more impacted than verbal, particularly visual reasoning, spatial conceptualization, visual organization, and spatial WM.[2,5,7] Many of these studies did not control for general cognitive abilities, and comparison groups had significantly higher cognitive abilities.[5,12] However, studies that have explored the relationship between EF and general intelligence have found only weak associations.[6] One study found children with a history of low birthweight performed more poorly than their normal birthweight peers on the

ROCF, even when controlling for cognitive ability (IQ > 85), providing support for a domain-specific impact of prematurity and low birthweight on EF.

Prematurity is also associated with greater risk for cerebral and subcortical injuries, such as intraventricular hemorrhage (IVH) and periventricular leukomalacia (PVL), that can further impact cognition and EF. Approximately 33% of children born premature or of extremely low birthweight (ELBW; i.e., birthweight under 1000 grams) experience IVH.[12] A study of very preterm (born at gestational age ≤ 28 weeks) and ELBW children at 8 years of age found that grade IV (most severe) IVH was associated with intellectual disability and impaired WM, planning, and spatial organization; there was a trend for children with grade III IVH to have EdF in the context of average intellect. Children with grades I and II IVH performed similarly to those with no history of IVH.[12] The EF deficits identified in more severe IVH may be related to anatomical compromise commonly noted in IVH, such as compression or thinning of cerebral white matter (especially the corpus callosum), damage to the projection pathways, and infarction to the motor, frontal, and posterior pathways.[12]

PVL occurs in approximately 3 to 4% of infants with very low birthweight (VLBW, or birthweight between 1000–1500 grams), and is characterized by focal or diffuse lesions in cerebral white matter.[13–15] Anatomical differences evident in the neonatal period include decreases in cerebral cortical gray matter, reductions in myelinated white matter volume, and compensatory increases in CSF compared with children born premature without PVL and full-term infants.[16] A study of 2 year-olds using a modified A-not-B task found toddlers with a history of prematurity took longer to learn the task and were twice as likely to make errors, suggesting a failure to encode and retain spatial information). Children with no history of IVH or PVL were six times more likely to successfully complete the task than those with IVH or PVL, highlighting the importance of localized connections for memory function.[17]

Neuroimaging studies exploring structural differences associated with prematurity and low birthweight have indicated decreased volume in the cerebral cortex, basal ganglia, amygdala, hippocampus, and corpus callosum, with increases in the lateral ventricles.[5,8,18,19] Differences remained in white matter structures, subcortical gray matter, and cerebellum even when controlling for whole brain volume, and were most pronounced for children of ELBW.[19] In a longitudinal study exploring brain growth from adolescence through early adulthood, cerebellar volumes decreased 3.11% by adulthood for those born very preterm (vs. remaining stable in full-term controls); cerebellar volume at adulthood was related to decision making capacity.[18]

Anoxia, hypoxia, and ischemia

Approximately 2.9 to 9 in 1000 infants experience ischemic insults during the perinatal period,[20] which can be secondary to direct hypoxia/anoxia, prematurity, or ELBW. In an autopsy study of 1152 infants who died by 3 months of age, there was evidence of brain hemorrhage in 40 to 50% of preterm infants and far fewer in full-term infants, white matter infarction (i.e., PVL) in 35 to 49% of preterm and 28% of full-term infants, and cortical damage in 14% of preterm and 37% of full-term infants.[21] Smaller and more recent autopsy studies report similar rates.[22,23] Prenatal risk factors for ischemia include twin pregnancies, placental dysfunction, prolonged labor, and premature birth; during the neonatal period, risks include cardiorespiratory resuscitation and surgical interventions.[20,24–26]

Ischemic events typically develop into neonatal encephalopathy.[27] In an animal model of neonatal encephalopathy, rats who experienced intermittent hypoxic insults during a critical period in development (equivalent to 32 to 36 weeks gestational age in humans) showed impairments in WM.[28] One human study showed that 7-year-olds with severe neonatal encephalopathy exhibited EdF (as measured by the NEPSY Attention/Executive Function tasks) relative to those with moderate encephalopathy and healthy controls; there was a trend for EdF in children with moderate neonatal encephalopathy relative to controls, suggesting a spectrum of EF depending on the severity of the infarction.[27] In addition to severity, age of insult also leads to variability in EF, as vascular insults occurring prior to 3 years of age result in more global and severe effects on EF than insults later in childhood.[29]

Spina bifida and related congenital anomalies

Spina bifida, one of the most common congenital malformations, occurs in approximately 1 in 1000 births.[30] Approximately 70 to 90% of individuals with spina bifida have myelo-meningocele (SBM),[30,31] where the spinal cord, meninges, and nerve roots protrude through an opening in the spine.[32] SBM affects the CNS well beyond the level of the lesion, and results in persisting effects throughout development. It is associated with a host of orthopedic, urinary/bowel, and neurologic complications.[33]

The most common brain anomaly in SBM is Arnold–Chiari Type II malformation, a deformity of the brainstem and cerebellum where the flow of CSF in the third and/or fourth ventricles becomes obstructed.[34] In 80 to 90% of cases this anomaly leads to congenital hydrocephalus that typically requires placement of a shunt.[35] The buildup of CSF can enlarge the ventricles, causing stretching of nearby white matter tracts. In particular, hydrocephalus frequently damages frontal-subcortical white matter tracts, circuitry crucial to EF that allows for communication between the PFC and other regions of the brain.[36,37] Hydrocephalus is also associated with thinning of the cortex, particularly the corpus callosum and posterior regions.[38,39] Malformations of the corpus callosum may also result from abnormal neuronal migration.[40] Partial agenesis (i.e., dysgenesis) of the corpus callosum occurs in nearly half of the cases of SBM;[34,41] complete agenesis is less common.[42]

SBM is associated with average to low-average intellect;[43] EdF is observed even when controlling for cognitive ability, including mental flexibility, problem-solving, WM (both verbal and visual domains), and attention focus and shifting.[32,36,44–49] Studies using the BRIEF parent report have found that adolescents with SBM often show deficits in meta-cognitive abilities (planning, WM, and organization) relative to healthy peers; however, these limitations may be subtle, as they do not fall in the clinically significant range relative to normative data.[32,33,42,50,51] Less consistent results have been found for behavioral regulation, with some studies indicating greater difficulty relative to healthy peers,[33,42] while others demonstrate no significant differences.[50] Children with SBM and ADHD were rated as more dysexecutive than those with SBM who did not have ADHD.[32] EdF has been associated with social adjustment difficulties in adolescents with SBM[51] and with delayed or absent attainment of milestones such as leaving home and attending college.[52]

The neurocognitive profile of SBM often is complicated by associated medical and environmental factors. Severity of EdF is related to a history of shunt-related proced-ures,[33,51,53,54] suggesting a link between impairment and potential damage to white matter association tracts and surrounding regions. History of CNS infection, oculomotor abnormalities, and agenesis of the corpus callosum are also related to EdF.[53] Hydrocephalus, regardless of the presence of SBM, is associated with EdF.[55] Environmental factors such as SES,[53] social adjustment,[51] and parental/familial stress[56–58] are related to the degree of EdF in SBM.

Because SBM and hydrocephalus are commonly associated with insults to the brainstem, cerebellum, and posterior brain regions,[59] researchers have suggested that executive limitations may be more attributable to dysfunction of broader arousal and attentional networks rather than frank insults to traditional "frontal" circuitry. Behavioral data support this theory; for example, children with SBM perform more poorly on the Stroop task due to speed of naming rather than inhibition. In addition, on tasks of problem solving such as the Tower of London or WCST, children with SBM do not differ from controls in their ability to complete the task, but rather demonstrate decreased efficiency in their problem-solving.[36]

Summary and future directions

The neonatal and perinatal period is an especially sensitive time for the development of early foundational networks that later give rise to EF. Insults during this time have specific and persistent effects on EF that remain even after adjusting for general cognitive abilities. The extent of impairment ranges from subtle to profound, creating a spectrum of EdF across conditions. EF tends to be more severely implicated for those born earlier and of lower birth weight, for cerebral injuries of greater severity (e.g., grade IV IVH), and for those with additional medical complications (as in the case of spina bifida). Across congenital anomalies, decreases in brain volume are noted, along with specific impairments in WM. EdF is pervasive across conditions, raising the question of whether there is one particular pattern of cognitive insult or rather several combinations of symptoms that can lead to a general disruption in EF. In addition, it is also important to consider bidirectional effects of EdF, as early deficits likely hinder future learning and cognitive development.

Several directions are important for future research. First, many of these conditions are intimately linked and serve as risk factors for later complications, making it particularly difficult to parse individual contributions to EdF (as in the case of IVH and ischemic events). In addition, ongoing medical treatments, such as shunt placements and revisions for SBM, further complicate the picture of executive decline. Future research will need to consider the relative contribution of these factors to executive development. Second, the majority of research on congenital and prenatal issues focuses on outcome in the school-age and adolescent years, overlooking early childhood and adulthood outcomes. With more children surviving into adulthood, there is a growing need to better understand the full developmental trajectory, particularly the impact of EdF on social and adaptive functioning. Finally, as discussed in Chapter 17, additional research should explore interventions most effective for overcoming executive weakness due to congenital and prenatal issues.

In summary, it is essential to consider the effects of congenital anomalies beyond simply general intelligence. Many subtle learning difficulties noted in these populations may be attributable to weaknesses in EF. EdF may manifest during the school-age and adolescent years as poor organization, difficulty following complex instruction, or struggling to acquire and integrate information. Due to the complex and often persistent nature of these conditions, consideration for the interplay of multiple medical and neurological complications is crucial. Congenital and prenatal insults occur in the earliest moments of development, and have long-lasting impacts on EF that persist throughout the lifespan.

References

1. Volpe J. *Neurology of the Newborn.* 4th edn. Philadelphia: Saunders; 2001.

2. Taylor HG, Minich N, Bangert B, Filipek PA, Hack M. Long-term neuropsychological outcomes of very low birth weight: associations with early risks for periventricular brain insults. *J Int Neuropsychol Soc* 2004; 10(7): 987–1004.

3. Taylor HG, Hack M, Klein N. Attention deficits in children wtih < 750 gm birth weight. *Child Neuropsychol* 1998; 4: 21–34.

4. Waber DP, McCormick MC. Late neuropsychological outcomes in preterm infants of normal IQ: selective vulnerability of the visual system. *J Pediatr Psychol* 1995; 20(6): 721–35.

5. Anderson PJ, Doyle LW, Group VICS. Executive functioning in school-aged children who were born very preterm or with extremely low birth weight in the 1990s. *Pediatrics* 2004; 114: 50–7.

6. Harvey JM, O'Callaghan MJ, Mohay H. Executive function of children with extremely low birthweight: a case control study. *Dev Med Child Neurol* 1999; 41(5): 292–7.

7. Luciana M, Lindeke L, Georgieff M, Mills M, Nelson CA. Neurobehavioral evidence for working-memory deficits in school-aged children with histories of prematurity. *Dev Med Child Neurol* 1999; 41(8): 521–33.

8. Isaacs EB, Lucas A, Chong WK, *et al.* Hippocampal volume and everyday memory in children of very low birth weight. *Pediatr Res* 2000; 47(6): 713–20.

9. Rose SA, Feldman JF. Memory and processing speed in preterm children at eleven years: a comparison with full-terms. *Child Dev* 1996; 67(5): 2005–21.

10. Ross G, Boatright S, Auld PA, Nass R. Specific cognitive abilities in 2-year-old children with subependymal and mild intraventricular hemorrhage. *Brain Cogn* 1996; 32(1): 1–13.

11. Vicari S, Caravale B, Carlesimo GA, Casadei AM, Allemand F. Spatial working memory deficits in children at ages 3–4 who were low birth weight, preterm infants. *Neuropsychology* 2004; 18(4): 673–8.

12. Sherlock RL, Anderson PJ, Doyle LW. Neurodevelopmental sequelae of intraventricular haemorrhage at 8 years of age in a regional cohort of ELBW/very preterm infants. *Early Hum Dev* 2005; 81(11): 909–16.

13. Leviton A, Paneth N. White matter damage in preterm newborns – an epidemiologic perspective. *Early Hum Dev* 1990; 24(1): 1–22.

14. Volpe JJ. *Neurology of the Newborn.* Philadelphia, PA: Saunders; 1995.

15. de Vries LS, Regev R, Dubowitz LM, Whitelaw A, Aber VR. Perinatal risk factors for the development of extensive cystic leukomalacia. *Am J Dis Child* 1988; 142(7): 732–5.

16. Inder TE, Huppi PS, Warfield S, *et al.* Periventricular white matter injury in the premature infant is followed by reduced cerebral cortical gray matter volume at term. *Ann Neurol* 1999; 46(5): 755–60.

17. Woodward LJ, Edgin JO, Thompson D, Inder TE. Object working memory deficits predicted by early brain injury and development in the preterm infant. *Brain* 2005; 128(11): 2578–87.

18. Parker J, Mitchell A, Kalpakidou A, Walshe M, Jung HY, Nosarti C, *et al.* Cerebellar growth and behavioural & neuropsychological outcome in preterm adolescents. *Brain* 2008; 131(Pt 5): 1344–51.

19. Taylor HG, Filipek PA, Juranek J, Bangert B, Minich N, Hack M. Brain volumes in adolescents with very low birth weight: effects on brain structure and associations with neuropsychological outcomes. *Dev Neuropsychol* 2011; 36(1): 96–117.

20. Tuor UI, Del Bigio MR, Chumas PD. Brain damage due to cerebral hypoxia/ischemia in the neonate: pathology and pharmacological modification. *Cerebrovasc Brain Metab Rev* 1996; 8(2): 159–93.

21. Terplan KL. Histopathologic brain changes in 1152 cases of the perinatal and early infancy period. *Biol Neonate* 1967; 11: 348–66.

22. Leech RW, Olson MI, Alvord EC, Jr. Neuropathologic features of idiopathic respiratory distress syndrome. *Arch Pathol Lab Med* 1979; **103**(7): 341–3.

23. Squier M, Keeling JW. The incidence of prenatal brain injury. *Neuropathol Appl Neurobiol* 1991; **17**(1): 29–38.

24. Nyakas C, Buwalda B, Luiten PG. Hypoxia and brain development. *Prog Neurobiol* 1996; **49**(1): 1–51.

25. Vannucci RC. Perinatal hypoxic/ischemic encephalopathy. *Neurologist* 1995; 1: 35–52.

26. Towbin A. Central nervous system damage in the human fetus and newborn infant. Mechanical and hypoxic injury incurred in the fetal-neonatal period. *Am J Dis Child* 1970; **119**(6): 529–42.

27. Marlow N, Rose AS, Rands CE, Draper ES. Neuropsychological and educational problems at school age associated with neonatal encephalopathy. *Arch Dis Child Fetal Neonatal Ed* 2005; **90**(5): F380–7.

28. Decker MJ, Hue GE, Caudle WM, Miller GW, Keating GL, Rye DB. Episodic neonatal hypoxia evokes executive dysfunction and regionally specific alterations in markers of dopamine signaling. *Neuroscience* 2003; **117**(2): 417–25.

29. Anderson V, Spencer-Smith M, Coleman L, *et al.* Children's executive functions: are they poorer after very early brain insult. *Neuropsychologia* 2010; **48**(7): 2041–50.

30. Charney E. Neural tube defects: Spina bifida and myelomeningocele. In Batshaw M, Perret Y, eds. *Children with Disabilities: A Medical Primer.* 3rd edn. Baltimore, MD: Brooks Publishing Company; 1992, 471–88.

31. Norman MG. *Congenital Malformations of the Brain: Pathologic, Embryologic, Clinical, Radiologic, and Genetic Aspects.* New York: Oxford University Press; 1995.

32. Burmeister R, Hannay HJ, Copeland K, Fletcher JM, Boudousquie A, Dennis M. Attention problems and executive functions in children with spina bifida and hydrocephalus. *Child Neuropsychol* 2005; **11**(3): 265–83.

33. Brown TM, Ris MD, Beebe D, *et al.* Factors of biological risk and reserve associated with executive behaviors in children and adolescents with spina bifida myelomeningocele. *Child Neuropsychol* 2008; **14**(2): 118–34.

34. Barkovich AJ. *Pediatric Neuroimaging.* 3rd edn. Philadelphia, PA: Lippincott Williams and Wilkins; 2000.

35. Reigel DH, Rotenstein D. Spina bifida. In Cheek WR, ed. *Pediatric Neurosurgery.* 3rd edn. Philadelphia, PA: Saunders, WB.; 1994, 51–76.

36. Fletcher JM, Brookshire BL, Landry SH, Bohan TP. Attentional skills and executive functions in children with early hydrocephalus. *Dev Neuropsychol* 1996; **12**(1): 53–76.

37. Denckla MB. A theory and model of executive function: a neuropsychological perspective. In Lyon GR, Krasnegor NA, eds. *Attention, Memory, and Executive Function.* Baltimore: Brookes; 1996, 263–78.

38. Fletcher JM, McCauley SR, Brandt ME, *et al.* Regional brain tissue composition in children with hydrocephalus. Relationships with cognitive development. *Arch Neurol* 1996; **53**(6): 549–57.

39. Fletcher JM, Dennis M, Northrup H. Hydrocephalus. In Yeates KO, Ris MD, Taylor HG, eds. *Pediatric Neuropsychology: Research, Theory, and Practice.* New York: Guilford Press; 2000, 25–46.

40. Wills KE. Neuropsychological functioning in children with spina bifida and/or hydrocephalus. *J Clin Child Psychol* 1993; **22**(2): 247–65.

41. Hannay HJ. Functioning of the corpus callosum in children with early hydrocephalus. *J Int Neuropsychol Soc* 2000; **6**(3): 351–61.

42. Tarazi RA, Zabel TA, Mahone EM. Age-related differences in executive function among children with spina bifida/hydrocephalus based on parent behavior ratings. *Clin Neuropsychol* 2008; **22**(4): 585–602.

43. Wills KE, Holmbeck GN, Dillon K, McLone DG. Intelligence and achievement in children with myelomeningocele. *J Pediatr Psychol* 1990; **15**(2): 161–76.

44. Brewer VR, Fletcher JM, Hiscock M, Davidson KC. Attention processes in children with shunted hydrocephalus versus attention deficit-hyperactivity disorder. *Neuropsychology* 2001; **15**(2): 185–98.

45. Holmbeck GN, Westhoven VC, Phillips WS, *et al.* A multimethod, multi-informant, and multidimensional perspective on psychosocial adjustment in preadolescents with spina bifida. *J Cons Clin Psychol* 2003; **71**(4): 782–96.

46. Landry SH, Robinson SS, Copeland D, Garner PW. Goal-directed behavior and perception of self-competence in children with spina bifida. *J Pediatr Psychol* 1993; **18**(3): 389–96.

47. Snow JH. Executive processes for children with spina bifida. *Children's Hlth Care* 1999; **28**(3): 241–53.

48. Yeates KO, Enrile BG, Loss N, Blumenstein E, Delis DC. Verbal learning and memory in children with myelomeningocele. *J Pediatr Psychol* 1995; **20**(6): 801–15.

49. Mammarella N, Cornoldi C, Donadello E. Visual but not spatial working memory deficit in children with spina bifida. *Brain Cogn* 2003; **53**(2): 311–14.

50. Mahone EM, Zabel TA, Levey E, Verda M, Kinsman S. Parent and self-report ratings of executive function in adolescents with myelomeningocele and hydrocephalus. *Child Neuropsychol* 2002; **8**(4): 258–70.

51. Rose BM, Holmbeck GN. Attention and executive functions in adolescents with spina bifida. *J Pediatr Psychol* 2007; **32**(8): 983–94.

52. Zukerman JM, Devine KA, Holmbeck GN. Adolescent predictors of emerging adulthood milestones in youth with spina bifida. *J Pediatr Psychol* 2010; **36**(3): 265–76.

53. Loss N, Yeates KO, Enrile BG. Attention in children with myelomeningocele. *Child Neuropsychol* 1998; **4**: 7–20.

54. Snow JH, Prince M, Souheaver G, Ashcraft E, Stefans V, Edmonds J. Neuropsychological patterns of adolescents and young adults with spina bifida. *Arch Clin Neuropsychol* 1994; **9**(3): 277–87.

55. Iddon JL, Morgan DJ, Loveday C, Sahakian BJ, Pickard JD. Neuropsychological profile of young adults with spina bifida with or without hydrocephalus. *J Neurol Neurosurg Psychiatry* 2004; **75**(8): 1112–18.

56. Carr J. The effect of neural tube defects on the family and its social functioning. In Tew B, Spastics Society, Bannister CM, eds. *Current Concepts in Spina Bifida and Hydrocephalus.* New York: Cambridge University Press; 1991.

57. Wallander JL, Varni JW, Babani L, Banis HT, DeHaan CB, Wilcox KT. Disability parameters, chronic strain, and adaptation of physically handicapped children and their mothers. *J Pediatr Psychol* 1989; **14**(1): 23–42.

58. Holmbeck GN. Toward terminological, conceptual, and statistical clarity in the study of mediators and moderators: examples from the child-clinical and pediatric psychology literatures. *J Cons Clin Psychol* 1997; **65**(4): 599–610.

59. Fletcher JM, Brookshire BL, Landry SH, *et al.* Behavioral adjustment of children with hydrocephalus: relationships with etiology, neurological, and family status. *J Pediatr Psychol* 1995; **20**(1): 109–25.

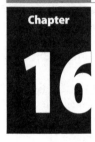

Chapter

16

Executive functions in acquired brain injury

Cynthia Salorio

Acquired brain injury (ABI) in children and adolescents can have many causes, including trauma, CNS infections like HIV (see Chapter 13), non-infectious disorders (epilepsy – see Chapter 11, hypoxia/ischemia, genetic/metabolic disorders – see Chapter 7), tumors (see Chapter 12), and stroke or other vascular abnormalities.[1] Identifying prognostic factors after brain injury is vital, in order to optimize interventions and provide appropriate education to family or caregivers for future planning. In children, early prediction of outcomes is critical, because targeted interventions must focus on assisting the child in re-gaining lost skills, and also promoting ongoing development. Predictors of outcome may differ depending on age, making generalization of adult findings to children difficult.

EF is commonly impacted after ABI, and researchers have identified multiple factors associated with better or worse EF, including variables related to the mechanism of injury, post-injury factors, and pre-injury or demographic factors. Many of the etiologies of ABI are covered in other chapters; as such, this chapter will focus on EF after traumatic, anoxic/ hypoxic, and vascular causes of ABI.

Traumatic brain injury

While there are many causes of ABI in children, traumatic brain injury (TBI) is by far the most common. More than 450,000 children under the age of 14 years are admitted to the emergency department each year for TBI.[2] As a result, the largest body of research examining EF after ABI in children focuses on TBI.

Executive dysfunction in TBI

Deficits in EF, as measured by both performance-based tasks and rating scales, are frequently observed after pediatric TBI. Deficits have been identified in numerous aspects of EF, including WM, inhibitory control, cognitive flexibility, abstract reasoning, judgment, and planning.[3]

Several injury-related variables have been associated with worse EF after TBI. In general, severity of injury is related to degree of deficit in EF. For example, children with more severe TBI, as measured by the earliest Glasgow Coma Scale (GCS) score, have worse WM on both performance based tasks and rating scales.[4] Performance on tests of verbal fluency, concept formation, abstract reasoning and cognitive flexibility has also been related to severity of TBI in children.[5–7] One study noted that between 18–38% of children with

Executive Function and Dysfunction, ed. Scott J. Hunter and Elizabeth P. Sparrow. Published by Cambridge University Press. © Cambridge University Press 2012.

moderate to severe TBI demonstrated clinically significant deficits in EF during the first year after injury, as measured by the BRIEF parent report, with more severe injuries associated with greater dysfunction.[8] Similarly, a study of adolescents and young adults between 7–10 years post-injury found that moderate TBI was associated with worse performance on tasks of cognitive flexibility, abstract reasoning, and goal setting relative to mild TBI.[9]

The literature on concussion has been mixed with regard to long term deficits. One study of soccer players suggested that increased frequency of "heading" during play was significantly related to decreased cognitive flexibility, and the number of head injuries sustained was inversely related to divided attention.[10] This is consistent with several DTI studies showing that concussion can cause axonal damage, and that reduced FA in the frontal regions is associated with aspects of EdF, such as poorer impulse control.[11] Studies using fMRI have also shown reduced activation in the DLPFC after concussion, which has been correlated with diminished processing speed and cognitive flexibility.[12] In contrast, another study of soccer players did not find that neuropsychological impairments were related to "heading" frequency or head injury incidence,[13] and a further study suggested that litigation was the only significant correlate to neuropsychological impairment at 3-months post-concussion.[14] Additional research is needed to clarify the impact of concussion on EF, and the factors associated with increased symptoms.

In addition to overall severity, several other injury-related variables have been studied. For example, the mechanism of injury appears to be important, and in general, children with inflicted (e.g., non-accidental) injuries have worse outcomes than do children with noninflicted (e.g., accidental) injuries.[15] Secondary complications have also been studied, and research has inconsistently shown that the development of seizures after TBI is associated with worse EF. For example, Anderson and colleagues[16] suggested that TBI-related seizures were associated with lower attentional control, but not with changes in goal setting, everyday EF, cognitive flexibility or WM. In contrast, another study by the same research group suggested that post-TBI seizures are associated with changes in verbal fluency, problem solving, cognitive flexibility and inhibition.[17] Brenner and colleagues[18] demonstrated that brain spectroscopy variables at 1–7 years post-pediatric TBI, such as lactate and Cho/Cre, were highly (inversely) correlated with measures of EF as measured by the NEPSY.

Some of the variability in findings may relate to the use of different measures of EF across studies. Rating scales and performance-based tests of EF are not strongly correlated[4,19] and some authors argue that performance-based measures have limited ecological validity, and therefore questionable utility in diagnosing deficits in EF.[20] Interestingly, Wilson, Donders, and Nguyen[21] compared responses on rating scales designed to measure real-world EF (BRIEF), and found that parent ratings of adolescents tended be reflect more dysfunction in EF than did the adolescents ratings about themselves, with greater discrepancies in those with more severe TBI. This highlights the potential impact of EdF on awareness of deficits in adolescents who have sustained TBI, which has implications for intervention success.

The neurological basis of executive dysfunction in TBI

EF is principally mediated by the frontal networks of the brain, with developmental increases in performance corresponding to maturation of these brain regions.[22,23]

The frontal lobes are particularly vulnerable to TBI, and, not surprisingly, frontal lobe lesions have been associated with deficits in EF.[24] Studies using sensitive neuroimaging techniques have also associated deficits in EF with dysfunction or damage to the frontal brain regions, specifically FA in the frontal regions,[25,26] but also reduced cortical thickness in both the frontal and parietal regions.[27] Several studies, however, have found that the volume of lesions outside the frontal areas (extra-frontal) is also significantly predictive of deficits in EF after TBI, above and beyond measures of severity, suggesting that in children, the integrity of the entire brain may be important for frontal lobe connectivity and EF.[7,28]

Age at injury is another important factor impacting EF after pediatric TBI. While younger children are felt to have greater brain plasticity, possibly allowing for better potential resilience after injury, research has shown that the developing brain may be particularly vulnerable to injury during critical periods. Because the frontal lobes have a protracted developmental trajectory, they are therefore at particular risk for disruption due to injury in childhood.[22] The relationship between age at injury and EF at follow-up is complex and appears to be nonlinear.[29,30] In fact, while adults tend to show deficits in EF immediately after moderate to severe TBI, children are more likely to "grow into" deficits, or begin to demonstrate weaknesses in EF as the demands for these skills increase with age and brain maturation.[31,32] Studies suggest that very young age at injury is associated with worse EF at follow-up, most notably for children under age 2–3 at the time of injury.[16,33] Interestingly, behavioral difficulties were more pronounced in children injured between 7–9 years, as opposed to younger children, suggesting that not all functions share the same critical periods of vulnerability.[33]

There are few longitudinal studies that evaluate EF after pediatric TBI. Sesma and colleagues[8] examined EF during the first year after injury and found no differences between TBI and controls in pre-injury EF on the BRIEF, but significantly worse EF at 3-months and 1-year post-injury relative to controls. Anderson and Catroppa[34] suggested that although some recovery is obvious at 2 years post-injury, deficits in EF are still evident. One study followed children with TBI for 7–10 years post-injury and found ongoing deficits in several domains of EF, including cognitive flexibility, abstract reasoning, as well as more global difficulties in EF as measured by parent ratings on the BRIEF.[35] There appears to be an interaction between severity and age at injury, such that in children with severe TBI, younger age (3–7) is associated with significantly less recovery than older age at injury (8–12), an effect that has been termed a "double hazard" model for early severe injury.[36] These findings highlight the need for parent education about the potential delayed effects after TBI in young children, and the importance of long term follow-up beyond the initial period of recovery in children after TBI.

Factors related to the individual have also been associated with outcome after TBI in children. For example, the presence of symptoms consistent with a diagnosis of ADHD following severe TBI is associated with worse EF at one-year.[37] In addition, family functioning appears to mediate deficits in EF following pediatric TBI, in a bidirectional manner.[38] A study of children with TBI at 5-years post injury found that greater deficits in EF were associated with increased parent distress, perceived family burden and worse overall family functioning.[39] In addition, Wade, Carey and Wolfe[40] demonstrated that improved family functioning increases outcomes and improves EF in adolescents following TBI. Pre-injury learning and behavior problems and limited family resources have also been associated with worse EF following severe TBI in children.[41]

Deficits in EF after pediatric TBI have been associated with impairments in several important areas of function, particularly the development of social skills. One study of children at 6-months post-TBI found that EF was a major determinant of social competence.[42] Another study found that EF, specifically cognitive control, was associated with social outcomes 1-year post-injury.[43] Additionally, the relationship between EF and social outcome appears to be sustained up to 10 years post-TBI.[35] In fact, 71% of children who sustained a TBI with damage in the PFC prior to age five had social deficits that persisted into adulthood.[44] EF has also been associated with other functional impairments, such as adaptive behavior and daily living skills.[45] Galvin and Mandalis[46] argue for a contextual framework for rehabilitation of children after TBI, in order to reduce the potential long-term impact of EF deficits on functioning.

Anoxia/hypoxia

While ABI in children most commonly results from trauma, anoxic/hypoxic injuries can also occur through events that eliminate or restrict oxygen delivery to the brain. Research suggests that children who experience an anoxic or hypoxic brain injury experience worse outcomes than those with TBI.[47] As with TBI, studies show that the more severe the injury, the worse the cognitive and motor outcomes are likely to be after anoxic brain injury.[48,49]

Executive dysfunction in anoxia/hypoxia

Hypoxia, or reduced oxygen availability to brain tissue, can result from a variety of causes, including near drowning, suffocation, strangulation, cardiac arrest, sleep disorder, carbon monoxide exposure, and respiratory disorders. Few studies have focused on EF in children following anoxic/hypoxic brain injury; however, given the high metabolic demands of the frontal brain regions and their broad networks, it is not unreasonable to assume that EF is vulnerable to reductions in oxygen availability to the brain.[50] A substantial body of research using animal models has supported this hypothesis[51] and recent studies in humans are also suggestive of a relationship between EdF and frontal lobe integrity after hypoxia.[52]

Most of the studies of cognitive sequelae of anoxic/hypoxic injury have been done in adults. A review article by Caine and Watson[53] indicated that deficits in EF, including behavioral and personality change, were reported in approximately 46% of cases of cerebral anoxia. A study by Garcia-Molina and colleagues[54] showed that, in adults, ischemic anoxia (i.e., anoxia due to cardiac abnormalities) resulted in more severe neuropsychological deficits, including EF, than hypoxemic anoxia (i.e., anoxia due to respiratory difficulties). Armengol[55] found particular EF deficits in self-regulation and establishing set in a group of adults who had experienced a severe anoxic event. Volpe and Pepito[56] reported specific deficits in abstract reasoning in two individuals after severe anoxia. Most of the literature in children focuses on overall intellectual functioning or motor skill;[57] however, given the rapid development of EF in children, it is reasonable to propose an increased vulnerability in younger age groups who experience anoxia/hypoxia. Of note, a recent study of children living in high altitude demonstrated specific deficits in EF, in the context of otherwise intact neuropsychological functioning.[58]

Younger age at injury (children vs. adults) is associated with better outcomes after hypoxic injury, when a full range of ages is examined. In one study, patients who were younger than 25 years of age at time of injury had better independent living skills than patients who were older.[59] While research is sparse, there is some literature to suggest that early injury (before 1 year of age) is associated with worse long-term neuropsychological outcome.[60]

The neurological basis of executive dysfunction in anoxia/hypoxia

The literature on carbon monoxide exposure (CO) suggests that EdF is one of the most prominent deficits following this type of anoxic/hypoxic injury, at least in adults. One study using diffusion tensor imaging found that EF deficits following CO intoxication were related to FA of the frontotemporal white matter.[61] Another study suggested that the EF deficits do not improve over the first year after exposure, and continue to be associated with the integrity of the white matter in the brain.[62] In addition to damage to the frontal brain regions, the integrity of the periventricular white matter and the centrum semiovale in particular appear to be associated with EF following CO poisoning.[63]

There is some pediatric literature in the area of sleep disordered breathing (SDB), which can be associated with reduced oxygen availability to the brain, and related to deficits in EF.[64,65] SDB has been associated with focal reductions in gray matter volume in the superior frontal gyrus, which are positively correlated with neuropsychological impairments in EF.[66] Specific EF deficits in children with SDB include cognitive flexibility, initiation, self-monitoring, and planning/organization.[67] Of note, while the actual oxygen deprivation may be relatively minor, it still appears to have a profound impact on cognition; deficits in EF have been found in children with even mild cases of SDB.[68] Some studies found that treatment of SDB results in amelioration of EF deficits, while other studies have not shown these improvements.[66,69]

Stroke and other vascular abnormalities

Stroke in children is relatively rare after the neonatal period. Strokes can be idiopathic, related to a specific disease process such as sickle cell disease (SCD), or related to vascular abnormalities such as arteriovenous malformations (AVM). Outcomes may vary by stroke type, extent of lesion, and location.[70]

Executive dysfunction after stroke and AVM

The development of seizures after stroke appears to be a marker for poor global outcome, but injury location has not been consistently associated with specific neurocognitive outcomes. Similar to findings in other types of ABI, age at time of stroke has been shown to predict outcomes. Children whose injury occurred early (before 12 months of age) have worse global outcomes than those whose injury occurred later.[70] That said, the specific association between age and EdF after pediatric stroke is less consistent in the literature. For example, Max and colleagues[71] found that children with early stroke (first year of life) generally had worse cognitive outcomes, but that the children who were older at the time of insult actually performed more poorly on two of three tests of EF. Westmacott and colleagues[72] studied children who sustained a stroke prior to age 16, and found times of peak vulnerability associated with different lesion locations, with subcortical strokes causing the most subsequent EF deficits when sustained in the perinatal period, and strokes in cortical areas more detrimental when sustained between ages 1 and 5 years. Interestingly, a recent study examining neonatal and childhood stroke found intact EF using the NEPSY (but impairments across other cognitive domains) in both stroke groups at follow-up.[73] Most studies of childhood stroke combine etiologies, making generalizability difficult.

The neurological basis of executive dysfunction with vascular issues

Max and colleagues[74] reported that children with stroke showed worse EF than healthy children, and larger lesions to the prefrontal attention/EF networks of the brain were associated with greater impairment. Focal lesions in the frontal lobes were more likely to be associated with deficits in EF on the BRIEF than more global processes.[75] In contrast, Long and colleagues[76] showed that insults involving both frontal and extra-frontal regions appeared to impact cognitive performance, with subcortical lesions having the greatest impact on everyday EF.

Sickle cell disease (SCD), a genetic disorder associated with an elevated risk of stroke, has been extensively studied. Research shows that children with SCD and stroke generally perform worse on tests of EF than children with SCD who have not had a stroke.[77] In addition, recurrent (as opposed to single episode) stroke has been associated with greater academic and cognitive difficulties in children with SCD.[78] Studies have also found that children with SCD who have a high neurological risk but no identified stroke demonstrate worse EF, particularly WM, than children with SCD and low neurological risk, regardless of age.[79] Given that the frontal watershed areas are particularly vulnerable to stroke in SCD, children are prone to "silent" infarcts that are not detected clinically.[80] These infarcts are typically associated with neurocognitive deficits, particularly EdF, even when their presence is not detected on physical exam.[81] Some providers have suggested that regular screening of neuropsychological status may be more efficient and sensitive to detect these silent strokes than imaging or neurological exams, with measures of EF being particularly helpful.[80]

In individuals with AVMs, the size and location of the lesion is a predictor of global outcomes. Lesion volume greater than 20 cm^3, deep drainage, and location in rolandic, inferior limbic, and insular locations have all been associated with greater complications, more severe morbidity and overall mortality.[82] Deficits in EF have been found in children with AVM regardless of location of the malformation.[83] Notably, neuropsychological deficits in children with AVMs are not consistently associated with location in the brain, possibly suggesting that shunting of blood flow away from other areas, rather than mass effect of the malformation itself, may play a role in the more specific cognitive outcomes.[83] There is some evidence that treatment of the AVM through surgical resection or embolization may improve EdF.[84]

Summary and future directions

In summary, EdF is a common area of difficulty after ABI in children. TBI has been most extensively studied, with deficits in EF reported in the areas of WM, behavioral regulation, cognitive flexibility, abstract reasoning, judgment, and planning. Reduced EF after pediatric TBI can be identified on both performance-based tasks and on rating scales, though these measures do not always correlate, and individuals with injuries may under-report EdF. Several factors are associated with worse EF, including younger age at injury, poor family functioning, frontal lobe (but also extra-frontal) pathology, and, less consistently, other medical factors, such as the development of seizures. Other causes of ABI, such as anoxia/hypoxia, are less well studied in children, but research also demonstrates EdF after these types of neurological insults. In children with SDB, even mild levels of hypoxia can be associated with EF deficits. Stroke in children has also been associated with EdF, and lesions in the frontal brain regions have been associated with worse EF. Location of vascular malformations, however, is not consistently related to deficits in EF. Screening with tests of EF can assist in identifying high-risk children with SCD who do not have clinically evident strokes. In children with early ABI, impairments in EF are often not evident until school-age or adolescence, but are associated with significant functional impairments in social and adaptive skill, and appear to persist over time. More research is needed to elucidate the mechanisms of EdF in children after brain injury, in order to design appropriate interventions, educate parents and teachers, and support ongoing development long after injury.

References

1. Tojo M, Nitta H. Clinico-etiological study of 116 children with acquired damage to the central nervous system during the last decade in Niigata Prefecture. *No To Hattasu* 2003; **35**(4): 292–6.

2. Langlois JA, Rutland-Brown W, Wald MM. The epidemiology and impact of traumatic brain injury: a brief overview. *J Head Trauma Rehabil* 2006; **21**: 375–8.

3. Levin HS, Hanten G. Executive function after traumatic brain injury in children. *Ped Neurol* 2005; **33**: 79–93.

4. Conklin HM, Salorio CF, Slomine BS. Working memory performance following paediatric traumatic brain injury. *Brain Injury* 2008; **22**(11): 847–57.

5. Levin HS, Song J, Scheibel RS, Fletcher JM, Harward H, Lilly M, Goldstein F. Concept formation and problem-solving following closed head injury in children. 1997. *Journal Int Neuropsychol Soc* 3: 598–607.

6. Levin HS, Song J, Ewing-Cobbs L, Chapman SB, Mendelsohn D. Word fluency in relation to severity of closed head injury associated frontal brain lesions and age at injury in children. *Neuropsychologia* 2001; **39**: 122–31.

7. Slomine BS, Gerring JP, Grados MA, Vasa R, Brady KD, Christensen JR, Denkla MB. Performance on measures of 'executive function' following pediatric brain injury. *Brain Injury* 2002; **169**: 759–72.

8. Sesma HW, Slomine BS, Ding R, McCarthy ML, and the Children's Health After Trauma (CHAT) Study. Executive functioning in the first year after pediatric traumatic brain injury. *Pediatrics* 2008; **121**: e1686–95.

9. Muscara F, Catroppa C, Anderson V. The impact of injury severity on executive function 7–10 years following pediatric traumatic brain injury. *Dev Neuropsychol* 2008; **335**: 623–36.

10. Rutherford A, Stephens R, Potter D, Fernie G. Neuropsychological impairment as a consequence of football soccer play and football heading: preliminary analyses and report on university footballers. *J Clin Exp Neuropsychol* 2005; **27**: 299–319.

11. Bazarian JJ, Zhong J, Blyth B, Zhu T, Kavcic V, Peterson D. Diffusion tensor imaging detects clinically important axonal damage after mild traumatic brain injury: a pilot study. *J Neurotrauma* 2007; **24**: 1447–59.

12. Chen J, Johnson KM, Collie A, McCrory P, Ptito A. A validation of the post-concussion symptom scale in the assessment of complex concussion using cognitive testing and functional MRI. *J Neurol Neurosurg Psychiatry* 2007; **78**: 1231–8.

13. Rutherford A, Stephens R, Fernie G, Potter D. Do UK university football club players suffer neuropsychological impairment as a consequence of their football soccer play? *J Clin Exp Neuropsychol* 2009; **316**: 664–81.

14. Belanger HG, Curtiss G, Demery JA, Lebowitz BK, Vanderploeg RD. Factors moderating neuropsychological outcomes following mild traumatic brain injury: a meta-analysis. *J Int Neuropsychol Soc* 2005; **11**: 215–27.

15. Keenan HT, Runyan DK, Nocera M. Child outcomes and family characteristics 1 year after severe inflicted or non-inflicted traumatic brain injury. *Pediatrics* 2006; **1172**: 317–24.

16. Anderson V, Spencer-Smith M, Coleman L, *et al.* Children's executive functions: are they poorer after very early brain insult? *Neuropsychologia* 2010; **48**: 2041–50.

17. Anderson V, Jacobs R, Spencer-Smith M, *et al.* Does early age predict worse outcome? Neuropsychological implications. *J Pediatr Psychol* 2010; **357**: 716–27.

18. Brenner T, Freier MC, Holshouser BA, Burley T, Ashwal S. Predicting neuropsychologic outcome after traumatic brain injury in children. *Pediatr Neurol* 2003; **28**: 104–14.

19. Vreizen ER, Pigott SE. The relationship between parental report on the BRIEF and performance-based measures of executive function in children with moderate to severe traumatic brain injury. *Child Neuropsychol* 2002; **84**: 296–303.

20. Gioia GA, Kenworthy L, Isquith PK. Executive function in the real world: BREIF lessons from Mark Ylvisake. *J Head Trauma Rehabil* 2010; **256**: 433–9.

21. Wilson KR, Donders J, Nguyen L. Self and parent report ratings of executive functioning after adolescent traumatic brain injury. *Rehabil Psychol* 2011; **562**: 100–6.

22. Levin HS, Culhane KAM, Hartmann JM, *et al.* Developmental-changes in performance on tests of purported frontal-lobe functioning. *Dev Neuropsychol* 1991; **7**: 377–95.

23. Rubia K, Smith AB, Wooley J, *et al.* Progressive increase of frontostriatal brain activation from childhood to adulthood during event-related tasks of cognitive control. *Hum Brain Mapping* 2006; **27**: 973–93.

24. Levin HS, Culhane KA, Mendelsohn D, *et al.* Cognition in relation to magnetic resonance imaging in head-injured children and mid adolescents. *Arch Neurol* 1993; **50**: 897–905.

25. Kurowski B, Wade SL, Cecil KM, *et al.* Correlation of diffusion tensor imaging with executive function measures after early childhood traumatic brain injury. *J Pediatr Rehabil Med* 2009; **2**: 273–83.

26. Wozniak JR, Krach L, Ward E, *et al.* Neurocognitive and neuroimaging correlates of pediatric brain injury: A diffusion tensor imaging DTI study. *Arch Clin Neuropsychol* 2007; **22**: 555–68.

27. Tamnes CK, Ostby Y, Walhovd KB, Westlye LT. Neuroanatomical correlates of executive functions in children and adolescents: a magnetic resonance imaging MRI study of cortical thickness. *Neuropsychologia* 2010; **48**: 2496–508.

28. Jacobs R, Harvey AS, Anderson V. Are executive skills primarily mediated by the prefrontal cortex in childhood? Examination of focal brain lesions in childhood. *Cortex* 2011; **47**: 808–24.

29. Horton AM, Soper H, Reynolds CR. Executive functions in children with traumatic brain injury. *Appl Neuropsychol* 2010; **17**: 99–103.

30. Jacobs R, Harvey AS, Anderson V. Executive function following focal frontal lobe lesions: Impact of timing of lesion on outcome. *Cortex* 2007; **43**: 792–805.

31. Eslinger PJ. Conceptualizing describing and measuring components of executive function: a summary. In: Lyon GR, Krasnegor NA, eds. *Attention Memory and Executive Function.* Baltimore MA: Paul H Brookes Publishing Co; 1996, 367–95.

32. Giza CC, Mink RB, Madikians A. Pediatric traumatic brain injury: not just little adults. *Curr Opin Crit Care* 2007; **13**: 143–52.

33. Anderson V, Spencer-Smith M, Leventer R, *et al.* Childhood brain insult: can age at insult help us predict outcome? *Brain* 2009; **132**: 45–56.

34. Anderson V, Catroppa C. Recovery of executive skills following paediatric traumatic brain injury TBI: A 2 year follow-up. *Brain Inj* 2005; **196**: 459–70.

35. Muscara F, Catroppa C, Anderson V. Social problem-solving skills as a mediator

between executive function and long-term social outcome following paediatric traumatic brain injury. *J Neuropsychol* 2008; **2**: 445–61.

36. Anderson V, Catroppa C, Morse S, Haritou F, Rosenfeld J. Functional plasticity or vulnerability after early brain injury? *Pediatrics* 2005; **1166**: 1374–82.

37. Slomine BS, Salorio CF, Grados MA, Vasa RA, Christensen JR, Gerring JP. Differences in attention executive functioning and memory in children with and without ADHD after severe traumatic brain injury. *J Int Neuropsychol Soc* 2005; **11**: 645–53.

38. Tonks J, Williams WH, Yates P, Slater A. Cognitive correlates of psychosocial outcome following traumatic brain injury in early childhood: Comparisons between groups of children aged under and over 10 years of age. *Clin Child Psychol Psychiatry* 2011; **162**: 185–94.

39. Mangeot S, Armstrong K, Colvin AN, Yeates KO, Taylor HG. Long-term executive function deficits in children with traumatic brain injuries: Assessment using the behavior rating inventory of executive function BRIEF. *Child Neuropsychol* 2002; **84**: 271–84.

40. Wade SL, Carey J, Wolfe CR. The efficacy of an online cognitive behavioral family intervention in improving child behavior and social competence following pediatric brain injury. *Rehabil Psychol* 2006; **513**: 179–89.

41. Wade SL, Taylor HG, Yeates KO, *et al.* Long-term parental and family adaption following pediatric brain injury. *J Pediatr Psychol* 2006; **3110**: 1072–183.

42. Ganesalingam K, Yeates KO, Taylor HG, Waltz NC, Stancin T, Wade S. Executive functions and social competence in young children 6 months following traumatic brain injury. *Neuropsychol* 2011; Advance online publication doi:101037/a0022768.

43. Levin HS, Hanten G, Li X. The relation of cognitive control to social outcome after paediatric TBI: Implications for intervention. *Devel Neurorehabil* 2009; **125**: 320–9.

44. Anderson SW, Wisnowski JL, Barrash J, Damasio H, Tranel D. Consistency of neuropsychological outcome following damage to prefrontal cortex in the first years of life. *J Clin Exp Neuropsychol* 2009; **312**: 170–9.

45. Schwartz L, Taylor HG, Drotar D, Yeates KO, Wade SL, Stancin T. Long-term behavior problems following pediatric traumatic brain injury: Prevalence predictors and correlates. *J Ped Psychol* 2003; **284**: 251–63.

46. Galvin J, Mandalis A. Executive skills and their functional implications: Approaches to rehabilitation after childhood TBI. *Devel Neurorehabil* 2009; **125**: 352–60.

47. Heindl UT, Laub MC. Outcome of persistent vegetative state following hypoxic or traumatic brain injury in children and adolescents. *Neuropediatrics* 1996; **27**: 94–100.

48. Kriel RL, Krach LE, Luxenberg MG, Jones-Saete C, Sanchez J. Outcome of severe anoxic/ischemic brain injury in children. *Pediatr Neurol* 1994; **10**: 207–12.

49. Habib DM, Tecklenburg FW, Webb SA, Anas NG, Perkin RM. Prediction of childhood drowning and near-drowning morbidity and mortality. *Pediatr Emerg Care* 1996; **12**: 255–8.

50. Biagas K. Hypoxic-ischemic brain injury: advancements in the understanding of mechanisms and potential avenues for therapy. *Curr Opin Pediatr* 1999; **113**: 223–8.

51. Kheirandish L, Gozal D, Pequignot JM, Pequignot J, Row BW. Intermittent hypoxia during development induces long-term alterations in spatial working memory monoamines and dendritic branching in rat frontal cortex. *Pediatr Res* 2005; **58**(3): 594–9.

52. Ayalon L, Ancoli-Israel S, Aka AA, McKenna BS, Drummond SPA. Relationship between obstructive sleep apnea severity and brain activation during a sustained attention task. *Sleep* 2009; **32**(3): 373–81.

53. Caine D, Watson JDG. Neuropsychological and neuropathological sequelae of cerebral

anoxia: a critical review. *J Int Neuropsychol Soc* 2000; **6**: 86–99.

54. Garcia-Molina A, Roig-Rovira T, Ensenat-Cantallops A, *et al.* Neuropsychological profile of persons with anoxic brain injury Differences regarding physiopathological mechanism. *Brain Inj* 2006; **20**(11): 1139–45.

55. Armengol CG. Acute oxygen deprivation: neuropsychological profiles and implications for rehabilitation. *Brain Inj* 2000; **143**: 237–50.

56. Volpe BT, Petito CK. Dementia with bilateral medial temporal lobe ischemia. *Neurology* 1985; **35**: 1793–7.

57. Bass JL, Corwin M, Gozal D, *et al.* The effect of chronic or intermittent hypoxia on cognition in childhood: A review of the evidence. *Pediatrics* 2004; **1143**: 805–16.

58. Virues-Ortega J, Bucks R, Kirkham FJ, Baldeweg T, Baya-Botti A, Hogan AM. Changing patterns of neuropsychological functioning in children living at high altitude above and below 4000 m: a report from the Bolivian Children Living at Altitude (BoCLA) study. *Devel Sci* 2011; **145**: 1185–93.

59. Groswasser Z, Cohen M, Costeff H. Rehabilitation outcome after anoxic brain damage. *Arch Phys Med Rehabil* 1989; **70**: 186–8.

60. Hopkins RO, Haaland KY. Neuropsychological and neuropathological effects of anoxic or ischemic induced brain injury. *J Int Neuropsychol Soc* 2004; **10**: 957–61.

61. Chang CC, Lee YC, Chang WN, *et al.* Damage of white matter tract correlated with neuropsychological deficits in carbon monoxide intoxication after hyperbaric oxygen therapy. *J Neurotrauma* 2009; **6**: 1263–70.

62. Chang C, Chang W, Lui C, *et al.* Longitudinal study of carbon monoxide intoxication by diffusion tensor imaging with neuropsychiatric correlation. *J Psychi Neurosci* 2010; **352**: 115–25.

63. Parkinson RB, Hopkins RO, Cleavinger HB, *et al.* White matter hyperintensities and neuropsychological outcome following carbon monoxide poisoning. *Neurology* 2002; **58**: 1525–32.

64. Beebe DW, Groesz L, Wells C, *et al.* The neuropsychological effects of obstructive sleep apnea: a meta-analysis of norm referenced and case-controlled data. *Sleep* 2003; **26**: 298–307.

65. Blunden S, Beebe DW. The contribution of intermittent hypoxia sleep debt and sleep disruption to daytime performance deficits in children: consideration of respiratory and non-respiratory sleep disorders. *Sleep Med Rev* 2006; **102**: 109–18.

66. Canessa N, Castronovo V, Cappa SF, *et al.* Obstructive sleep apnea: Brain structural changes and neurocognitive function before and after treatment. *Am J Resp Crit Care Med* 2011; **183**: 1419–26.

67. Beebe DW, Wells CT, Jeffries J, Chini B, Kalra M, Amin R. Neuropsychological effects of pediatric obstructive sleep apnea. *J Int Neuropsychol Soc* 2004; **10**: 962–75.

68. Halbower AC, Mahone EM. Neuropsychological morbidity linked to childhood sleep-disordered breathing. *Sleep Med Rev* 2006; **10**: 97–107.

69. Ferini-Strambi L, Baietto C, Di Gioia MR, *et al.* Cognitive dysfunction in patients with obstructive sleep apnea OSA: partial reversibility after continuous positive airway pressure CPAP. *Brain Res Bull* 2003; **61**: 87–92.

70. Lynch JK, Han CJ. Pediatric stroke: what do we know and what do we need to know? *Sem Neurol* 2005; **254**: 410–23.

71. Max JE, Bruce M, Keatley E, Delis D. Pediatric stroke: plasticity vulnerability and age of lesion onset. *J Neuropsychiatry Clin Neurosci* 2010; **22**: 30–9.

72. Westmacott R, Askalan R, MacGregor D, Anderson P, Deveber G. Cognitive outcome following unilateral arterial ischaemic stroke in childhood: effects of age at stroke and lesion location. *Dev Med Child Neurol* 2010; **52**: 386–93.

73. Kolk A, Ennok M, Laugesaar R, Kaldoja M, Talvik T. Long-term cognitive outcomes

after pediatric stroke. *Pediatr Neurol* 2011; **44**: 101–9.

74. Max JE, Robin DA, Taylor HG, *et al.* Attention function after childhood stroke. *J Int Neuropsychol Soc* 2004; **10**: 976–86.

75. Anderson VA, Anderson P, Northam E, Jacobs R, Mikiewicz O. Relationships between cognitive and behavioral measures of executive function in children with brain disease. *Child Neurol* 2002; **84**: 231–40.

76. Long B. Spencer-Smith MM, Jacobs R, *et al.* Executive function following child stroke: the impact of lesion location. *J Child Neurol* 2011; **263**: 279–87.

77. Schatz J, Finke RL, Kellett JM, Kramer JH. Cognitive functioning in children with sickle cell disease: a meta-analysis. *J Pediatr Psychol* 2002; **278**: 739–48.

78. Schatz J, Brown RT, Pascual JM, Hsu L, DeBaun MR. Poor school and cognitive functioning with silent cerebral infarcts and sickle cell disease. *Neurology* 2001; **56**: 1109–11.

79. Schatz J, Roberts CW. Neurobehavioral impact of sickle cell disease in early childhood. *J Int Neuropsychol Soc* 2007; **13**: 933–43.

80. Gold JI, Johnson CB, Treadwell MJ, Hans N, Vichinsky E. Detection and assessment of stroke in patients with sickle cell disease: neuropsychological functioning and magnetic resonance imaging. *Pediatr Hemat Oncol* 2008; **25**: 409–21.

81. Kral MC, Brown RT, Hynd GW. Neuropsychological aspects of pediatric sickle cell disease. *Neuropsychol Rev* 2001; **114**: 179–96.

82. Pasqualin A, Barone G, Cioffi F, Rosta L, Scienza R, DaPian R. The relevance of anatomic and hemodynamic factors to a classification of cerebral arteriovenous malformations. *Neurosurgery* 1991; **28**: 370–9.

83. Whigham KB, O'Toole K. Understanding the neuropsychologic outcome of pediatric AVM within a developmental framework. *Cogn Behav Neurol* 2007; **204**: 244–57.

84. Baker RP, McCarter RJ, Porter DG. Improvement in cognitive function after right temporal arteriovenous malformation excision. *Br J Neurosurg* 2004; **185**: 541–4.

Chapter

17

Empirical status regarding the remediation of executive skills

Beth Slomine, Gianna Locascio, and Megan Kramer

As has been discussed in previous chapters, EdF is a frequent consequence of neurodevelopmental and acquired neurological conditions, and often warrants intervention. At this time, there are several approaches available for the treatment of EdF. Treatment can involve cognitive, behavioral, or pharmacologic approaches. While there is a paucity of research on the efficacy of interventions to address EdF in children,[1,2] there is a solid literature describing the theoretical considerations and models for remediation of EF in children.[3–5] In this chapter, the current empirical literature describing cognitive and behavioral interventions for EdF are reviewed, with a brief discussion of the efficacy of pharmacologic treatments for EdF.

Examining efficacy of interventions

It has been proposed that the best context for EdF intervention is through everyday functional activities, using everyday people and routines. According to this theoretical model, teaching cognitive processes in an entirely decontextualized manner is not likely to be effective.[5] Instead, it is believed necessary to teach and support EF skills in the context of everyday routines. These skills emerge through a process of sequential mastery; slowly introducing new EF demands into daily routines (such as expecting the child to initiate each step independently) or alternating the sequence of steps to achieve a goal more efficiently is the typical approach taken to ensure successful acquisition. As such, interventions should be integrated into the child's home routine and educational program and implemented by caregivers, teachers, and therapists.[4]

While complex, holistic intervention approaches (with the components described above) are preferable for the treatment of EdF, designing studies to adequately examine the efficacy of these interventions has been challenging. Because complex interventions have multiple components, it can be challenging to isolate active components of the intervention. Fortunately, there is a growing research literature composed of studies with good experimental designs, such as those that examine the impact of a specific neuropsychological intervention on individual components of EF. These focused interventions, however, can have limited generalizability to the real world.

Developmental issues are also particularly challenging to address when studying EF interventions for children, as age at time of intervention may impact the appropriateness of interventions utilized, as well as treatment efficacy. Given the changes in cognitive skill

Executive Function and Dysfunction, ed. Scott J. Hunter and Elizabeth P. Sparrow. Published by Cambridge University Press. © Cambridge University Press 2012.

Table 17.1. *Definition of classification of evidence for intervention studies*

Classification	Definitions for Classification of Evidence
Class I	Prospective, randomized controlled clinical trial with masked outcome assessment in a representative population. The primary outcome, inclusion criteria and exclusion criteria must be clearly defined. Dropouts and crossover to the other group are minimal. Baseline characteristics must be similar between groups.
Class II	Prospective matched group cohort study in a representative population with masked outcome or a randomized controlled trial has one significant flaw (e.g., primary outcome not clearly defined).
Class III	All other controlled trials (including well defined natural history controls or patients serving as own controls) in a representative population where outcome is independently assessed or independently derived by objective outcome measurement.
Class IV	Evidence from uncontrolled studies, case series, case reports, or expert opinion.

Based on Edlund W, Gronseth G, Yuen So *et al.* (2004) *Clinical Practice Guideline Process Manual.*

and functional expectations that occur in typically developing children, effective interventions for children with EdF vary depending on the age of the child.[1] For example, scaffolding and supervision are often naturally in place to help younger children establish and maintain simplified, consistent routines. Older children may not naturally have this level of daily adult supervision, and therefore may need more supports than are typical for a child of their age, or may benefit from other interventions (such as massed practice training).

While individual studies are important to consider when examining treatment efficacy, meta-analyses and systematic reviews provide vital information necessary for developing evidence-based practice guidelines. Meta-analyses explore the effect size of specific treatments across group studies. Meta-analyses, however, do not allow consideration of single-case studies or small case series that do not include a control group. While group studies are considered methodologically stronger, single-case studies and small case series also have the potential to provide useful information about EF interventions that may lead to improved competency.[6] In fact, Prigatano has commented that "careful clinical observation of patients who benefit from rehabilitation programs compared with those who fail is the most important method for advancing knowledge in this field."

Given this rationale, systematic reviews of the literature may provide a superior analysis of the extant literature, allowing for examination of both group and case studies. In a systematic review, studies are identified through a rigorous search of existing databases and each individual study is classified based on the strength of the study design. A summary of how intervention studies are classified based on the strength of the study design according to one commonly used classification system[7] is provided in Table 17.1. Based on the strength of the evidence, practice standards, guidelines, or options can be generated. While each classification system varies slightly in how the strength of the evidence is translated into suggestions for practice, one common approach is provided in Table 17.2.[8]

Table 17.2. *Definition of recommendations levels*

Practice standard	Based on at least one well-designed class I study with an adequate sample, with support from class II or class III evidence, that directly addresses the effectiveness of the treatment in question, providing substantive evidence of effectiveness to support a recommendation that the treatment be specifically considered for people with acquired neurocognitive impairments and disability.
Practice guideline	Based on one or more class I studies with methodologic limitations, or well-designed class II studies with adequate samples, that directly address the effectiveness of the treatment in question, providing evidence of probable effectiveness to support a recommendation that the treatment be specifically considered for people with acquired neurocognitive impairments and disability.
Practice option	Based on class II or class III studies that directly address the effectiveness of the treatment in question, providing evidence of possible effectiveness to support a recommendation that the treatment be specifically considered for people with acquired neurocognitive impairments and disability.

From Cicerone *et al.* (2011).

Empirical literature on interventions for executive deficits

For the remainder of this chapter, we will review the empirical literature on EF interventions for children with a variety of neurodevelopmental disabilities (NDD), including ADHD, LD, TBI, and other types of ABI. The few systematic reviews and meta-analyses that have been conducted in children with EdF will also be highlighted. Because there are several well-designed studies examining the efficacy of EF interventions in adults, major findings from this body of literature are also reviewed. While we recognize that there are multiple ways of conceptualizing EF skills, in this chapter, we will address the domains of attention/WM, initiation, problem solving, and inhibitory control.

Attention and working memory

Attention has been divided into components including focus, sustain, select, alternate, and divide,[9] while WM, related to attention, refers to temporary storage ("holding") and active processing ("manipulating") of information.[10] Interventions to support, enhance, or remediate attention and WM deficits typically emphasize massed practice training. Many interventions employ computerized training of these skills using repeated and hierarchically ordered tasks or games.

For remediation of attentional deficits, including difficulties with WM, Sohlberg and Mateer[11,12] developed attention process training (APT), based on a multidimensional model of attention that includes the components mentioned above. Their program incorporates massed practice with groups of hierarchically organized remediation tasks. As patients demonstrate success on easier levels, difficulty increases within each dimension. Many studies have examined APT in adults with brain injuries. In fact, in their most recent systematic review on cognitive rehabilitation in adults with TBI and stroke, Cicerone and colleagues[8] included as a practice standard the remediation of attention during post-acute rehabilitation, specifically via use of direct attention training and metacognitive training of compensatory strategies. Additionally, Cicerone and colleagues suggested that computer-based interventions be considered as a practice option, but only when used in addition to treatment guided by a clinician. Accordingly, they specifically caution against computer-based intervention without the oversight or involvement of a trained professional. Similarly, in their meta-analysis of a smaller sample of studies examined in Cicerone and colleagues' previous reviews,[8,13] Rohling and colleagues[14] concluded that attention training research has resulted in sufficient evidence for the effectiveness of attention training after TBI in adults.

There is also a recommendation for attention remediation to be a practice guideline to assist recovery in children and adolescents with ABI.[15] Moreover, since that guideline was suggested, even stronger evidence for the efficacy of attention remediation in children has emerged. Attention remediation studies in children are summarized below. (See Chapter 16 for discussion of ABI in children.)

In one study, van't Hooft and colleagues[16] evaluated use of the Amsterdam memory and attention training for children program (AMAT-C), based on a model of attention including sustained and selective attention and mental tracking. Children with brain injury due to a variety of etiologies (including trauma, infection, or brain tumor) used the program 30 minutes per day over a 17-week period. A group of control participants receiving only adult interaction and support for the same amount of time was compared to the intervention group. Researchers were not blinded, but groups were randomized. The intervention group improved on measures of sustained and selective attention. In another study employing the Amat-C, Sjo and colleagues[17] studied seven children (8–16 years) with ABI. The authors delivered the intervention within a school setting, with the goal of transferring skills to the children's everyday learning context. They included modifications to the program intended to increase motivation. Results revealed that children and parents were satisfied with the program, and that children remained motivated throughout the intervention. Statistically significant improvements were noted on formal measures of attention, speed, learning, memory, and EF skills. Parents, however, did not report significant improvements in EdF.

The cognitive remediation program (CRP) is a similar intervention program that involves massed practice of attention exercises along with metacognitive and psychotherapeutic (e.g., cognitive and behavioral) strategies. In a non-randomized pilot study, Butler and Copeland[18] studied the efficacy of CRP in 21 children who had undergone radiation treatment for cancer, some of whom had undergone brain tumor resection. (See Chapter 12 for additional information about EF and pediatric cancer.) When compared with ten control participants who did not receive the intervention, participants had improved attention span and vigilance, but no significant change in performance of mathematical calculations. In a follow-up randomized study examining effectiveness of attention training, 161 children ages 6–17 years with cancer-related ABI were assigned to a 20-session program or waitlist control group.[19] All children had attentional deficits as documented by scores on a CPT and parent rating form. Results indicated that the experimental group improved on parent report of attention, and statistically significant increases were noted in their academic achievement. However, no statistically significant differences in neurocognitive functioning were reported.

Galbiati[19] also evaluated an attention remediation training program. The authors evaluated 65 children and adolescents (6–18 years) who had sustained severe brain injuries and who demonstrated marked attentional deficits; 40 were administered the intervention, which included attention-specific neuropsychological training, tabletop tasks, and computerized tasks (the Rehacom program or the Attenzione e Concentrazione program). Sessions lasted 45 minutes, and occurred four times per week for 6 months. Twenty-five control participants did not receive the intervention. At 1-year follow-up, the experimental group showed improved scores on formal cognitive and attention measures, as well as decreased scores on measures of impulsivity.

Children with ADHD have been shown to have EdF (see chapter 5);[20–22,23] thus, the efficacy of computerized programs to promote attention and WM has also been examined in children with ADHD. In one randomized controlled study of 14 children using a computerized, massed practice program addressing attention and WM, spatial span improved.[23] This computer-based training program was designed to resemble a video game, and targeted different components of WM. A subsequent study completed with a larger group confirmed improvements in spatial WM, as well as improved response inhibition.[24] Additionally, exposure to this program was associated with reductions on parent/caregiver ratings of inattention, hyperactivity, and impulsivity. Importantly, these improvements remained apparent three months after the training ended. Support for the same computerized intervention was reported by Beck and colleagues,[25] who found that in a group of children with ADHD (ages 7–17) and comorbid diagnoses, post-intervention parent ratings of attention, ADHD symptoms, and WM were improved when compared to a waitlist control group. These findings were noted both immediately after the intervention and at 4-month follow-up. After subsequently receiving the same intervention, similar findings were reported in the group of children initially waitlisted as controls. The computerized intervention used in these studies is now a commercially available program called *Cogmed* (see Table 17.3).

The efficacy of *Cogmed* for attentional difficulties has also been examined in a group of ELBW children. (See Chapter 15 for information about EdF in ELBW children.) Løhaugen and colleagues[26] evaluated effects on EF skills in adolescents with history of ELBW and associated EdF. The authors included children with lower levels of intellectual functioning (i.e., WISC-3 FSIQ scores < 80). Sixteen children with ELBW and 19 typically developing controls participated in the training. Results indicated improved WM scores in both children with ELBW and the control group. Results for children in the ELBW group remained stable at 6-month follow-up.[27]

More recently, Rabiner and colleagues[28] published a randomized-controlled trial evaluating two commercially available products, *Captain's Log* (Braintrain®; see Table 3), a computerized attention training program (CAT) and *Destination Reading and Math*, a computer assisted instruction (CAI) program. In that study, 77 first grade students with attentional difficulties were randomly assigned to groups that received CAT ($n = 25$), CAI ($n = 27$), or no intervention (waitlist controls, $n = 25$). Students receiving either intervention were more likely than controls to show a moderate decline in teacher-rated attention problems; however, these improvements in attention were no longer evident (relative to controls) at the beginning of the next school year. Post-hoc analyses suggested better maintenance of positive effects for those children who had the most symptoms of inattention at baseline.

Additional support for *Captain's Log* has been demonstrated in children with HIV and malaria. (See Chapter 13 for information on EdF in HIV.) In an initial study conducted by Bangirana and colleagues[29] in Uganda, authors evaluated the program in 62 children (ages 7–12) with histories of cerebral malaria and subsequently impaired attention and memory. Children were randomly assigned to either intervention or control groups, although authors were not blinded. Significant improvements were noted among intervention group children in the areas of visuospatial processing on a WM/learning task, as well as on a

Table 17.3. Commercially available computer-based intervention programs

Program	Publisher	Description	Age Range	Cost	Format
Attention Process Training –3 (APT-3)	Lash & Associates Publishing/Training Inc., 2009 www.lapublishing.com	Attention exercises for individuals with history of ABI and related attentional impairments. Targeted areas include sustained attention and executive control processes related to WM, selective attention, and suppression and alternating attention. Administered by a clinician along with related strategy training and generalization activities.	Adolescents and adults	$850	Computer
Pay Attention!	Lash & Associates Publishing/Training Inc., 2009 www.lapublishing.com	Therapeutic attentional activities for children with TBI, ADHD, and ABI	4–10yo	$375	Computer
Cogmed Working Memory Training	Pearson; www.cogmed.com	Computerized, massed practice trials of tasks involving attention and WM. Designed to resemble a video game, which features different components of WM.	Pre-school (Cogmed JM), middle school/ adolescent (Cogmed RM), and adult (Cogmed QM)	$300–500 per use; $600 for clinician training	Computer
Captain's Log	Brain Train; braintrain.com	Multilevel "brain-training" exercises designed to help develop and improve a variety of cognitive skills, including memory, attention, mental processing speed, impulse control, listening skills, problem solving, and more.	"5–105"yo	$1995–$5495	Computer
Lumosity	Lumos Labs; Lumosity.com	Online "training" games intended to increase WM, attention, and a variety of other cognitive domains. Several condition-specific activities are available on an experimental basis (e.g., TBI, ADHD).	"Any age"	$6.70 per month; $299 for lifetime	Computer and iPhone app (Braintrainer)

measure of processing speed, while performance of control group children did not improve significantly. In a subsequent study, Boivin and colleagues[30] examined *Captain's Log* computerized cognitive rehabilitation therapy (CCRT), specifically configured for attention and memory skills. The authors randomly assigned 60 Ugandan children with HIV to 10 sessions of the intervention or a no-intervention control group. On post-testing, children in the intervention group demonstrated greater improvement on measures of attention and processing speed, as compared to the control group. Authors reported a 95% adherence rate to training sessions, important since the program was designed to be administered over ten total sessions.

Similarly, Kerns and colleagues[31] used a computerized measure of attention training in ten children ages 6–15 with FASD and associated attentional problems. (See Chapter 14 for information about EdF and FASD.) These children completed a 9-week training program with the *Computerized Progressive Attention Training* (CPAT). Results from post-intervention evaluation indicated increased scores on measures of sustained and selective attention, as compared to pre-intervention findings. Researchers also reported increased scores on associated measures of spatial WM, math fluency, and reading, suggesting generalization of improved attention to other cognitive tasks.

Preliminary research on *Lumosity*, a commercially available internet-based cognitive training program, has involved small samples. In a study of 12 girls diagnosed with Turner's syndrome who participated in *Lumosity*, Kesler[32] reported significant improvements in processing speed, numeration, and mental flexibility, with a trend toward improvement in WM. Subsequently, Kesler and colleagues[33] developed an eight week, 40 session curriculum also based upon *Lumosity*. The curriculum was administered to a group of 17 children and adolescents aged 7–19 years with EdF associated with a history of ALL or posterior fossa brain tumors (including medulloblastomas, fourth ventricle ependymomas, and pineal tumors) who had undergone radiation and/or chemotherapy (see Chapter 12 for information about EdF associated with these conditions). Participants demonstrated significantly improved performance on measures of processing speed, verbal and visual declarative memory, and cognitive flexibility after the intervention, even after controlling for practice effects. WM and visual attention did not improve, however. No control group was included for comparison with either study.

Overall, there is a growing literature of reasonably well-designed studies examining attention and WM in children. Studies highlighted above provide support for the use of these interventions in children with deficits resulting from a variety of etiologies. While rigorous study of commercially available products is limited, their availability holds promise for the practical translation of research findings to clinical treatment.

Initiation

Initiation has been described as the ability to independently and spontaneously start and carry out a task. Children with initiation deficits may have the skills necessary to complete a particular task, but require extensive cueing to fully engage with and accomplish the task.[34] As such, interventions to address initiation deficits typically emphasize aspects of cueing. Cues can be provided verbally, visually (e.g., pictorial cues such as signs or notes placed in strategic locations), and physically (e.g., a gentle shoulder tap). External devices such as timers, alarms, pagers, or personal digital assistants (PDAs) can provide cues. Cueing can be used for many aspects of task completion, including alerting an individual if a task has not been completed by a designated time, prompting an individual to begin a previously mastered activity or task, prompting specific components of a multistep task, and signaling a transition between activities.

Recently, researchers have begun to investigate use of self-operated prompting systems as tools for increasing independence and decreasing reliance on external prompts delivered by support individuals e.g.,[35-37] PDAs and smartphone devices have some utility in supporting children and adolescents with initiation deficits, as they provide programmable reminder functions.

Prior to the advent of smartphones, there was promising research exploring the utility of paging systems. Wilson and colleagues examined the use of *NeuroPage*, a paging system where individuals are sent reminder messages regarding tasks they should complete, in a group of individuals ages 8–83 with a history of TBI, stroke, and other non-progressive ABIs.[38] (See Chapter 16 for information about EdF in ABI.) The study used a block-randomized control crossover design that included a 2-week baseline and a 7-week intervention period that occurred immediately following baseline or following a 7-week waiting period. Eighty percent of participants were significantly more successful in carrying out everyday activities with the use of the pager.[38] A later report described the results from the subset of 12 children and adolescents (7 of whom had ABIs and 5 with NDDs) in greater depth.[39] All children showed a significant increase in task achievement with use of the pager compared to baseline. Additionally, the group of children who received the intervention first and were then monitored following return of the pager continued to demonstrate significantly improved performance compared to baseline, although at a level below their performance with the pager.[39]

In a recent group study, thirty-five children with either TBI or ID participated in an 8-week trial of three organizational aids: a daily planner and two different types of PDAs.[40] (See chapters 7 and 16 for information about EdF in these conditions.) Each week, the students were required to complete eight scheduled tasks on time with the assistance of the organizational aid, which was changed each week of the trial. Results indicated that participants had the highest rate of on-time task completion using the Palm PDA reminder system, and the lowest performance using the daily planner, but no information was provided regarding baseline task performance. In a follow-up case report of six children (the best and worst performing participants in the original trial), the researchers met with each child and a support person to provide individualized instruction on the PDA device and its features in order to support continued use of the device in daily life situations for 5–8 weeks.[35] In this case description, the authors reported that several factors impacted success with the device including student motivation, the presence of an audible alarm, adult support for programming and troubleshooting, ability for customization of device, and direct instruction with the device.[35] At 1-year follow-up, all six students continued using the devices and qualitatively reported that they felt more independent in their daily functioning.

There is also a growing literature of case studies demonstrating the efficacy of PDAs to improve initiation of functional skills in children with NDDs and associated initiation difficulties. In two independent single-case studies, use of the alarm feature of a PDA was effective in improving independent and on-task behavior in children with autism spectrum disorders.[41,42] Epstein and colleagues[43] reported on a 10-year-old child with ADHD who improved in taking medication on time, getting books ready, and putting homework away with the use of a vibrating pager that was programmed to prompt up to ten tasks each day.

(See chapter 5 for information about EdF in ADHD.) Two case reports of adolescents with spina bifida found that the use of an external alarm with a displayed message (e.g., "time to catheterize") was useful in increasing parent satisfaction with independent initiation of self-care tasks.[44,45] (See Chapter 15 for information about EdF and SBM.) Cihak and colleagues[36] found that the use of a PDA as a prompting system facilitated independent transitions from task to task in a community-based vocational instructional site for four adolescents with moderate and severe ID; successful use of the device was maintained at the 9-week follow-up.[36] Separate case series have also demonstrated the use of PDAs to increase independent performance of a multistep cooking recipe in adolescents with ID[37] or autism,[46] using antecedent video, pictorial, and auditory prompts. Cihak and colleagues recently demonstrated successful use of an iPod to deliver video-modeling procedures that led to improved independent transitions within the school environment for four elementary school children with autism.[47] (See chapters 6 and 7 for information about EdF in these populations.)

In sum, studies highlighted above provide support that alarmed electronic systems programmed specifically to help children achieve a specific goal are useful in improving initiation. While there are several studies demonstrating that older technologies such as pagers and PDAs are useful, technology in this area is emerging rapidly. As smartphones and devices with multiple applications, such as handheld data devices or personal tablets, are more readily available, there is great potential for use of these devices to improve initiation in the daily lives of children with EdF. Nevertheless, adoption of a device to promote initiation in children with EdF requires careful assessment, planning, customization, instruction, and systematic implementation by clinicians and teachers.[35] Children with EdF will also require ongoing assistance with programming and troubleshooting[35] in order to be successful in the use of these devices. Lastly, difficulties with attention and engagement may compromise the successful use of such devices in some children with EdF, although preliminary research indicates that multifunction devices are more likely to be used by children.[36]

Problem solving

Problem solving skills include the ability to appropriately strategize and manage task demands in order to set and achieve a goal. Problem solving requires organization, planning, sequencing, multistep task performance, identifying and applying an appropriate strategy, as well as monitoring one's own performance towards goal attainment. In the pediatric neuropsychology literature, there have been several theoretical papers emphasizing the need to explicitly teach children problem solving strategies.[1,3,5] Marlowe (2000) emphasized that children with EdF can be taught the steps of problem solving, including identifying a goal to be accomplished, identifying potential strategies to accomplish the goal, selecting the best strategy, developing a sequential series of planning steps, identifying and collecting materials to complete the task, beginning the task according to plan, monitoring for accuracy, modifying as necessary throughout the task, and cleaning up. The model presented by Marlowe also emphasizes that it is important to engage children in familiar routines and provide only as much external support as needed to complete a task.

While approaches to teaching problem solving strategies to children with EdF have been outlined,[1,3,5] there have been few well-designed studies examining the efficacy of such instruction in children with EdF. In contrast, the adult neuropsychology literature provides much stronger support for these interventions. For example, training in formal problem solving strategies and their application to everyday activities is considered a practice guideline for adults with TBI.[8] Currently, however, there is not enough evidence available in the literature to make a similar clinical recommendation for younger age groups.[48]

Training in one aspect of problem solving (metacognitive skills) has very strong support in the adult literature. Metacognition is the knowledge about the nature and content (including strengths and weaknesses) of one's own cognitive skills. It involves the ability to reflect and act on the knowledge of one's own cognitive capacities, in order to modify ineffective processes and strategies.[49] Metacognition includes active regulation, self-monitoring, and self-evaluation of ongoing cognition, by which the child gradually gains conscious control of learning.[50] Metacognitive strategy training is recommended as a practice standard for EdF after TBI in adults and as a component of interventions for deficits in other areas such as attention and memory.[8]

Until recently, there have been few studies highlighting the effectiveness of problem solving training and/or metacognitive skill development in children. Efficacy of a problem solving training program was examined in a small group of children following ABI.[50] Results revealed that this training technique contributed to improved performance on a computer-based problem-solving task. Moreover, participants, parents, and teaching staff reported generalization of the training program. There is also evidence from case series reports that children have been observed to improve functional life skills when they are taught to identify causes of success and failure, and when they are provided explicit feedback about their performance.[51–53]

A pilot study was conducted evaluating a problem-solving skills training program in 12 survivors of childhood cancer who had cognitive deficits.[54] (See Chapter 12 for information about EdF in pediatric cancer.) This clinic-based training program (60 to 90 minutes, once a week for 15 consecutive weeks) was designed to improve daily problem solving, attention and memory, and academic performance by providing instruction in five core components: (1) a general problem-solving framework; (2) behavioral study skills and metacognitive strategies; (3) mnemonic techniques; (4) compensatory techniques focusing on improving academic mastery; and (5) collaborative contact with child's parents and teachers. The majority of children completed 70% of sessions, although not all within the 3- month time limit. Parents reported that missed sessions were related to difficulty traveling to the clinic after school hours. Improvements were observed on objective measures and parent ratings of perceived problem solving. While differences were noted between pre- and post-testing, the study did not include a control group and no follow-up data were obtained.

A randomized, controlled trial examined explicit instruction of problem solving training (based on metacognitive principles) in children with ABI in Hong Kong.[55] (See Chapter 16 for information about EdF in ABI.) Participants included 32 children with ABI who were enrolled in a mainstream educational setting and had impaired problem solving. The average time from ABI onset to initiation of problem solving training was 3 years. Children were matched as pairs based on demographic factors and then randomly assigned to the problem solving training group or a waitlist control group. Intervention included 14 group sessions comprised of 5–6 children, meeting twice per week, for 3 hours each. The program focused on teaching children how to identify problems in a systematic and structured way, generate alternative solutions, identify a goal to fix the problem, and monitor their progress, allowing them to modify behavior based on feedback that arose from the consequences of a chosen action. Although the experimental group had better functioning than the comparison group at baseline, results revealed that children in the experimental group made greater improvements between pre- and post-testing in their abstract reasoning, metacognitive skills, and functional behavior in the home and social situations relative to the comparison group. Of note, the therapists who provided the intervention also performed the pre- and post-testing, and neither therapists nor parents were blinded to intervention assignment. Additionally, no follow-up data were obtained, so maintenance was not evaluated.

There is a developing body of literature suggesting that teaching specific problem solving strategies to children and their families is efficacious. In a randomized controlled trial, a psychotherapeutic intervention to help families of children with TBI develop problem solving strategies resulted in reduced behavioral problems.[56] In that study, 32 families of school-aged children with moderate to severe TBIs were randomly assigned to a family-centered problem solving (FPS) intervention or usual care during a six month period. The FPS intervention consisted of seven biweekly core sessions and up to four individualized sessions focusing on problem solving and didactic training to address unresolved stressors of the individual families. The problem solving skills framework involved a five-step process: "Aim, Brainstorm, Choose, Do It, and Evaluate." Sessions took place in a clinic or in the family's home. Fifteen of the 19 families receiving intervention attended the seven core sessions. Results indicated significant improvement in child internalizing behavior problems for the FPS group relative to the usual care group. The intervention, however, did not address the varying developmental levels and consequent learning needs of all the participating children (Wade, SL. Email sent to: Beth Slomine. 12th August 2011), hampering generalizability.

To focus more closely on the problem solving difficulties common in adolescents with EdF, Wade and colleagues[57,58] conducted a preliminary study designed specifically for families of adolescents with TBI. Nine families of adolescents injured less than 24 months prior to the intervention participated. The Teen Online Problem Solving (TOPS) program consisted of ten core web-based sessions and up to four supplemental web-based sessions designed to target EF skills that are essential for adult functioning. After an initial in-home session with a therapist, sessions included self-guided web exercises and a videoconference therapy session. Both parent- and self-report measures indicated improvement in the adolescent's internalizing behavior and mood.[57] In a larger follow-up study of 41 families randomly assigned to either TOPS or an internet resources comparison group, self-report indicated improvements in EF after TOPS, but parent-report did not reveal significant improvement between treatment groups.[58] Another report from that intervention study revealed less parent-reported parent–teen conflict at follow-up in the TOPS group, with moderating effects of SES and injury severity observed on improvements in behavior problems.[59] These findings suggest that intervention efficacy may vary in response to patient characteristics. Importantly, in this series of studies, children were not required to have problem-solving difficulties or other EdF to be eligible to participate; treatment effects may have been minimized as children without EdF were less likely to show improvement on the outcome measures.

Explicit instruction in problem solving has also been evaluated in the classroom. From the educational literature, there is evidence for the use of the teaching technique called Direct Instruction for enhancing skills in children with a variety of special learning needs. Direct Instruction is a systematic instructional approach that has many components in common with explicit instruction in problem solving strategies, including explicit instruction and practice, consistent instructional routines, introduction and modeling of component skills, use of guided practice, teaching of generalizable strategies, and frequent and cumulative review.[60] In a large meta-analysis, direct instruction combined with explicit instruction in problem solving strategies was shown to be the most effective instructional approach for teaching children with LD[61] among all approaches considered. (See Chapter 9 for information about EdF in LD.)

Graham and Harris have developed self-regulated strategy development (SRSD), an intervention that combines strategy instruction and the development of self-regulation skills including goal setting, self-instruction, self- monitoring, and self-reinforcement. SRSD has been employed in several academic domains, with its largest body of evidence seen in the area of writing instruction. A meta-analysis of 18 single-case and small-group studies indicated that SRSD led to significant improvement in writing skills among a variety of elementary to high school aged students with diagnoses of LD, students at risk for difficulties, and students without disabilities.[62]

In summary, explicit instruction of problem-solving strategies is useful for promoting day-to-day EF and reducing difficulties in children with EdF. As demonstrated in the adult literature, there is some evidence to suggest that explicit instruction of one particular aspect of problem solving skills – metacognitive skills – may be particularly important in helping children with EdF. While instruction in metacognitive skills is a practice standard for adults with EdF secondary to TBI, research on the efficacy of metacognitive skill instruction in children is lacking, although accumulating evidence is promising. In addition, studies are showing that involving families and teachers is a crucial component of many problem solving interventions for children. Teaching problem solving strategies, however, can be time intensive and some studies of clinic-based interventions describe a notable rate of missed sessions. As a result, online and school-based problem solving programs may be more practical.

Inhibitory control

Inhibitory control is the ability to resist an impulse or stop one's own behavior. Deficits in inhibitory control often present as disruptive behavior or impaired social–emotional regulation. As such, strategies used by behavior specialists are often helpful when promoting inhibitory control. In adults with TBI, problem solving strategy training typically includes explicit instruction of verbal self-regulation strategies to promote emotional regulation. In line with this, practice guidelines for training in formal problem solving to improve everyday functioning emphasize that strategies to promote emotional regulation are a necessary component.[8]

Several intervention programs have been designed to reduce behavioral problems and improve social competence in both typically developing children and children at risk for behavioral and academic difficulties. These programs include parent and/or classroom interventions, and facilitate self-regulation by promoting social-emotional development and competence.[63] For example, randomized controlled studies that included over 300 children in each trial showed that the promoting alternative thinking strategies (PATHS) curriculum (a curriculum-based intervention that focuses on social skills, aggression control, and conflict management) improved inhibitory control on cognitive tests in typically developing second and third graders[64] and in at-risk preschool children enrolled in Head Start.[65] Similarly, another educational intervention, Tools of the Mind, led to improved performance on EF tests in 85 typically-developing preschoolers. Tools of the Mind promotes EF with strategies like self-regulatory private speech, dramatic play, and memory and attention aids.[66]

A similar educational intervention was also found to be efficacious for children who display disruptive behaviors. In a randomized controlled study, over 200 kindergarten through third grade students identified as having difficulties with behavior, social–emotional functioning, and on-task behavior were assigned to a 4-month school-based intervention or a waitlist control group.[67] The intervention consisted of working with a mentor to learn and practice behavioral and cognitive skills focused on improving self-regulation and school adaptation. Compared with waitlist controls, children who participated in the intervention demonstrated significantly reduced teacher-rated problems in the areas of behavioral control, social skills, social withdrawal, and off-task behaviors, and demonstrated a reduction in disciplinary referrals.[67] For a comprehensive review of curriculum- and educational-based interventions, the reader is referred to Chapter 18 in this volume.

Much of the available information regarding interventions to improve inhibitory skills in clinical populations comes from research on ADHD and behavior disorders, as inhibitory control deficits are one of the core defining features of ADHD[69] (see chapter 5 for additional information about EdF in ADHD). In general, the existing research, including the results of the NIMH-funded multimodal treatment of attention deficit hyperactivity disorder (MTA) study[68] suggests that combined behavioral and pharmacological treatment is the most effective approach for reducing overall ADHD symptoms (e.g., inattention and distractibility, impulsivity, and motor restlessness). Behavioral interventions in the home and school environment that target task engagement and disruptive behavior have also resulted in improvements in parent ratings and observed behavior.[70] In a review of the literature on psychosocial and behavioral interventions for children with ADHD, Pelham and Fabiano concluded that behavioral parent training, behavioral classroom management, and intensive summer program peer interventions are well supported as evidence-based treatments for ADHD in children.[71] Additionally, review of psychosocial treatments for child and adolescent disruptive behavior, including ODD and CD, identified 16 treatments, including both parent- and child-training programs (e.g., Parent Management Training Oregon Model, Parent-Child Interaction Therapy, and Anger Control Training) as efficacious evidence-based treatments.[72] (See chapter 5 for information about EdF in ODD and CD.)

Interventions for either increasing or decreasing target behaviors (e.g., off-task behavior, impulsive or disinhibited behavior, and disruptive behavior) have also been examined in children with TBI (see Chapter 16 for additional information about EdF in TBI). Specifically, there are several case studies and case series suggesting that providing support and routine in the child's everyday environment through the use of context-sensitive, cognitive behavioral scripts is promising. For example, in a series of eight single-subject reversal designs,[73–76] Feeney and Ylvisaker demonstrated that a combined behavioral, cognitive, and EF intervention delivered in a public school setting reduced the frequency and intensity of aggressive behaviors and increased the amount of work accomplished. The participants were children aged 6–7[73–75] and 10 and 17[76] who demonstrated significant self-regulatory difficulties after TBI. The intervention employed graphic organizers (i.e., photographic cues), a structured daily routine, and cognitive and behavioral strategies within each student's everyday classroom setting.

In another case study, a comprehensive behavioral program with several antecedent management strategies reduced the frequency of challenging and disruptive behaviors and increased school task completion in two adolescents with a history of TBI (ages 12 and 13) in their residential school placement.[77] Similarly, participation in a structured after-school behavioral treatment program with clear rules/routines and a token economy system resulted in a decrease in disruptive behavior in three children with ABI aged 8, 6, and 14.[78] In a small-case series, on-task behavior improved during independent math assignments in three adolescents with ABI who were explicitly taught to self-monitor their attention, productivity, and accuracy in school.[79] All three adolescents displayed increased on-task behavior during treatment (relative to baseline), and improvements were maintained during follow-up.

Although behavioral reinforcement can improve inhibitory control in children with EdF, the effectiveness of reinforcement may vary across specific population groups. For example, children with ADHD require stronger incentives to improve their inhibitory control on an inhibition task (relative to typically developing children).[80] Similarly, reward contingencies are not as effective in improving inhibition for children with TBI compared with children with ADHD or unaffected controls.[81] This has led some researchers to suggest that antecedent control should be emphasized over manipulation of consequences when working to modify behavior in children with significant inhibitory control deficits as a result of ABI or other NDDs.[82]

In summary, there is growing support that interventions incorporating behavioral, environmental, and cognitive supports can improve aspects of inhibitory control in both typically developing children and children with EdF. Evidence suggests that these interventions are particularly effective in the educational setting, where children are supported by the teachers in their everyday environment. However, further research is necessary to better understand the efficacy of specific interventions to promote inhibitory control in specific population groups.

Pharmacological interventions

Pharmacology has emerged as one of the primary methods used to treat EdF (particularly inattention) in a variety of populations (e.g., ADHD, ABI). Across multiple studies, stimulants have been shown to have reasonably strong evidence for their use to improve attention, particularly in ADHD where stimulants such as d-amphetamine and methylphenidate are the first-line choice. These drugs enhance dopamine release from presynaptic dopamine terminals, which is believed to contribute to greater availability of dopamine to support regulatory neural networks. An additional form of amphetamine (l-amphetamine) releases norepinephrine in addition to dopamine,[83] and is believed to support enhanced attentional control. Cholinesterase inhibitors, including donepezil, have also shown promise in the improvement of attention, including divided attention, as well as with memory and processing speed.[84–86] In addition, several neuroleptics have been used with some success to address attentional insufficiency,[87–90] albeit not without controversy given their side effect profiles. Finally, other medications with less understood mechanisms of action (e.g., amantadine) have also show promise in improvement of EdF. Below is a brief review of the efficacy of pharmacological agents for treatment of various aspects of EdF.

In the aforementioned MTA study, the long-term effects of stimulant medications and behavioral therapy were evaluated. In the initial phase, children aged 7–10 were assigned to one of four treatment arms: intensive behavioral therapy, intensive medication management (with individual titration of dosage), a combination of the two, or routine community care. After 14 months, results indicated that children in the combination group and medication management group both showed significantly greater reduction of

ADHD symptoms than children assigned to either the behavior therapy or routine community care groups.[68] While findings persisted at 24 months, effect sizes were reduced.[91] Of note, after 36 months, with significant changes observed in medication use patterns (e.g., children in the combination group discontinuing medication; children in the behavior group initiating medication) differences in symptom reduction between the original groups were no longer apparent. However, all groups showed improvement from baseline.[92]

More recently, Rowles and Findling[93] reviewed the literature on the efficacy of stimulant medications in children with developmental disabilities and "ADHD-like symptoms." Populations reviewed included children with impaired intelligence, PDD, genetic disorders (including FraX, DS, tuberous sclerosis, NF-1, and WS), and children who had been exposed in utero to alcohol. (See Chapters 6, 7, and 14 for information about EdF in these conditions.) In general, the authors found that similar effectiveness with stimulants is obtained in children with or without developmental disorders; however, the authors noted that risk and side effect profiles may be greater in children with developmental disabilities, as compared to typically-developing children with EdF.

In the ABI population, methylphenidate has been shown to have a positive effect on attention, concentration, and vigilance.[94] Additionally, while other dopaminergic agents have been less frequently studied in children and adolescents with ABI, evidence has been shown for increased attention in patients prescribed amantadine after TBI.[95] However, variability in effects of medications intended to improve attention has been seen as well, including evidence of worse attentional performance in adults prescribed bromocriptine after TBI;[96] no significant improvements with amantadine as compared to placebo;[97] and significant dose-related attentional improvements with bromocriptine in a TBI case study.[98] Williams[99] reviewed the literature on the use of amantadine after TBI in children and found significant improvements in the areas of alertness and arousal. However, no significant improvements were observed on performance-based measures of attention or EF, while improved parental ratings of inhibitory control, flexibility, and emotional modulation were reported.

Cholinergic medications have also been evaluated in the ADHD and ABI populations. In a case report of eight children and adolescents (ages 10–17) with PDD, ADHD-like symptoms, and other psychiatric comorbidity, severity of ADHD-like symptoms decreased with donepezil treatment.[100] However, in a double-blind, placebo-controlled trial of 34 children and adolescents (ages 8–17) with ASD, both the treatment and control groups improved, and no statistically significant between-group differences were reported.[101] When donepezil was administered to three teenagers after severe TBI, participants demonstrated increased learning and immediate recall, but no improvement in delayed recall. The authors interpreted this as evidence of improved EF (e.g., attention and WM) as opposed to memory.[102] Families of the participants reported "real-world" improvements in WM (e.g., remembering instructions to get something in another room).

Neuroleptics have also been studied in children with ADHD and comorbid DBD (e.g., ODD, CD; see chapter 5). Gunther and colleagues[103] did not find significant risperidone-related improvement relative to controls or to pre-treatment baseline on a Go/No-Go task in their evaluation of 23 children with ADHD who had at least one comorbid DBD. However, improvements were observed on clinician ratings of inattention/hyperactivity and aggression. While other studies of neuroleptics have shown some efficacy in addressing aspects of inhibitory control, including behavioral control and aggression,[87–90] many of these studies have focused on adults after ABI. Overall, the use of neuroleptics to treat behavioral dyscontrol after ABI (e.g., agitation, behavioral disturbance) is not well researched; and much of the available information regarding their use in this population comes from case reports. Significant adverse effects such as extrapyramidal side effects significantly limit the acceptability of neuroleptics to patients and their families.

Currently, methylphenidate, dopaminergic agents, and some of the neuroleptics hold the most promise for treatment of individuals with EdF. However, more research and the development of clear practice standards are necessary in formulating the best treatment planning for children with a variety of etiologies of EdF.

Translating research to practice

In order to translate research into practice, clinicians need to be aware of the current literature and also have access to successful research interventions. In the past, many research-validated programs were not commercially available or were cost-prohibitive, limiting their use. However, as access to computers, the internet, handheld data phones, and personal tablets has increased, availability of validated interventions, including external reminder aides, monitoring devices, and training programs has also increased. At the same time, multiple online programs and applications (i.e., "apps") for electronic devices are now readily available, claiming "brain training" or "brain fitness" properties. Unfortunately, however, many of these new programs and apps have little research behind them, and, as such, are extremely limited in terms of reliability and validity data to support their consideration for clinical use. Further research into more readily available and cost-effective programs is both warranted and sorely needed.

Access to research-based attention and WM interventions, and solid empirical support for their use has increased significantly. A few of the currently available products are described below, and summarized in Table 3. Sohlberg and Mateer's[11,12] evidence-based APT model has been adapted and developed into a commercially available computer-based product. The most recently released and updated product, *APT-3* (see Table 17.3), includes a range of attention exercises appropriate for adolescents and adults with history of ABI and related attentional impairments. Targeted areas include sustained attention and executive control processes related to WM, selective attention, and suppression and alternating of attention. The program is administered by a clinician along with related strategy training and generalization activities. Similarly, for pediatric populations with history of ABI or ADHD, The *Pay Attention!* (see Table 17.3) system includes activities for remediation of attention in children aged 4–10. Both of these programs are adaptations of the original[11] APT model.

Cogmed Working Memory Training is another evidence-based computer-administered product developed to train attention and WM. It is commercially available through Pearson for three age groups (pre-school, middle school/adolescent, and adult). The currently available version is based upon the WM training program originally developed by Klingberg.[23]

Lumosity (see Table 17.3) offers fee-based online "training" games through their website, as well as via an iPhone/iPad application called *Brain Trainer*. Activities are intended to increase WM, attention, and a variety of other cognitive domains. Several condition-specific activities are available online on an "experimental" basis.

Access to devices which can be used to improve initiation in children with EdF has also increased. Currently, many children and adolescents have their own cell phones, smartphones, mp3 players, or personal data tablets, all of which can be easily programmed to make use of the alarm or calendar features or by downloading relevant applications that may support organization. Many are available for free or a minimal fee. Although formally researched products (e.g., *NeuroPage*) are less accessible, such devices often rely upon SMS (text message) technology to send task reminders. Children in need of prompts or cues could easily receive text or video messages from caregivers, parents, or teachers at certain times throughout the day.

Manualized treatment programs offer effective ways to translate specific research protocols into useful interventions for clinicians. Many manualized programs have been published to support behavior management and extend opportunities for behavior control, including Barkley's *Defiant Children*.[104]

Involvement of caregivers, parents, and teachers has emerged as a common theme in effective treatments for children and adolescents with EdF, particularly in regard to problem-solving skills. Incorporating families and educators consistently into interventions and treatment is an easy way for clinicians to translate research into practice, particularly when addressing problem solving deficits found in a variety of clinical conditions. Using reminding devices across settings, implementing an individualized intervention program within the child's school setting, and developing curriculum-based interventions all hold great promise for building EF skills in children.

Taken together, future efforts should focus on translating researched interventions into programs which are commercially available, easily accessible via small personal devices, affordable, and can be implemented by children and supported by parents, clinicians, and teachers.

Summary and future directions

In this chapter, we explored the developing literature examining computer-based training for attention and WM skills, the use of external cueing systems to promote initiation, metacognitive skill development and support to improve organization, planning, and problem solving, as well as behavior management techniques to address difficulties with inhibitory control. A basic review of common pharmacologic interventions was also provided. Although the literature on cognitive and behavioral interventions for children with EdF is currently limited, the research exploring the efficacy of these interventions is growing rapidly. As new technologies allow for increased utilization of EdF interventions by clinicians, educators, and the lay public, it is essential that our research efforts stay ahead of the curve in order to inform the use of these technologies and interventions. Further research needs to be conducted to examine the effectiveness of interventions in children of various ages with EdF as a result of differing etiologies in order to appropriately tailor the intervention to the child.

References

1. Mahone EM, Slomine BS. Managing dysexecutive disorders. In Hunter S, Donders J, eds. *Pediatric Neuropsychological Intervention*. Cambridge, UK: Cambridge University Press; 2007.

2. Slomine B, Locascio G. Cognitive rehabilitation for children with acquired brain injury. *Dev Disabil Res Rev* 2009; 15(2): 133–43.

3. Marlowe WB. An intervention for children with disorders of executive functions. *Dev Neuropsychol* 2000; 18(3): 445–54.

4. Ylvisaker M, Szekeres SF, Haarbauer-Krupa J. Cognitive rehabilitation: organization, memory and language. In: Ylvisaker M, ed. *Traumatic Brain Injury Rehabilitation: Children and Adolescents* (Revised Edition). Boston: Butterworth-Heinemann; 1998; 181–220.

5. Ylvisaker M, Turkstra LS, Coelho C. Behavioral and social interventions for individuals with traumatic brain injury: a summary of the research with clinical implications. *Semin Speech lang* 2005; **26**(4): 256–67.

6. Prigatano GP. Challenging dogma in neuropsychology and related disciplines. *Arch Clin Neuropsychol* 2003; **18**(8): 811–25.

7. Edlund W, G.G, So Y, Franklin G. *AAN Clinical Practice Guideline Process Manual.* St Paul: American Academy of Neurology; 2004.

8. Cicerone KD, Langenbahn DM, Braden C, *et al.* Evidence-based cognitive rehabilitation: updated review of the literature from 2003 through 2008. *Arch Phys Med Rehabil* 2011; **92**(4): 519–30.

9. Sohlberg MM, Mateer CA. *Theory and Remediation of Attention Disorders. Introduction to Cognitive Rehabilitation: Theory and Practice.* New York: Guilford Press; 1989. 110–13.

10. Baddeley A, Logie R, Bressi S, Della Sala S, Spinnler H. Dementia and working memory. *Quart J Exp Psychol A* 1986; **38**(4): 603–18.

11. Sohlberg MM, Mateer CA. *Attention Process Training (APT).* Puyallup, WA: Association for Neuropsychological Research and Development; 1986.

12. Sohlberg MM, Mateer CA. Effectiveness of an attention training program. *Journal of Clinical and Experimental Neuropsychology* 1987; **9**(2): 117–30.

13. Cicerone KD, Dahlberg C, Malec JF, *et al.* Evidence-based cognitive rehabilitation: updated review of the literature from 1998 through 2002. *Arch Phys Med Rehab* 2005; **86**(8): 1681–92.

14. Rohling ML, Faust ME, Beverly B, Demakis G. Effectiveness of cognitive rehabilitation following acquired brain injury: A meta-analytic re-examination of Cicerone *et al.*'s (2000, 2005) systematic reviews. *Neuropsychology* 2009; **23**(1): 20–39.

15. Laatsch L, Harrington D, Hotz G, *et al.* An evidence-based review of cognitive and behavioral rehabilitation treatment studies in children with acquired brain injury. *J Head Trauma Rehab* 2007; **22**(4): 248–56.

16. Van't Hooft I, Andersson K, Bergman B, Sejersen T, Von Wendt L, Bartfai A. Beneficial effect from a cognitive training programme on children with acquired brain injuries demonstrated in a controlled study. *Brain Inj* 2005; **19**(7): 511–18.

17. Sjo NM, Spellerberg S, Weidner S, Kihlgren M. Training of attention and memory deficits in children with acquired brain injury. *Acta Paediatr* 2010; **99**(2): 230–6.

18. Butler RW, Copeland DR. Attentional processes and their remediation in children treated for cancer: a literature review and the development of a therapeutic approach. *J Int Neuropsychol Soc* 2002; **8**(1): 115–24.

19. Galbiati S, Recla M, Pastore V, *et al.* Attention remediation following traumatic brain injury in childhood and adolescence. *Neuropsychology* 2009; **23**(1): 40–9.

20. Martinussen R, Hayden J, Hogg-Johnson S, Tannock R. A meta-analysis of working memory impairments in children with attention-deficit/hyperactivity disorder. *J Am Acad Child Adolesc Psychiatry* 2005; **44**(4): 377–84.

21. Seidman LJ, Biederman J, Valera EM, Monteaux MC, Doyle AE, Faraone SV. Neuropsychological functioning in girls with attention-deficit/hyperactivity disorder with and without learning disabilities. *Neuropsychology* 2006; **20**(2): 166–77.

22. Willcutt EG, Sonuga-Barke EJ, Nigg JT, Sergeant JA. Recent developments in neuropsychological models of childhood psychiatric disorders. In Banaschewski T, Rohde LA, eds. *Biological Child Psychiatry: Recent Trends and Developments.* Basel, Switzerland: Karger; 2008, 195–226.

23. Klingberg T, Forssberg H, Westerberg H. Training of working memory in children with ADHD. *J Clin Exp Neuropsychol* 2002; **24**(6): 781–91.

24. Klingberg T, Fernell E, Olesen PJ, *et al.*
    Computerized training of working memory
    in children with ADHD – a randomized,
    controlled trial. *J Am Acad Child Adolesc
    Psychiatry* 2005;
    44(2): 177–86.

25. Beck SJ, Hanson CA, Puffenberger SS,
    Benninger KL, Benninger WB.
    A controlled trial of working memory
    training for children and adolescents with
    ADHD. *J Clin Child Adolesc Psychol* 2010;
    39(6): 825–36.

26. Lohaugen GC, Antonsen I, Haberg A, *et al.*
    Computerized working memory training
    improves function in adolescents born at
    extremely low birth weight. *J Pediatr* 2011;
    158(4): 555–61.e4.

27. Thorell LB, Lindqvist S, Bergman Nutley S,
    Bohlin G, Klingberg T. Training and
    transfer effects of executive functions in
    preschool children. *Dev Sci* 2009;
    12(1): 106–13.

28. Rabiner DL, Murray DW, Skinner AT,
    Malone PS. A randomized trial of two
    promising computer-based interventions
    for students with attention difficulties.
    J Abnorm Child Psychol 2010; **38**(1):
    131–42.

29. Bangirana P, Giordani B, John CC,
    Page C, Opoka RO, Boivin MJ.
    Immediate neuropsychological and
    behavioral benefits of computerized
    cognitive rehabilitation in Ugandan
    pediatric cerebral malaria survivors.
    J Dev Behav Pediatr 2009; **30**(4):
    310–18.

30. Boivin MJ, Busman RA, Parikh SM, *et al.*
    A pilot study of the neuropsychological
    benefits of computerized cognitive
    rehabilitation in Ugandan children
    with HIV. *Neuropsychology* 2010;
    24(5): 667–73.

31. Kerns KA, Macsween J, Vander Wekken S,
    Gruppuso V. Investigating the efficacy of
    an attention training programme in
    children with foetal alcohol spectrum
    disorder. *Dev Neurorehabil* 2010; **13**(6):
    413–22.

32. Kesler S. Cognitive intervention and
    neuroplasticity in children with

    neurodevelopmentally based executive
    function deficits. *J Int Neuropsychol Soc*
    2008; **14**(S1): 179.

33. Kesler SR, Lacayo NJ, Jo B. A pilot study of
    an online cognitive rehabilitation program
    for executive function skills in children
    with cancer-related brain injury. *Brain Inj*
    2011; **25**(1): 101–12.

34. Loring DW, Meador KJ, eds. *INS
    Dictionary of Neuropsychology*. New York:
    Oxford University Press; 1998.

35. DePompei R, Gillette Y, Goetz E,
    Xenopoulos-Oddsson A, Bryen D, Dowds
    M. Practical applications for use of PDAs
    and smartphones with children and
    adolescents who have traumatic brain
    injury. *NeuroRehabilitation* 2008; **23**(6):
    487–99.

36. Cihak D, Kessler K, Alberto PA. Use of a
    handheld prompting system to transition
    independently through vocational tasks for
    students with moderate and severe
    intellectual disabilities. *Educ Train Dev
    Disab* 2008; **43**(1): 102–10.

37. Mechling LC, Gast DL, Seid NH.
    Evaluation of a personal digital assistant as
    a self-prompting device for increasing
    multi-step task completion by students
    with moderate intellectual disabilities. *Educ
    Train Autism Dev Disabi* 2010; **45**(3):
    422–39.

38. Wilson BA, Emslie HC, Quirk K, Evans JJ.
    Reducing everyday memory and planning
    problems by means of a paging system: a
    randomised control crossover study.
    J Neurol Neurosurg Psychiatry 2001;
    70(4): 477–82.

39. Wilson BA, Emslie H, Evans JJ, Quirk K,
    Watson P, Fish J. The NeuroPage system
    for children and adolescents with
    neurological deficits. *Dev Neurorehabil*
    2009; **12**(6): 421–6.

40. Gillette Y, DePompei R. The potential of
    electronic organizers as a tool in the
    cognitive rehabilitation of young people.
    NeuroRehabilitation 2004; **19**(3):
    233–43.

41. Ferguson H, Myles BS, Hagiwara T. Using
    a personal digital assistant to enhance the
    independence of an adolescent with

Asperger syndrome. *Educ Train Dev Disab* 2005; **40**(1): 60–7.

42. Alberto PA, Taber TA, Fredrick LD. Use of self-operated auditory prompts to decrease aberrant behaviors in students with moderate mental retardation. *Res Dev Disabil* 1999; **20**(6): 429–39.

43. Epstein J, Willis M, Conners C, Johnson D. Use of a technological prompting device to aid a student with attention deficit hyperactivity disorder to initiate and complete daily tasks: an exploratory study. *J Special Educ Technol* 2001; **16**(1): 19–28.

44. Flannery MA, Butterbaugh GJ, Rice DA, Rice JC. Reminding technology for prospective memory disability: a case study. *Pediatr Rehabil* 1997; **1**(4): 239–44.

45. Zabel TA, Kirk JK, Mahone EM, *et al.* The use of electronic devices to cue self-catheterization for adolescents with Spina Bifida [abstract]. *Cereb Fluid Res* 2004; **1** (Suppl 1) (S57).

46. Mechling LC, Gast DL, Seid NH. Using a personal digital assistant to increase independent task completion by students with autism spectrum disorder. *J Autism Dev Disord* 2009; **39**(10): 1420–34.

47. Cihak D, Fahrenkrog C, Ayres KM, Smith C. The use of video modeling via a video iPod and a system of least prompts to improve transitional behaviors for students with autism spectrum disorders in the general education classroom. *J Positive Behav Interventions* 2010; **12**(2): 103–15.

48. Kennedy MRT, Coelho C, Turkstra L, *et al.* Intervention for executive functions after traumatic brain injury: a systematic review, meta-analysis and clinical recommendations. *Neuropsychol Rehabil* 2008; **18**(3): 257–99.

49. Dennis M, Barnes MA, Donnelly RE, Wilkinson M, Humphreys R. Appraising and managing knowledge: Metacognitive skills after childhood head injury. *Dev Neuropsychol* 1996; **12**: 77–103.

50. Suzman KB, Morris RD, Morris MK, Milan MA. Cognitive-behavioral remediation of problem solving deficits in children with acquired brain injury.

J Behav Ther Exp Psychiatry 1997; **28**(3): 203–12.

51. Gureasko-Moore S, Dupaul GJ, White GP. The effects of self-management in general education classrooms on the organizational skills of adolescents with ADHD. *Behav Modif* 2006; **30**(2): 159–83.

52. Snyder MC, Bambara LM. Teaching secondary students with learning disabilities to self-manage classroom survival skills. *J Learn Disab* 1997; **30**(5): 534–43.

53. Crowley JA, Miles MA. Cognitive remediation in pediatric head injury: a case study. *J Pediatr Psychol* 1991; **16**(5): 611–27.

54. Patel SK, Katz ER, Richardson R, Rimmer M, Kilian S. Cognitive and problem solving training in children with cancer: a pilot project. *J Pediatr Hematol Oncol* 2009; **31**(9): 670–7.

55. Chan DY, Fong KN. The effects of problem-solving skills training based on metacognitive principles for children with acquired brain injury attending mainstream schools: a controlled clinical trial. *Disab Rehabil* 2011; **33**: 2023–32.

56. Wade SL, Michaud L, Brown TM. Putting the pieces together: preliminary efficacy of a family problem-solving intervention for children with traumatic brain injury. *J Head Trauma Rehab* 2006; **21**(1): 57–67.

57. Wade SL, Walz NC, Carey JC, Williams KM. Preliminary efficacy of a Web-based family problem-solving treatment program for adolescents with traumatic brain injury. *J Head Trauma Rehabil* 2008; **23**(6): 369–77.

58. Wade SL, Walz NC, Carey J, Williams KM, Cass J, Herren L, *et al.* A randomized trial of teen online problem solving for improving executive function deficits following pediatric traumatic brain injury. *J Head Trauma Rehabil* 2010; **25**(6): 409–15.

59. Wade SL, Walz NC, Carey J, *et al.* Effect on behavior problems of teen online problem solving for adolescent TBI: A Randomized Clinical Trial. *Pediatrics* 2011; **128**(4): e947–53.

60. Glang A, Ylvisaker M, Stein M, Ehlhardt L, Todis B, Tyler J. Validated instructional practices: application to students with traumatic brain injury. *J Head Trauma Rehab* 2008; **23**(4): 243–51.

61. Swanson HL, Hoskyn M. Experimental intervention research on students with learning disabilities: a meta-analysis of treatment outcomes. *Rev Educ Res* 1998; **68**: 277–321.

62. Graham S, Harris KR. Students with learning disabilities and the process of writing: a meta-analysis of SRSD studies. In Swanson HL, Harris KR, Graham S, Swanson HL, Harris KR, Graham S, eds. *Handbook of Learning Disabilities.* New York, NY, USA: Guilford Press; 2003, 323–44.

63. Blair C, Diamond A. Biological processes in prevention and intervention: the promotion of self-regulation as a means of preventing school failure. *Dev Psychopathol* 2008; **20**(3): 899–911.

64. Riggs NR, Greenberg MT, Kusche CA, Pentz MA. The mediational role of neurocognition in the behavioral outcomes of a social-emotional prevention program in elementary school students: effects of the PATHS Curriculum. *Prev Sci* 2006; **7**(1): 91–102.

65. Bierman KL, Nix RL, Greenberg MT, Blair C, Domitrovich CE. Executive functions and school readiness intervention: impact, moderation, and mediation in the Head Start REDI program. *Dev Psychopathol* 2008; **20**(3): 821–43.

66. Diamond A, Barnett WS, Thomas J, Munro S. Preschool program improves cognitive control. *Science* 2007; **318**(5855): 1387–8.

67. Wyman PA, Cross W, Hendricks Brown C, Yu Q, Tu X, Eberly S. Intervention to strengthen emotional self-regulation in children with emerging mental health problems: proximal impact on school behavior. *J Abnorm Child Psychol* 2010; **38**(5): 707–20.

68. Group MC. A 14-month randomized clinical trial of treatment strategies for attention-deficit/hyperactivity disorder. The MTA Cooperative Group. Multimodal Treatment Study of Children with ADHD. *Arch Gen Psychiatry* 1999; **56**(12): 1073–86.

69. Barkley RA. Behavioral inhibition, sustained attention, and executive functions: constructing a unifying theory of ADHD. *Psychol Bull* 1997; **121**(1): 65–94.

70. Chronis AM, Jones HA, Raggi VL. Evidence-based psychosocial treatments for children and adolescents with attention-deficit/hyperactivity disorder. *Clin Psychol Rev* 2006; **26**(4): 486–502.

71. Pelham WE, Jr, Fabiano GA. Evidence-based psychosocial treatments for attention-deficit/hyperactivity disorder. *J Clin Child Adolesc Psychol* 2008; **37**(1): 184–214.

72. Eyberg SM, Nelson MM, Boggs SR. Evidence-based psychosocial treatments for children and adolescents with disruptive behavior. *J Clin Child Adolesc Psychol* 2008; **37**(1): 215–37.

73. Feeney TJ, Ylvisaker M. Context-sensitive behavioral supports for young children with TBI: short-term effects and long-term outcome. *J Head Trauma Rehabil* 2003; **18**(1): 33–51.

74. Feeney T, Ylvisaker M. Context-sensitive cognitive-behavioural supports for young children with TBI: a replication study. *Brain Inj* 2006; **20**(6): 629–45.

75. Feeney TJ, Ylvisaker M. Context-sensitive cognitive-behavioral supports for young children with TBI: a second replication study. *J Positive Behav Interventions* 2008 04;**10**(2): 115–28.

76. Feeney TJ. Structured flexibility: the use of context-sensitive self-regulatory scripts to support young persons with acquired brain injury and behavioral difficulties. *J Head Trauma Rehabil* 2010; **25**(6): 416–25.

77. Gardner RM, Bird FL, Maguire H, Carreiro R, Abenaim N. Intensive positive behavior supports for adolescents with acquired brain injury: long-term outcomes in community settings. *J Head Trauma Rehabil* 2003; **18**(1): 52–74.

78. Mottram L, Berger-Gross P. An intervention to reduce disruptive behaviours in children with brain injury. *Pediatr Rehabil* 2004; 7(2): 133–43.

79. Selznick S, Savage RC. Using self-monitoring procedures to increase on-task behavior with three adolescent boys with brain injury. *Behav Intervent* 2000; 15(3): 243–60.

80. Slusarek M, Velling S, Bunk D, Eggers C. Motivational effects on inhibitory control in children with ADHD. *J Am Acad Child Adolesc Psychiatry* 2001; 40(3): 355–63.

81. Konrad K, Gauggel S, Manz A, Scholl M. Lack of inhibition: a motivational deficit in children with attention deficit/hyperactivity disorder and children with traumatic brain injury. *Child Neuropsychol* 2000; 6(4): 286–96.

82. Ylvisaker M, Feeney T. Apprenticeship in self-regulation: supports and interventions for individuals with self-regulatory impairments. *Dev Neurorehabil* 2009; 12(5): 370–9.

83. Stahl S. *Essential Psychopharmacology*. 2nd edn. New York: Cambridge University Press; 2000.

84. Khateb A, Ammann J, Annoni JM, Diserens K. Cognition-enhancing effects of donepezil in traumatic brain injury. *Eur Neurol* 2005; 54(1): 39–45.

85. Zhang L, Plotkin RC, Wang G, Sandel ME, Lee S. Cholinergic augmentation with donepezil enhances recovery in short-term memory and sustained attention after traumatic brain injury. *Arch Phys Med Rehabil* 2004; 85(7): 1050–5.

86. Masanic CA, Bayley MT, VanReekum R, Simard M. Open-label study of donepezil in traumatic brain injury. *Arch Phys Med Rehabil* 2001; 82(7): 896–901.

87. Michals ML, Crismon ML, Roberts S, Childs A. Clozapine response and adverse effects in nine brain-injured patients. *J Clin Psychopharmacol* 1993; 13(3): 198–203.

88. Noe E, Ferri J, Trenor C, Chirivella J. Efficacy of ziprasidone in controlling agitation during post-traumatic amnesia. *Behav Neurol* 2007; 18(1): 7–11.

89. Kim E, Bijlani M. A pilot study of quetiapine treatment of aggression due to traumatic brain injury. *J Neuropsychiatry Clin Neurosci* 2006; 18(4): 547–9.

90. Chatham Showalter PE, Kimmel DN. Agitated symptom response to divalproex following acute brain injury. *J Neuropsychiatry Clin Neurosci* 2000; 12(3): 395–7.

91. MTA Cooperative Group. National Institute of Mental Health Multimodal Treatment Study of ADHD follow-up: 24-month outcomes of treatment strategies for attention-deficit/hyperactivity disorder. *Pediatrics* 2004; 113(4): 754–61.

92. Jensen PS, Arnold LE, Swanson JM, *et al.* 3-year follow-up of the NIMH MTA study. *J Am Acad Child Adolesc Psychiatry* 2007; 46(8): 989–1002.

93. Rowles BM, Findling RL. Review of pharmacotherapy options for the treatment of attention-deficit/hyperactivity disorder (ADHD) and ADHD-like symptoms in children and adolescents with developmental disorders. *Dev Disabil Res Rev* 2010; 16(3): 273–82.

94. Chew E, Zafonte RD. Pharmacological management of neurobehavioral disorders following traumatic brain injury – a state-of-the-art review. *J Rehabil Res Dev* 2009; 46(6): 851–79.

95. Terplan KL, Krauss RF. Histopathologic brain changes in association with ataxia-telangiectasia. *Neurology* 1969; 19: 446–54.

96. Whyte J, Vaccaro M, Grieb-Neff P, Hart T, Polansky M, Coslett HB. The effects of bromocriptine on attention deficits after traumatic brain injury: a placebo-controlled pilot study. *Am J Phys Med Rehabil* 2008; 87(2): 85–99.

97. Schneider WN, Drew-Cates J, Wong TM, Dombovy ML. Cognitive and behavioural efficacy of amantadine in acute traumatic brain injury: an initial double-blind placebo-controlled study. *Brain Inj* 1999; 13(11): 863–72.

98. Ben Smail D, Samuel C, Rouy-Thenaisy K, Regnault J, Azouvi P. Bromocriptine in traumatic brain injury. *Brain Inj* 2006; 20(1): 111–15.

99. Williams SE. Amantadine treatment following traumatic brain injury in children. *Brain Inj* 2007; **21**(9): 885–9.

100. Doyle RL, Frazier J, Spencer TJ, Geller D, Biederman J, Wilens T. Donepezil in the treatment of ADHD-like symptoms in youths with pervasive developmental disorder: a case series. *J Atten Disord* 2006; **9**(3): 543–9.

101. Handen BL, Johnson CR, McAuliffe-Bellin S, Murray PJ, Hardan AY. Safety and efficacy of donepezil in children and adolescents with autism: neuropsychological measures. *J Child Adolesc Psychopharmacol* 2011; **21**(1): 43–50.

102. Trovato M, Slomine B, Pidcock F, Christensen J. The efficacy of donepezil hydrochloride on memory functioning in three adolescents with severe traumatic brain injury. *Brain Inj* 2006; **20**(3): 339–43.

103. Gunther T, Herpertz-Dahlmann B, Jolles J, Konrad K. The influence of risperidone on attentional functions in children and adolescents with attention-deficit/ hyperactivity disorder and co-morbid disruptive behavior disorder. *J Child Adolesc Psychopharmacol* 2006; **16**(6): 725–35.

104. Barkley RA. *Defiant Children: A Clinician's Manual.* New York: The Guilford Press; 1997.

Chapter 18

Educational implications of executive dysfunction

Lisa A. Jacobson and E. Mark Mahone

As has been discussed throughout this volume, EF is a broad term describing the range of skills required for purposeful, goal-directed activity, socially appropriate conduct, and independent regulation of action and affect.[1,2] EF skills can be considered a "domain of neurocognitive competence"[1] that sets the stage for learning, academic achievement, and rule-governed behavioral functioning. In practical terms, EF involves developing and implementing an approach to performing a task that has not been habitually performed.[3] When skills become overlearned through practice and thus automatized, they require less executive or "top-down" control.

In performance-based activities, implementation of EF occurs after perception but before action, thus involving a preparedness to respond.[4] The central components of EF are those that facilitate a "pause" that occurs after perception but before action, that allows for appropriate response preparation. These components include response inhibition, attention regulation, WM, and planning.[5] Expanded definitions of EF also include problem solving skills, organization of behavior, mental flexibility, set-shifting, and the capacity to delay gratification.[2,6] These sub-components are considered separable from the specific cognitive domains and modalities in which they are assessed, but are nevertheless crucial to performance, and critical for remediation of learning difficulties of all kinds.[4]

Terminology for these fundamental skills often varies as a function of discipline-specific literature. For example, the developmental psychology literature refers to these skills as self-regulation and/or effortful control, although assessment of these skills has often relied upon measures tapping very similar types of skills (e.g., inhibition, cognitive control, WM) within cognitive, behavioral, affective, and/or temperamental domains.

EF skills required for the cognitive control of behavior and affect show a protracted (but uneven) developmental trajectory (see Chapters 2 and 3 in this volume for a more detailed discussion of this developmental process). These skills develop throughout childhood and into young adulthood, concurrent with the development of neural synapses, myelination of brain regions, and recruitment and consolidation of neural networks.[7,8] During early childhood, the internalization of standards, the ability to delay gratification, and behavioral and cognitive self-regulatory skills are consolidated and applied to learning and social situations.[9,10] The preschool years provide a critical window in the development of foundational EF skills during the period of rapid neurological, cognitive, and social-behavioral growth.[11] Although various EF skills show different growth rates and trajectories throughout development, many skills emerge by early childhood.[12,13] These include planning and

Executive Function and Dysfunction, ed. Scott J. Hunter and Elizabeth P. Sparrow. Published by Cambridge University Press. © Cambridge University Press 2012.

problem solving,[14] sustained attention,[15] inhibition or switching attention,[16,17] and self-regulation for compliance.[18] Thus, core EF skills such as planning, attentional control, and behavioral self-regulation are evident as early as the pre-school years, with improvement and refinement in these skills throughout childhood and into adulthood.[19]

Contributions to outcomes

Deficits or delays in attaining core EF skills can interfere with a child's ability to successfully manage and complete daily tasks and to navigate social interactions. EdF puts children at risk for ineffective interactions with the environment, leading to significant and lasting cognitive, academic, and social difficulties.[20,21] Problem solving and planning skills are necessary for self-regulation of behavior and affect and for negotiating social interactions where understanding others' behavior in context and responding appropriately becomes important.[13] Not surprisingly then, problems with developing early competence in executive control have been shown to predict children's social problems, with later EF predictive of a variety of psychosocial outcomes in adolescents.[22,23] Similarly, difficulty with behavioral self-regulation may result in a child's failure to develop important social competencies, including compliance with requests, delaying gratification, and managing appropriate behavior in social and educational settings – all skills required for successful school entry.[24] Additionally, deficits in early foundational self-regulatory behaviors may compromise later development of social and behavioral problem-solving skills by significantly impeding academic, adaptive, and social competence.[25,26]

Readiness and availability for learning. EF skills represent an important prerequisite for learning, and provide the cognitive, affective, and behavioral foundation for a student's readiness (globally) and availability (moment-to-moment) for learning. Early school readiness includes not just knowledge of basic pre-academic concepts, but also the ability to behave as a learner. Kindergarten and first grade students are expected to listen attentively, sit still when required, take turns, follow directions, get along with others, and inhibit impulsive actions or irrelevant responses. Early behavioral dysregulation can significantly affect children's functioning during the transition into formal schooling.[27] Data from a national sample of kindergarten teachers indicate that many of the children entering school do not have adequate "learning to learn" skills and show behavioral regulation problems that substantially limit their availability for early learning.[28] In fact, one study found that children's cooperation and self-control significantly predicted kindergarten retention rates.[29] According to teachers, work-related skills such as compliance with directives and listening to instructions were considered the most important skills for kindergarten success, even above pre-academic skills,[30] and can be considered to set the stage for future academic success.

Behavioral regulation. Early behavioral regulation in the classroom has been shown to predict a variety of later school-related behavioral outcomes, including social interaction skills and interpersonal behavior,[31] as well as academic and work-related behaviors.[32,33] For example, at the kindergarten level, children's performance on tasks requiring inhibition, cognitive control, and emotional self-regulation at school entry significantly predicted teachers' reports of children's behavioral self-control, cognitive self-control, and work habits in the spring of the kindergarten year.[34] Blair and Diamond[35] suggested that children who begin school with EdF are at risk for experiencing a "negative feedback loop," in which difficulty with tasks and poor interactions with others lead to changes in self-concept and levels of arousal, which in turn impact cognitive and affective control. These changes reduce children's motivation and investment in the academic process, increase their resistance to school, increase the potential for dropout, and may contribute to the increasing achievement gap between children with and without adequate EF skills.[35]

Cognitive control. Sustained attention and inhibition of impulsive responding have been shown to predict children's cognitive functioning and academic achievement.[36] These skills are important developmentally because academic success depends upon the ability to stay with a task long enough to complete it while avoiding distractions.[37] Not surprisingly, inhibitory control and WM in particular have been shown to be critical to young children's intellectual development[38] and academic success.[39] In very young children, early EdF, within the context of otherwise typical cognitive development, has been hypothesized as a marker of increased risk for early developing psychopathology and LD.[40]

Early EF skills have been shown to predict not only school readiness, but also later academic success.[41,42] For example, early work-related skills assessed at the start of kindergarten predicted reading and math skills during kindergarten and beyond.[43] More broadly, skills involved in executive control are positively correlated with children's academic achievement scores, teacher-rated competence, and academic grades.[44,45] In fact, early EF skills assessed prior to school entry have been shown to predict academic success and psychosocial functioning during the transition into middle school.[33] Specifically, inhibition, effortful control, and nonverbal problem solving skills predict mathematics achievement in kindergarten and beyond. Inhibition made the strongest contribution to early math abilities, while set-shifting, WM, and problem solving all contributed to achievement of later (more conceptually complex) math skills.[41,46,47] Spatial WM in particular has been shown to relate to children's early counting ability[48] and to mathematics achievement as late as middle school.[49]

EF skills have also been implicated in the development of language-related academic skills, including reading (decoding, fluency, comprehension) and written expression.[47,50] For example, WM, inhibition, and planning are associated not only with pre-reading skills in preschool, but also with reading achievement in later elementary school years.[41] In particular, WM and planning have also been shown to be uniquely associated with reading comprehension (over and above the contributions of vocabulary, decoding and reading fluency) in school-aged children,[51] suggesting a link between EdF and late-onset reading comprehension difficulties among children who may not present initially with deficits in basic word decoding skills.[52,53]

Processing speed. Children who struggle to meet these increasingly complex classroom demands are at greater risk of being identified by teachers and even parents as "lazy" or "unmotivated," particularly when they are slower to complete their work or require additional time to complete tasks.[62] In fact, there is increasing evidence that children with EdF may actually require more time to complete tasks; cognitive processing speed is significantly slower for many children who demonstrate EdF.[63] As a result, slowed processing of incoming information can cause affected children to miss aspects of classroom instruction, limiting their capacity to respond to additional incoming information, and delaying their ability to generate a reasonable approach to tasks and events. Furthermore, processing speed influences the efficiency of other academic tasks, including reading fluency[64] as well as more complex tasks such as reading comprehension. For example, children with ADHD tend to show slower reading fluency compared to controls even in the absence of comorbid reading or language disorders.[63,65] These children, although less likely to present with overt behavioral problems, are apt to forget quickly and thus struggle with multiple aspects of classroom functioning related to both implementation of procedures and acquisition of specific academic skills.

Social functioning. Finally, as children progress through school, the complexity of their social interactions increases. Social exchanges demand not only more inferential language and nonverbal communication skills, but also the ability to regulate affect and behavior to meet the demands of the situation. For many children, social interactions that take place within the classroom or broader school setting can be especially challenging. These exchanges may involve some type of conflict, whether teasing, power-struggles, or explicit aggression, circumstances which require the child to regulate emotions, inhibit immediate actions and reactions in order to comply with school expectations and rules, and initiate other methods for dealing with their peers as well as their own reactions. Such situations place a high demand on aspects of EF that some have labeled "hot EF;" these are circuits linking medial and orbital frontal regions with other brain areas (see Chapters 1 and 3). These circuits have been specifically implicated in decision-making under emotionally salient conditions.[66] There is a growing body of work suggesting that EF is a product of complex orchestration of regions in the brain that also process emotion and affective responses to social cues.[67,68] Not surprisingly, EF has been strongly linked to social behavioral problems and psychopathology in children.[33,69]

Executive functions in school

The child–environment interaction. Development of EF occurs within a complex environmental context (see Chapters 2 and 3). Given the prolonged period of postnatal development and maturation of these skills, EF may be especially sensitive to environmental influences.[5,54] The frontostriatal brain systems that support EF have a protracted period of development – and are vulnerable to disruption through a variety of etiologies – which may be why so many children referred clinically present with concerns involving EdF.[55] Accordingly, functional academic difficulties related to EdF may be observed immediately, or, more often across time, such that the full range of functional deficits may not manifest until later in life even though the neurobiological basis of the condition is present earlier (see Chapter 19).[56]

Environmental factors that potentially influence EF development include family SES, parenting styles, parental language competence, and genetic influences,[57,58] among others. Multiple school factors also play an important role in supporting the development of EF skills. The elementary school setting demands an increasingly complex array of executive skills from children, including attentional regulation (i.e., attending to instruction and ignoring distractions), inhibition of impulsive responding, verbal WM (i.e., multi-tasking or remembering multistep instructions), and task approach skills (i.e., determining how to initiate a task or to break more complex tasks into manageable pieces). At the same time, contextual supports for executive control of behavior are typically reduced in later elementary years, leading to a mismatch in some students between skill development and environmental demands.[59] As such, the role of the teacher becomes critical in structuring the classroom, setting daily routines, and providing lessons in a manner that maximizes each child's availability for learning by reducing extraneous EF demands (e.g., multitasking, speeded activities, taking notes from lectures).[60]

Early elementary years. Even in the early elementary grades, certain academic tasks place a high demand on children's developing EF skills. There are particularly heavy demands for inhibition and WM, not only for "readiness" and "availability" behaviors, but also in the actual acquisition of early reading and mathematics skills. In the early grades, academic success is based on concrete, rote learning of new information and skills that become automatized over time through repetition and practice. Examples include learning the alphabet, sound–symbol relationships, sight words, letter formation, and math facts. As children progress through school, learning becomes more integrative. Children are asked to arrange single words (using rules) to make sentences and paragraphs and to apply basic math facts to solve long division problems. By third and fourth grade, instruction shifts from a "learning to read" model to a model requiring application and integration of prior knowledge ("reading to learn"). By fourth grade, assignments routinely require multiple steps, narrative responses, integrating of oral language and writing, and inferential ("beyond the text") thinking.[61] Unlike texts for beginning readers, fourth grade textbooks typically rely on expository language, with no explicit template to aid comprehension and recall. These more complex reading comprehension assignments place an increased demand on children's developing EF skills, especially verbal WM, which facilitates holding information in mind long enough to complete the passage, recall the main idea or relevant information, and answer related questions. Further, by fourth grade, poor reading fluency can increase demands on other cognitive processes (e.g., WM), leading to a competition with word decoding for time-limited resources, thus creating a bottleneck that is associated with rapid forgetting. Writing tasks also increase in complexity by the end of elementary school, as longer essay-type assignments require not only WM, but also organization, self-monitoring, and problem solving.

Late elementary years. As children reach upper elementary grades, expectations increase sharply for independent management of materials, assignments, work completion, and belongings. The structure of the classroom in the primary grades is often explicitly designed to support children's developing ability to transition smoothly between activities and events: teachers provide clear advance warning of upcoming transitions, give specific reminders of expected behavior, and anticipate areas of difficulty and plan accordingly. Often, these behavioral strategies are accompanied by concrete language, single-step directions, wait time between tasks, and assistance as needed. All these supports serve to reduce concurrent EF demands and increase students' readiness. By later elementary school, however, academic demands predominate and classrooms are structured in such a way as to increase the executive demands placed on children. For example, academic tasks increase in complexity; longer assignments must be completed in shorter amounts of time; assignments require more lengthy written output; multiple small groups may take place within the same classroom; lessons involve fewer hands-on materials and greater reliance on a lecture format; instructions frequently consist of multiple steps involving a variety of materials; and multiple transitions across the day take children outside of the classroom.

Furthermore, children are expected to independently monitor their progress on tasks relative to the time remaining, remember to turn in their completed homework, remember to copy the next homework assignment, and plan ahead to collect materials needed to complete upcoming homework. At the same time, expectations in the upper elementary grades and beyond often include the ability to appropriately begin, plan for, and carry out longer-term projects involving multiple steps. Such projects require initiation, problem solving, segmentation (breaking complex tasks into component parts), generating ideas, identifying an efficient approach, and carrying out the plan in a logical order. All of these demands rely heavily on children's EF skills and place children who enter school with EdF at significant risk for diminished academic achievement and negative school outcomes.

Middle school transition. EF skills continue to play an important role in successful academic and social functioning as children progress beyond the primary grades. As academic expectations increase, some children can experience a "regression" in self-regulation during early adolescence.[67] Increases in behavioral dysregulation during early adolescence are seen particularly in children at greatest risk for EdF.[70] At the same time as this developmental dysregulation, most children transition from an elementary school setting into a middle or junior high school setting, adding increasing demands on their still-developing EF skills.[71] The transition into middle school involves a physical change of location, changes in school perspective and instructional formats, increases in the number of different teachers, decreases in perceived teacher support, increases in class size, changes in peer networks, increased expectations for individual responsibility, and increased exposure to the potential for delinquent behavior.[72,73] Each of these new challenges places increasing demands on the child's developing EF skills, as the increased workload, class changes, and larger peer groups require greater self-regulation and WM than were required in an elementary school setting.[74] The changes in expectations and responsibilities at sixth grade are more apparent for those students who make a school transition than for those who remain in an extended elementary school; thus, self-regulation and other EF skills may play more of a role in their academic and social competence.[33,73]

Most students do navigate this transition successfully;[75] however, some children experience substantially greater difficulty, resulting in decreased self-worth, increased psychological distress, and increased school disengagement, as well as increased involvement in potentially risky behavior.[76,77] Stressful transitions to middle school can have long-term consequences, with greater negative impact on low-achieving children and children already at risk due to social factors.[77,78] For these children, this transition can produce significant reductions in achievement and effort and increases in behavioral and social–emotional problems.[78,79] African American students in particular have tended to experience greater declines in grades following the transition to middle school, compared with children from other ethnic groups.[80,81] Low-achieving students and those with LD tend to show more negative effects of transition to middle schools than higher achieving students.[82] Thus, the middle school transition can significantly impact children's adjustment and academic outcomes, with this transition posing even greater challenges to children already at risk for poor outcomes.

The ability to successfully manage the middle school transition depends on multiple factors, including personal maturity and coping skills, characteristics of the new school environment, and the level of preparation and social support available to the student both before and after the transition.[83] Individual coping skills include the ability to solve problems effectively and demonstrate self-control within a variety of classroom and social situations: in other words, intact EF. For example, children with ADHD[84] show an increase in parent reports of problem behaviors[70] following their transition into middle school. Given these findings, it is critical to consider the level of support provided to children during important school transitions, as well as following specific shifts in developmental expectations (e.g., mid-elementary school, etc.). The level and quality of support available to children prior to and during these transitions has the potential to significantly improve children's functioning.

School-based intervention

There are significant implications for children entering school without the self-regulatory and executive control skills needed to function competently and learn productively within the school setting.[28] Although most children learn and develop these skills over the course of elementary school, EdF persists in many children and contributes to less successful academic and social outcomes. There are a variety of classroom-based strategies that have been employed to address young students' social and emotional competence, which therefore have implications for improving EF. Unfortunately, fewer interventions have been examined for supporting children within the upper elementary grades and beyond. Strategies that have been proposed include improving the quality of instruction, strengthening teacher–student interactions, developing curricula targeting development of specific social and behavioral regulation skills, implementing individualized instruction to address particular children's needs, and providing problem-focused and skill-based strategy coaching in the schools. Proposed interventions vary in their focus; however, each shows promise for supporting development of the EF skills shown to be critical for school readiness, academic performance, and later life success.

Current educational policy (e.g., the reauthorization of IDEA and "No Child Left Behind") focuses on improving teacher quality broadly, emphasizing teacher pre-service training and educational qualifications. Proximal measures of classroom quality, including measures of the quality of specific teacher–child interactions and the use of specific instructional pedagogy and management strategies, have been shown to substantially affect children's academic and behavioral functioning.[85] For example, children in kindergarten classrooms in which teachers used proactive approaches to classroom management and a variety of instructional strategies demonstrated better behavioral and cognitive self-control in the spring of the kindergarten year and were observed to be more engaged in learning activities throughout the school year, compared with children in classrooms with teachers who used less proactive approaches.[34]

For children deemed most at-risk for early academic and behavioral dysfunction, high levels of instructional and emotional support within the classroom have been shown to result in less behavioral dysregulation and better academic outcomes.[85,86,87] Consistent with these findings regarding teacher practices, individualized student-focused instruction and consistent use of student-focused planning was found to improve self-regulation skills in children initially showing poorer inhibitory skills prior to the intervention.[88] These studies suggest that children's learning and behavioral regulation skills are fostered in classrooms where teachers provide coherent, consistent, and caring structure, including well-planned activities, proactive behavior management strategies, clear organization of transitions, individualized instructional feedback, and individualized interactions with students. It is very likely that the mechanisms involved in these associations relate to teachers' use of proactive behavior management strategies within a warm and caring environment that explicitly support children's developing EF skills and self-regulatory capabilities.

Large-scale problem-focused interventions have been evaluated for supporting development of behavioral self-regulation in children specifically identified as at-risk for behavioral and emotional problems. *The Chicago School Readiness Project*[89] was designed to improve teachers' abilities to provide classroom instructional and emotional support to their students through a combination of interventions used with children participating in Head Start. (Note: In general, children participating in Head Start programs are at risk for behavioral dysregulation and academic difficulty.) Teacher training and coaching were combined with one-on-one, child-focused, mental health consultation for up to five children per classroom, with a goal of improving teacher practices designed to support child self-regulation in children at risk for academic and behavioral difficulty. Results of intent-to-treat analyses from this randomized clinical trial revealed that this combination of supports resulted in substantial improvements in teacher responsiveness to individual student needs, better classroom monitoring, more proactive prevention of misbehavior, and less use of harsh or negative discipline practices.[89] These findings suggest that such environmental supports may better scaffold children's developing executive skills.

The *Rochester Child Resilience Project*[90] similarly targeted children at risk for social and behavior problems who were enrolled in kindergarten through third grade. Interventions involved up to 14 sessions with school-based mentors, including individualized skill-based instruction addressing specific components of EF and reactivity (e.g., monitoring of emotions, self-control, and emotion regulation). Additional support for classroom generalization and practice was included. Children participating in the program were rated by their teachers as showing improvements in behavior regulation, appropriately assertive behavior, and on-task learning behaviors, as well as fewer disciplinary referrals and out-of-school suspensions.[90] A notable element of this program was its use of in-classroom mentoring to provide opportunities for children to practice using specific self-regulatory skills within emotionally charged situations as they arose.

With these strategies in mind, a number of preschool and elementary curricula have been developed as universal prevention programs which focus on supporting development of children's self-regulation skills and executive control in order to promote early school readiness skills and better academic outcomes. Examples include *Promoting Alternative Thinking Strategies (PATHS*[91]*)*, *Tools of the Mind (Tools*[92,93]*)*, the *Incredible Years Teacher Classroom Management and Child Social and Emotion Curriculum (Incredible Years*[94,95]*)*, *I Can Problem Solve (ICPS*[96]*)*, and the *Open Circle Program (OCP*[97]*)*. Empirical work examining these curricula has demonstrated that use of targeted instructional strategies has the potential to improve children's EF within the classroom setting. Although some of these curricula explicitly focus on the self-regulatory skills considered to be critical to children's academic and social outcomes (e.g., *PATHS*, *Tools*, *ICPS*), others focus more broadly on training teachers to use more effective classroom management strategies in order to prevent or reduce problematic behavior and increase prosocial behavior (e.g., *Incredible Years*). In many cases, even when the focus of the program is on student behaviors, there is a clear emphasis on creating a positive, prosocial learning environment, involving some level of additional teacher consultation or training. (Editor's note: several of these intervention programs are also discussed in Chapter 17, with regard to their broader use outside of the school environment.)

Tools of the Mind[92] is based upon Luria and Vygotsky's theories of cognitive development and emphasizes both behavioral regulation (e.g., social self-regulation and cognitive control of attention and behavior) and specific academic skills within a framework of activities designed to support children's executive control. Use of the *Tools* curriculum in preschool for one to two academic years was associated with better performance on performance-based measures of inhibition as well as pre-reading skills.[98] In a randomized trial of the *Tools* curriculum, strategies designed to intentionally support development of self-regulation of behavior and emotions through play were found to reduce both internalizing and externalizing behavior problems (as measured by teacher reports) and improve performance on multiple measures of EF, with observations of teachers indicating improvements in classroom organization/productivity and more sensitive instructional teacher-child interactions.[93,98]

The *PATHS* curriculum[91] is a universal school-based prevention curriculum designed to reduce behavioral problems by promoting development of social–emotional and self-regulatory competence. *PATHS* provides specific instruction across multiple social skill domains through a developmental sequence spanning preschool through elementary school ages, with a focus on emotional regulation, conscious strategies for self-control (e.g., verbal mediation, inhibitory control), and supporting the child's innate ability to solve social problems effectively. In addition to specific lessons teaching self-control and social skills, the program includes detailed extension activities and strategies for helping teachers create an environment that promotes children's learning of social-emotional skills. A randomized trial of the preschool *PATHS* curriculum in Head Start classrooms found significant group effects on children's emotional knowledge and teacher-reported social competence, social withdrawal, and anxiety, but failed to find specific group differences on performance-based measures of inhibitory control, attention, or problem solving.[99] In contrast, elementary school-aged children in classrooms using the *PATHS* curriculum for one school year demonstrated not only fewer teacher-reported internalizing and externalizing behavior problems, but also improvements in performance-based measures of inhibitory control and verbal categorical fluency, compared with children in control classrooms.[100] Additionally, in children identified as eligible for special education support, effects of *PATHS* on externalizing and internalizing behaviors persisted at least 2 years after implementation of the curriculum.[101]

The *Open Circle Program* (*OCP*[97]) is a classroom-based intervention program that focuses primarily on improving social problem-solving and decision-making skills for early elementary students through a combination of specific, skill-focused lessons and on-site teacher consultation. Participation in the *OCP* during fourth grade was found to be associated with better student social skills and fewer problem-behavior scores (compared to fourth grade children in similar schools that did not implement *OCP*);[102] children attending school in urban areas showed the greatest gains. Similarly, middle school students who had participated in *OCP* for at least two years of elementary school demonstrated better social skills and interpersonal adjustment following their transition into middle school (relative to children from schools not implementing this program).[103] Although this study was conducted by the curriculum's creator, it is notable for its focus on the middle school transition, a period that demands greater executive control and during which difficulty is observed for many students (not only those with EdF) across both academic and behavioral domains. The data suggest that interventions at the elementary school level have the potential to scaffold development of the exact EF skills that are required for successful transition into middle school.

Unlike the *PATHS* and *Tools* curricula, the *Incredible Years* curriculum was originally designed for clinically referred children with early onset behavioral regulation difficulties, and showed promise in improving these children's problem behaviors across settings.[94] The original clinic-based model was adapted for use as a preventative preschool and early elementary universal intervention (the Dinosaur School curriculum). The *Incredible Years* Dinosaur School preschool curriculum and the associated teacher training in effective classroom management strategies and ways to promote children's executive control were found to result in significant improvements in emotional self-regulation, distractibility, peer interaction skills, and child conduct problems.[95] Follow-up evaluations of the program for children from low SES families who were at-risk educationally and behaviorally revealed a significantly larger impact on school readiness for students with greater initial difficulty with emotional and behavioral self-regulation skills.

Conclusions and implications for practice

EF involves a set of multidimensional skills that develop over a protracted period of time and set the stage for academic, behavioral and social competencies that are crucial for success in school and life. EF skills are founded on a complex cortico-striatal-thalamo-cerebellar network that develops over time, with functional outcomes mediated (positively and negatively) by environmental factors. EF skills are fundamental to the development of competence in children, especially those who may be vulnerable as a function of poverty, health problems, learning difficulty/LD, or societal stress. Attainment of appropriate EF skills is critical for school success, and children who have EF delays or deficits are more prone to learning difficulties, behavior problems, school withdrawal, and psychopathology. Despite having intact intelligence, many children with EdF fail to adequately develop the requisite skills to interact productively and effectively with the world. School-based interventions appear to facilitate growth in children's functional EF skills, and may ameliorate the risk in those most vulnerable. Individuals working with children need a framework for approaching EdF that includes an understanding of how the child's physical and brain development interacts with his/her environment and how these interactions change over time.

The most successful models and programs targeting EF development are those that integrate knowledge from child development, neuroscience, psychology, and education. Classroom teachers play a critical role in promoting EF skill development in children. A challenge exists, however, because many of the classroom demands that exacerbate EdF are hidden and not explicitly addressed. Such demands include the need for speed during academic work, multi-tasking during class activities, simultaneous writing and listening, and the challenge of an unpredictable school day. For example, while many middle and high schools employ a rotating daily class schedule to avoid having certain classes consistently in the afternoon (or morning), the inconsistency in daily schedules adds to the organizational demands already inherent in the curriculum and can adversely affect children who are vulnerable to organizational difficulties. A similar concern exists in using block scheduling in which classes are taken only every other day. Despite the benefits, block scheduling also places an additional organizational burden on students, in that they must spread homework assignments over days without direct instruction.

Continued research and intervention in this area will require collaboration between clinical researchers in the neurosciences, psychology, and education, with a goal of implementing training in the understanding and treatment of EdF in teacher preparation programs. At the same time, core child clinical psychology training should include coursework to facilitate a better understanding of the school setting and the issues facing children as they navigate the academic, social, and behavioral demands within schools and classrooms.

References

1. Denckla, MB. Measurement of executive function. In Reid Lyon, G, ed. *Frames of Reference for Assessment of Learning Disabilities*. Baltimore: Paul H. Brookes; 1994.

2. Lezak MD. Newer contributions to the neuropsychological assessment of executive functions. *J Head Trauma Rehab* 1993; 8(1): 24–31.

3. Mahone EM, Cirino PT, Cutting LE, *et al.* Validity of the behavior rating inventory of executive function in children with ADHD and/or Tourette syndrome. *Arch Clin Neuropsychol* 2002; 17(7): 643–62.

4. Denckla, MB. Biological correlates of learning and attention: what is relevant to learning disability and attention-deficit/hyperactivity disorder? *J Dev Behav Pediatr* 1996; 17(2): 114–19.

5. Blair C. School readiness. Integrating cognition and emotion in a neurobiological conceptualization of children's functioning at school entry. *Am Psychol* 2002; **57**(2): 111–27.

6. Barkley, RA. Behavioral inhibition, sustained attention, and executive functions: constructing a unifying theory of ADHD. *Psychol Bull* 1997; **121**(1): 65–94.

7. Stevens MC, Skudlarski P, Pearlson GD, Calhoun VD. Age-related cognitive gains are mediated by the effects of white matter development on brain network integration. *NeuroImage* 2009; **48**(4): 738–46.

8. Tau GZ, Peterson BS. Normal development of brain circuits. *Neuropsychopharmacology* 2009; **35**(1): 147–68.

9. Kochanska G. Beyond cognition: expanding the search for the early roots of internalization and conscience. *Dev Psychol* 1994; **30**(1): 20–2.

10. Shoda Y, Mischel W, Peake PK. Predicting adolescent cognitive and self-regulatory competencies from preschool delay of gratification: Identifying diagnostic conditions. *Dev Psychol* 1990; **26**(6): 978–86.

11. McCabe LA, Cunnington M, Brooks-Gunn J. The development of self-regulation in young children: Individual characteristics and environmental contexts. In Baumeister, RF, Vohs D, eds. *Handbook of Self-regulation*. New York: Guilford Press; 1994.

12. Dowsett SM, Livesey DJ. The development of inhibitory control in preschool children: effects of "executive skills" training. *Dev Psychobiol* 2000; **36**(2): 161–74.

13. Zelazo PD, Carter A, Reznick JS, Frye D. Early development of executive function: a problem-solving framework. *Rev Gen Psychol* 1997; **1**(2): 198–226.

14. Welsh MC. Rule-guided behavior and self-monitoring on the tower of hanoi disk-transfer task. *Cog Dev* 1991; **6**(1): 59–76.

15. Weissberg R, Ruff HA, Lawson KR. The usefulness of reaction time tasks in studying attention and organization of behavior in young children. *J Dev Behav Pediatr* 1990; **11**(2): 59–64

16. Diamond A, Taylor C. Development of an aspect of executive control: Development of the abilities to remember what I said and to "Do as I say, not as I do". *Dev Psychobiol* 1996; **29**(4): 315–34.

17. Gerstadt CL, Hong YJ, Diamond A. The relationship between cognition and action: Performance of children 3-1/2-7 years old on a Stroop-like day-night test. *Cognition* 1994; **53**: 129–53.

18. Vaughn BE, Kopp CB, Krakow JB. The emergence and consolidation of self-control from eighteen to thirty months of age: normative trends and individual differences. *Child Dev* 1984; **55**(3): 990–1004.

19. Pennington BF. The working memory function of the prefrontal cortices: Implications for developmental and individual differences in cognition. In Haith M, Benson JB, Roberts J, Pennington, BF, eds. *Future-oriented Processes in Development*. Chicago: University of Chicago Press; 1994.

20. Clark C, Prior M, Kinsella G. The relationship between executive function abilities, adaptive behaviour, and academic achievement in children with externalizing behaviour problems. *J Child Psychol Psychiatry* 2002; **43**(6): 785–96.

21. Pascualvaca DM, Anthony BJ, Arnold LE, et al. Attention performance in an epidemiological sample of urban children: the role of gender and verbal intelligence. *Child Neuropsychol* 1997; **3**(1): 13–27.

22. Galambos NL, MacDonald SWS, Naphtali C, Cohen A-L, de Frias CM. Cognitive performance differentiates selected aspects of psychosocial maturity in adolescence. *Dev Neuropsychol* 2005; **28**(1): 473–92.

23. Santor DA, Ingram A, Kusumakar V. Influence of executive functioning difficulties on verbal aggression in adolescents: Moderating effects of winning and losing and increasing and decreasing levels of provocation. *Aggressive Behav* 2003; **29**(6): 475–88.

24. Houck GM, Lecuyer-Maus EA. Maternal limit setting during toddlerhood, delay of gratification, and behavior problems at age five. *In Mental Hlth J* 2004; **25**(1): 28–46.

25. Denham SA, Blair KA, DeMulder E, *et al.* Preschool emotional competence: pathway to social competence? *Child Dev* 2003; 74(1): 238–56.

26. Hughes C, Ensor R. Does executive function matter for preschoolers' problem behaviors? *J Abnorm Child Psychol.* 2008; 36(1): 1–14.

27. Brock LL, Rimm-Kaufman SE, Nathanson L, Grimm KJ. The contributions of 'hot' and 'cool' executive function to children's academic achievement, learning-related behaviors, and engagement in kindergarten. *Early Child Res Quart* 2009; 24(3): 337–49.

28. Rimm-Kaufman SE, Pianta RC, Cox MJ. Teachers' judgments of problems in the transition to kindergarten. *Early Child Res Quart.* 2000; 15(2): 147–66.

29. Agostin TM, Bain SK. Predicting early school success with developmental and social skills screeners. *Psychol Schools* 1997; 34(3): 219–28.

30. Foulks B, Morrow RD. Academic survival skills for the young child at risk for school failure. *J Educ Res* 1989; 82(3): 158–65.

31. Wahlstedt C, Thorell LB, Bohlin G. ADHD symptoms and executive function impairment: Early predictors of later behavioral problems. *Dev Neuropsychol* 2008; 33(2): 160–78.

32. Brocki K, Eninger L, Thorell L, Bohlin G. Interrelations between executive function and symptoms of hyperactivity/impulsivity and inattention in preschoolers: a two year longitudinal Study. *J Abnorm Child Psychol* 2010; 38(2): 163–71.

33. Jacobson LA, Williford AP, Pianta RC. The role of executive function in children's competent adjustment to middle school. *Child Neuropsychol* 2011; 17(3): 255–80.

34. Rimm-Kaufman SE, Curby TW, Grimm KJ, *et al.* The contribution of children's self-regulation and classroom quality to children's adaptive behaviors in the kindergarten classroom. *Dev Psychol* 2009; 45(4): 958–72.

35. Blair C, Diamond A. Biological processes in prevention and intervention: The promotion of self regulation as a means of preventing school failure. *Dev Psychopathol* 2008; 20(03): 899–911.

36. Barkley RA, Grodzinsky G, DuPaul GJ. Frontal lobe functions in attention deficit disorder with and without hyperactivity: a review and research report. *J Abnorm Child Psychol* 1992; 20(2): 163–88.

37. Ruff HA, Rothbart MK. *Attention in Early Development: Themes and Variations.* New York: Oxford University Press; 1996.

38. Hongwanishkul D, Happaney KR, Lee WSC, Zelazo PD. Assessment of hot and cool executive function in young children: Age-related changes and individual differences. *Dev Neuropsychol* 2005; 28(2): 617–44.

39. Blair C, Razza RP. Relating effortful control, executive function, and false belief understanding to emerging math and literacy ability in kindergarten. *Child Dev* 2007; 78(2): 647–63.

40. Riggs NR, Blair CB, Greenberg MT. Concurrent and 2-year longitudinal relations between executive function and the behavior of 1st and 2nd grade children. *Child Neuropsychol* 2004; 16;9(4): 267–76.

41. Bull R, Espy KA, Wiebe SA. Short-term memory, working memory, and executive functioning in preschoolers: Longitudinal predictors of mathematical achievement at age 7 years. *Dev Neuropsychol* 2008; 33(3): 205–28.

42. Razza RA, Blair C. Associations among false-belief understanding, executive function, and social competence: a longitudinal analysis. *J Applied Dev Psychol* 2009; 30(3): 332–43.

43. McClelland MM, Morrison FJ, Holmes DL. Children at risk for early academic problems: the role of learning-related social skills. *Early Child Res Quart* 2000; 15(3): 307–29.

44. Gumora G, Arsenio WF. Emotionality, emotion regulation, and school performance in middle school children. *J School Psychol* 2002; 40(5): 395–413.

45. Kurdek LA, Sinclair RJ. Psychological, family, and peer predictors of academic outcomes in first- through fifth-grade children. *J Educ Psychol* 2000; 92(3): 449–57.

46. Clark CAC, Pritchard VE, Woodward LJ. Preschool executive functioning abilities predict early mathematics achievement. *Dev Psychol* 2010; **46**(5): 1176–91.

47. Swanson HL, Jerman O. The influence of working memory on reading growth in subgroups of children with reading disabilities. *J Exp Child Psychol* 2007; **96**(4): 249–83.

48. Holmes J, Adams JW. Working memory and children's mathematical skills: Implications for mathematical development and mathematics curricula. *Educ Psychol* 2006; **26**(3): 339–66.

49. Jarvis HL, Gathercole, SE. Verbal and non-verbal working memory and achievements on National Curriculum tests at 11 and 14 years of age. *Educ Child Psychol*. 2003; **20**(3): 123–40.

50. St Clair-Thompson HL, Gathercole SE. Executive functions and achievements in school: Shifting, updating, inhibition, and working memory. *Quart J Exp Psychol* 2006; **59**(4): 745–59.

51. Sesma HW, Mahone EM, Levine T, Eason SH, Cutting LE. The contribution of executive skills to reading comprehension. *Child Neuropsychol* 2009; **15**(3): 232–46.

52. Cutting L, Materek A, Cole C, Levine T, Mahone E. Effects of fluency, oral language, and executive function on reading comprehension performance. *Ann Dyslexia* 2009; **59**(1): 34–54.

53. Locascio G, Mahone EM, Eason SH, Cutting LE. Executive dysfunction among children with reading comprehension deficits. *J Learn Disabil* 2010; **43**(5): 441–54.

54. Lewis C, Koyasu M, Oh S, Ogawa A, Short B, Huang Z. (2009). Culture, executive function, and social understanding. In Lewis C, Carpendale JIM, eds. *Social Interaction and the Development of Executive Function: New Directions in Child and Adolescent Development* 2009;123: 69–85.

55. Mahone EM, Slomine BS. Managing dysexecutive disorders. In Hunter S, Donders J, eds.*Pediatric Neuropsychological Intervention*. Cambridge: Cambridge University Press; 2007.

56. Rudel R. Residual effects of childhood reading disabilities. *Ann Dyslexia* 1981; **31**(1): 89–102.

57. Bernier A, Carlson SM, Whipple N. From external regulation to self-regulation: Early parenting precursors of young children's executive functioning. *Child Dev* 2010; **81**(1): 326–39.

58. Sarsour K, Sheridan M, Jutte D, Nuru-Jeter A, Hinshaw, S, Boyce WT. Family socioeconomic status and child executive functions: The roles of language, home environment, and Single Parenthood. *J Int Neuropsych Soc* 2011; **17**(1): 120–32.

59. Bernstein J, Waber D. Developmental neuropsychological assessment: The systemic approach. In Boulton A, Baker G, Hiscock M, eds. *Neuromethods: Neuropsychology*. Clifton: Humana Press; 1990.

60. Meltzer L, Pollica LS, Barzillai M. Executive function in the classroom: Embedding strategy instruction into daily teaching practices. In Meltzer L, ed. *Executive Function in Education: From Theory to Practice*. New York: Guilford Press; 2007.

61. Holmes JM. Natural histories in learning disabilities: Neuropsychological difference/environmental demand. In Ceci SJ, ed. *Handbook of Cognitive, Social and Neuropsychological Aspects of Learning Disabilities*. Hillsdale: Lawrence Erlbaum Associates; 1987.

62. Jacobson LA, Murphy-Bowman SC, Pritchard AE, Tart-Zelvin A, Zabel, TA, Mahone, EM. (in press). Factor structure of a sluggish cognitive tempo scale in clinically-referred children. *J Abn Child Psychol*

63. Jacobson LA, Ryan M, Martin RB, *et al.* Working memory influences processing speed and reading fluency in ADHD. *Child Neuropsychol* 2011; **17**(3): 209–24.

64. Rucklidge JJ, Tannock R. Neuropsychological profiles of adolescents with ADHD: effects of reading difficulties and gender. *J Child Psychol Psychiatry* 2002; **43**(8): 988–1003.

65. Willcutt EG, Pennington BF, Olson RK, DeFries JC. Understanding comorbidity: A twin study of reading disability and

attention-deficit/hyperactivity disorder. *Am J Med Genet* 2007; **144B**(6): 709–14.

66. Castellanos FX, Tannock R. Neuroscience of attention-deficit/hyperactivity disorder: the search for endophenotypes. *Nat Rev Neurosci* 2002; **3**(8): 617–28.

67. Anderson P. Assessment and development of executive function (EF) during childhood. *Child Neuropsychol* 2002; **8**(2): 71–82.

68. Bush G, Luu P, Posner MI. Cognitive and emotional influences in anterior cingulate cortex. *Trends Cogn Sci* 2000; **4**(6): 215–22.

69. Morgan AB, Lilienfeld SO. A meta-analytic review of the relation between antisocial behavior and neuropsychological measures of executive function. *Clin Psychol Rev* 2000; **20**(1): 113–36.

70. Langberg JM, Epstein JN, Altaye M, Molina BSG, Arnold LE, Vitiello B. The transition to middle school is associated with changes in the developmental trajectory of ADHD symptomatology in young adolescents with ADHD. *J Clin Child Adolescent Psychol* 2008; **37**(3): 651–63.

71. Luna B, Sweeney JA. Emergence of collaborative brain function: fMRI studies of the development of response inhibition. In Dahl RE, ed. *Adolescent Brain Development: Vulnerabilities and Opportunities*. NY: New York Academy of Sciences; 2004.

72. Akos P, Queen, JA, Lineberry C. *Promoting a Successful Transition to Middle School.* Larchmont, New York: Eye on Education; 2005.

73. Rudolph KD, Lambert SF, Clark AG, Kurlakowsky KD. Negotiating the transition to middle school: the role of self-regulatory processes. *Child Dev.* 2001; **72**(3): 929–46.

74. Harter S, Whitesell NR, Kowalski P. Individual differences in the effects of educational transitions on young adolescents' perceptions of competence and motivational orientation. *Am Educ Res J* 1992; **29**(4): 777–807.

75. Parker AK. Elementary organizational structures and young adolescents' self-concept and classroom environment perceptions across the transition to middle school. *J Res Child Educ* 2009; **23**: 325–39.

76. Carnegie Council on Adolescent Development. *Great transitions: Preparing adolescents for a new century: Concluding report of the Carnegie Council on Adolescent Development.* New York: Carnegie Corporation; 1995.

77. Eccles JS, Lord SE, Roeser RW, Barber BL, Jozefowicz D. The association of school transitions in early adolescence with developmental trajectories through high school. In Schulenberg J, Maggs, JL, Hurrelman K, eds. *Health Risks and Developmental Transitions during Adolescence.* New York: Cambridge University Press; 1997.

78. Burchinal MR, Roberts JE, Zeisel SA, Rowley SJ. Social risk and protective factors for African American children's academic achievement and adjustment during the transition to middle school. *Dev Psychol* 2008; **44**(1): 286–92.

79. Alspaugh JW. Achievement loss associated with the transition to middle school and high school. *J Educ Res* 1998; **92**(1): 20–5.

80. Gutman LM, Midgley C. The role of protective factors in supporting the academic achievement of poor African American students during the middle school transition. *J Youth Adolesce* 2000; **29**(2): 223–49.

81. Simmons RG, Black A, Zhou Y. African-American versus white children and the transition into junior high school. *Am J Educ* 1991; **99**(4): 481–520.

82. Anderman EM. The middle school experience. *J Learn Disabil* 1998; **31**(2): 128–38.

83. Crockett LJ, Petersen AC, Graber JA, Schulenberg JE, Ebata A. School transitions and adjustment during early adolescence. *J Early Adolesc.* 1989; **9**(3): 181–210.

84. Doyle AE. Executive functions in attention-deficit/hyperactivity disorder. *J Clin Psychiat* 2006; **67** Suppl 8: 21–6.

85. Cadima J, Leal T, Burchinal M. The quality of teacher-student interactions: Associations with first graders' academic

and behavioral outcomes. *J School Psychol* 2010; **48**(6): 457–82.

86. Hamre BK, Pianta RC. Can Instructional and emotional support in the first-grade classroom make a difference for children at risk of school failure? *Child Dev* 2005; **76**(5): 949–67.

87. Downer JT, Rimm-Kaufman SE, Pianta RC. How do classroom conditions and children's risk for school problems contribute to children's behavioral engagement in learning? *School Psychol Rev* 2007; **36**(3): 413–32.

88. Connor CM, Ponitz CC, Phillips BM, Travis QM, Glasney S, Morrison FJ. First graders' literacy and self-regulation gains: The effect of individualizing student instruction. *J School Psychol* 2010; **48**(5): 433–55.

89. Raver CC, Jones SM, Li-Grining CP, Metzger M, Champion KM, Sardin L. Improving preschool classroom processes: preliminary findings from a randomized trial implemented in Head Start settings. *Early Child Res Quart* 2008; **23**(1): 10–26.

90. Wyman P, Cross W, Hendricks Brown C, Yu Q, Tu X, Eberly S. Intervention to strengthen emotional self-regulation in children with emerging mental health problems: Proximal impact on school behavior. *J Abnorm Child Psychol* **38**(5): 707–20.

91. Kusche CA, Greenberg MT. *The PATHS Curriculum*. South Deerfield: Channing-Bete; 1994.

92. Bodrova E, Leong DJ. *Tools of the Mind: The Vygotskian Approach to Early Childhood Education*. Upper Saddle River: Prentice-Hall; 1996.

93. Barnett WS, Jung K, Yarosz DJ, *et al.* Educational effects of the Tools of the Mind curriculum: a randomized trial. *Early Child Res Quart* 2008; **23**(3): 299–313.

94. Webster-Stratton C, Hammond M. Treating children with early-onset conduct problems: a comparison of child and parent training interventions. *J Consult Clin Psychol* 1997; **65**(1): 93–109.

95. Webster-Stratton C, Jamila Reid M, Stoolmiller M. Preventing conduct problems and improving school readiness: evaluation of the Incredible Years Teacher and Child Training Programs in high-risk schools. *J Child Psychol Psychiatry* 2008; **49**(5): 471–88.

96. Shure MB, Spivack G. Interpersonal problem-solving in young children: a cognitive approach to prevention. *Am J Commun Psychol* 1982; **10**(3): 341–56.

97. Siegle P, Lange L, Macklem G. *Open Circle Curriculum. The Stone Center*, Wellesley College, Wellesley, MA; 1997.

98. Diamond A, Barnett WS, Thomas J, Munro S. Preschool Program Improves Cognitive Control. *Science* 2007; **318**(5855): 1387–8.

99. Domitrovich C, Cortes R, Greenberg M. Improving young children's social and emotional competence: A randomized trial of the preschool curriculum. *J Primary Prev* 2007; **28**(2): 67–91.

100. Riggs N, Greenberg M, Kusché, Pentz M. The mediational role of neurocognition in the behavioral outcomes of a social-emotional prevention program in elementary school students: Effects of the PATHS curriculum. *Prev Sci* 2006; **7**(1): 91–102.

101. Kam C, Greenberg MT, Kusché CA. Sustained effects of the PATHS curriculum on the social and psychological adjustment of children in special education. *J Emot Behav Disord* 2004; **12**(2): 66–78.

102. Hennessey, BA. Promoting social competence in school-aged children: The effects of the open circle program. *J School Psychol* 2007; **45**(3): 349–60.

103. Taylor CA, Liang B, Tracy AJ, *et al.* Gender differences in middle school adjustment, physical fighting, and social skills: Evaluation of a social competency program. *J Primary Prev* 2002; **23**(2): 259–72.

Chapter 19

Executive functions, forensic neuropsychology, and child psychiatry: opinions, cautions, and caveats

Scott J. Hunter, Niranjan S. Karnik, and Jennifer P. Edidin

There has been substantial discussion in the research literature and public press over the past decade about the growing body of knowledge concerning brain development across childhood and adolescence, and its impact on our thinking about responsibility, judgment, and choice.[1-3] Of note has been the range of television, newspaper and magazine articles, and commentaries and opinion pieces that have attempted to wrestle with concerns of judgment, decision making, and culpability for juveniles and young adults in the criminal and civil justice arenas.[4-7] The Supreme Court of the United States has grappled with this issue – particularly with regard to whether youth (with typical or atypical development) are capable of understanding the intentions and outcomes of their choices and actions, and how we as a society can address this concern through prevention and intervention (cf., Atkins v. Virginia, the 2002 decision regarding the diminished culpability of the intellectually disabled, ruling that the death penalty is inappropriate for such individuals; and Roper v. Simmons, the 2005 decision ruling that the death penalty for youth under 18 years of age is "cruel and unusual punishment").[8,9] This discussion is intimately intertwined with the unfolding body of research about EdF. It is within the area of EF perhaps more than anywhere else that we have been asked to provide guidance and direction to the legal, political, educational, and public safety systems to help them better understand the underlying neuropsychology of such concerns as "bad behavior" and "poor decision making" and how they impact broader society.

Although we have increased our understanding of the structure–function relationships that underlie and define cognition and behavioral regulation, we remain at a limited point in our knowledge base. We can now explicitly challenge the common notion that adult level understanding and behavioral control are present in adolescence, but we remain uncertain about when the "turning point" between youth and fully culpable adulthood occurs.[10] Data from multiple studies have suggested that the brain is not yet fully formed and at an adult level of functioning even by 18 years old; brain development, particularly with regard to the components most responsible for higher order EF, is protracted, perhaps even into the mid-20s.[11] Mature control of impulses and emotional response emerges across late adolescence and into young adulthood, with variation seen across individuals at both the environmental and biological levels. In tandem with this, we have come to recognize that not all individuals reach the same functional level of EF; nor do they reach adult milestones at similar rates.

Executive Function and Dysfunction, ed. Scott J. Hunter and Elizabeth P. Sparrow. Published by Cambridge University Press. © Cambridge University Press 2012.

While this realization may seem matter-of-fact to those who work with children, adolescents, and even young adults clinically, it remains less evident within the broader community, including among law enforcement professionals, individuals working in juvenile justice systems, educators, and parents. This lack of a common understanding about when and how a mature brain exists to support adult level choices and responsibilities hampers efforts to make effective decisions regarding when to hold youth and young adults legally responsible for their actions. Current knowledge in our field does not definitively support a clear guideline at this time (although see Steinberg[3] for a more thorough discussion); thus, we offer a set of caveats and cautions regarding EF and culpability. These cautions influence how we as clinicians and researchers guide appropriate public policy and legal decisions.[3] They are offered in an effort to encourage dialog and continued investigation regarding how to reasonably and effectively think about this issue of culpability in tandem with current developmental models of EF; to encourage further attention to implications for the forensic arena where neuropsychological and psychiatric expertise play a significant role. We present three examples of developmental issues involving EdF, to illustrate how the concepts and findings that have been discussed in earlier chapters in this book can be reasonably considered and applied in a neuro-psycho-legal context.

Case 1: "Growing into deficit" – Early childhood neurologic insult

A common discussion in the pediatric neuropsychologist's office concerns the longitudinal impact of early illness or brain injury on a child's cognitive development. As discussed in this volume, the effects of a brain insult in early childhood or developmental disorder often emerge over time. This is particularly relevant when considering the protracted emergence of self-control and problem solving skills, and evaluating how expected trajectories of capability may be altered after early neurologic insult. This is often described as "growing into deficit," based on research findings and clinical observations that, despite early indications of intact skill attainment and learning, an affected individual often shows later struggles and inefficiencies as she fails to make expected developmental gains. The pattern of deficit is particularly seen educationally as children are expected to learn more independently and handle increasingly complex tasks over time. Although the concept of "growth into deficit" has been documented in the literature, it remains less familiar to many individuals who work with youth, both educationally and in the professional helping fields.[12,13] Yet, this principle, that increasing difficulty emerges across time for many individuals who are neurodevelopmentally impacted, is critical in education and juvenile justice. In fact, it is often because of this principle of "growth into deficit" that a neuropsychologist is requested to serve as a consultant to schools or the courts – to consider and then describe how an early brain insult may come to hamper later emergence of intellectual, adaptive, and vocational success. As well, "growth into deficit" is a quite common underlying concern when longitudinal prediction is required as part of a consultation for schools or the court.

With current advances in medical diagnostics and treatment, more children are surviving childhood illness, injury, and neurodevelopmental disorders. However, the increased rates of survivorship often come with an associated cost: significant alterations in EF capacity and skill that may unfold across time for an individual child, as a result of disease or her neurological injury. In other words, there is a decrement in developmental potential that emerges with increasing age. Degree of loss typically, but not always, reflects the extent of neurologic injury and the treatment approach taken, as both can have a substantial impact on the developing brain and cognition (for example, see childhood cancers as discussed in Chapter 12).

To illustrate "growing into EdF," consider a child with a significant perinatal insult like hypoxic–ischemic encephalopathy (HIE). The long-term sequelae of such an early injury to the brain, which is encountered when prenatal or perinatal oxygen supply is compromised, often in a complicated pregnancy and delivery, is a particular concern that can lead an attorney, physician, or the child's parents to seek guidance from a pediatric neuropsychologist. Often, the consultation is sought to determine how a child's capacity to learn, and to do so independently, may be impacted, both currently and in the future. This seemingly simple question, posed by worried parents or an attorney representing an affected child, has many potential responses. Unfortunately, the literature regarding the impact of such an event on perinatal and postnatal status is mixed in its findings, and the outcome for any particular infant or young child across time is, in and of itself, potentially quite variable. As a result, the scientifically supported answer is frequently less specific, and perhaps more uncertain, than the law (and its practitioners) desire. The forensic neuropsychologist is challenged to convey this uncertainty, while simultaneously attempting to make sense of a specific child's issues in the context of the available scientific literature.

When asked to explain how EdF develops and how that applies to a particular child within a forensic context, it is important that the consultant make a good effort to present empirical evidence as well as research-based hypotheses. In the case of a problematic pregnancy/delivery resulting in a child with documented HIE, the consultant must explain that, although medical care for the affected infant substantially improved chances for physical survival, the child was left with increased risks of co-occurring cognitive and behavioral dysfunction. This specific situation is a particularly important example of what is meant by "growing into deficit." As discussed in Chapter 15, long-term survivors of early neurodevelopmental difficulties associated with premature birth and VLBW often display significant late cognitive and behavioral effects from their failure to meet developmental expectations and their individual response to treatment. The pattern of emerging deficits can include cognitive (e.g., thinking, problem solving, reasoning, decision-making, attention, memory), psychosocial (e.g., behavioral, emotional, social adjustment), and biological (i.e., hormonal, physical growth) abnormalities, which may not manifest for many years following the initial insult. The pattern of deficits observed is often chronic and progressive for the most vulnerable infants born prematurely, specifically those with significantly low birth weight and a more limited gestation. Although overall general intellectual capability, as measured by global IQ, may only show moderate evidence of deficit across time, a detailed assessment of EF and functional capability can show deficits that significantly increase with time, and progressively impact adaptation and learning. A prototypical pattern of EdF for such children is one of increasing inefficiency and ineffectiveness in problem solving, which can result in academic failure and even the inability to graduate from high school. As these developmentally impacted youth become adults, their deficits can affect their capacity for employment, level of income, ability for independent living, likelihood they will marry, emotional health, and ultimately, overall quality of life.

Despite the increased possibility of deficits among these youth, not all affected individuals experience the same form of difficulty or severity of impairment. Further, improved opportunities for developmentally based interventions across time can moderate the severity of EdF that may be experienced. Returning to the case of the child who sustained HIE, the consulting neuropsychologist must consider how initial medical support and subsequent developmental interventions (e.g., special education, physical therapy, occupational therapy) may have positively impacted functioning. Through neuropsychological assessment, the consultant can describe the child's current functioning relative to age-based expectations (i.e., normative data), discuss how current deficits may relate to the earlier adverse event, and provide recommendations for intervention (both current and future needs) to facilitate ongoing acquisition of skills and independence. The neuropsychological evaluation can also offer estimates regarding anticipated levels of functioning in adulthood.

Nonetheless, specifying individual probable outcomes can be difficult. Group research data provide a composite of possibilities; what is gleaned from the results of a series of studies across varied outcomes is not a definitive statement of what can or will happen for one specific affected child. Research has shown that our best predictions are made in the context of significant impairment.[14,15] For example, when considering a child with a history of severe neurodevelopmental impairment (e.g., moderate to severe ID, clear motor deficits, and severe self-regulation difficulties), it is more readily possible to make an accurate prediction about the impact of EdF on independence across time, even with added variables such as ongoing treatment and special education.

When a child shows ongoing gains in development, moderating factors such as the presence of strong early intervention, good financial resources, and an enriched environment must be considered. It is harder to predict outcome in such a situation, as compared to a child with clear and severe continuing impairment after neurologic insult. Through intensive intervention and support, even a child with substantial early impairment may develop improved independent living and learning skills.

In contrast, a child who initially appears to have good recovery from neurologic insult may later exhibit significant impairment, perhaps secondary to physical complications (e.g., developing lung or kidney problems), premature cessation of intervention, or living in a socio-economically impoverished environment. Because legal decisions concerning outcome typically occur within a circumscribed period of childhood, the consultant is faced with the challenge of predicting future needs with incomplete data for that child. A strong reliance on available research concerning potential outcomes across development is necessary, with the recognition that what is considered likely in the aggregate may differ for any given child, either positively or negatively. The consulting neuropsychologist must use available data for the individual child in the context of group data for similar children to determine the range of possible outcomes.

It is critical to recognize and emphasize that EdF emerges within an individual context, and can be both subtle and insidious in its effects. Time does not heal all wounds equally; this is clearly the case when considering early brain trauma and its subsequent course. For many youth impacted by a developmental insult, such as the case of our child who experienced HIE, it is usually the observation that "the true impact" of the injury emerges over time; i.e., the child "grows" into his or her deficits. This emergence of deficit can create changes in opportunity and an increased need for accommodation at stages when support and scaffolding are typically removed. Despite early intervention and opportunity, any individual child presenting with neurodevelopmental compromise has the potential for diminished success with increasing challenge and expectation; when this occurs, outcomes are often more limited. Quantifying this outcome requires that the neuropsychologist remain vigilant and engaged, reminding the child's support team of this potential, and guiding and monitoring efforts put in place to maximize the best outcome possible. To put it simply, early neurologic insult can limit future potential, with EdF appearing as the child fails to develop age-appropriate EF, literally "growing into EdF." In such situations, it is important to consider potential future losses as well as current levels of functioning.

Case 2: Socio-environmental factors and executive dysfunction – homelessness in youth

Socio-environmental variables can be either protective or risk factors for EdF. Socio-economic deprivation can be conceptualized as a chronic lack of appropriate stimuli from the social world that exists around developing youth.[16] Social supports and opportunities that contribute to development include good educational experiences, early exposure to language, participation in after school activities, time with positive role models, access to nutritious foods, and adequate financial resources.[17] However, there are many other elements (e.g., good parent practices, access to medical care) that define a positive child-hood, and together they form an axis along which positive cognitive development can occur.[18] This is not to say that without these elements a child is destined for negative outcomes, but certainly research has consistently demonstrated that positive early child-hood experiences increase the likelihood of good developmental outcomes.[19–21]

To illustrate the impact of socioenvironmental factors on EF, consider the issue of homelessness in youth. Homelessness among youth is more pervasive than realized by most communities. Relative to the general population, homeless youth are drawn disproportion-ately from the foster care system.[22,23] Their biologic families have elevated rates of violence, abuse, drug use and psychiatric disorders.[24–26] Ongoing poverty, poor nutrition, and reduced educational support are commonly observed in this population.[27] These factors contribute to adversity, including negative neurodevelopmental and behavioral outcomes. In this respect, we can see homeless youth as a case study of the chronic effects of socio-environmental risk factors. There is increasing empirical support that these factors negatively impact the developmental trajectory of EF, both in the USA and across the globe.[16,28]

Educational disruption, another socio-environmental factor, occurs when youth fail to make appropriate progress in their learning due to factors like inconsistent attendance at school, poor-quality teaching, and limited educational supports. Studies indicate that educational factors may contribute to poor EF development.[28] Intrinsic educational dis-abilities, such as ADHD and LD, can limit a youth's ability to absorb and retain academic knowledge. External stressors, such as the lack of a consistent place to live, can be associated with the development of academic problems.[29,30] School-based factors, such as failure to provide adequate services to youth with special education needs, may also take their toll. Educational disruption negatively impacts youth in the present, in terms of failing to make progress, in the immediate future in that they lack earlier educational building blocks to reach advanced conceptual levels, and in the potential future, as they are less likely to take advantage of supports and opportunities that may be provided. The longer a youth is off track, the lower the likelihood that he will be able to resume his education successfully.

This pattern of educational disruption has been noted to impact homeless youth.[31,32] Traditionally, school is difficult for homeless youth to access for logistic as well as cognitive reasons. While federal law guarantees youth access to education, the lack of stable housing and challenges in meeting basic needs lead to increased stress in trying to meet educational goals in school. Even when homeless youth are attending school, it is difficult to concentrate on academics while worrying about food, shelter, and safety. It is also challenging to complete homework and projects without appropriate materials and a workspace. Innovative education programs for homeless youth have created non-traditional options like drop-in shelters that provide educational instruction at an individually paced level for school credit or allow youth to work toward a graduate equivalency diploma (GED).[33] Yet, one of the significant consequences of being a homeless youth is that opportunities for pursuing education will be missed unless strong effective scaffolding is provided.

Homeless adolescents often find themselves at risk for involvement with the legal system, given their marginalized status and choices they make to survive. Across the USA, many youth who are homeless exist outside of the structured systems developed to support individuals without a home.[34] Given their lack of a fixed residence, many of these youth fail to regularly attend classes and find little available opportunity for employment, given their age, lack of a permanent address, and lack of consistent education.[35,36] This can contribute to a reliance on survival behaviors that could be considered symptoms of CD or oppositionality, resulting in increased likelihood of negative interactions with the legal system. Choices such as shoplifting food or engaging in prostitution to obtain shelter can place these youth at risk for arrest, exploitation, and injury. Consequently, the trajectory of diminished opportunity for homeless youth, whether they have recently become homeless or have lived on the streets for an extended period of time, serves to challenge even the most resilient of individuals. This level of adversity during a period of significant change and growth in brain organization and executive skill development highlights a particular, substantial neurodevelopmental risk.[37]

The consistent lack of access to nutritious foods can lead to poor brain and physical development.[38] Thiamine, Folate, Vitamin B12, and a number of micronutrients are known to be essential for brain development. In addition, an appropriate balance of protein, carbohydrates, and fat are elements of a good diet that further serve to support the brain's energy and nutritional requirements. A consistent lack of any of these foundational nutrients serves to impact multiple aspects of neural patterning,[16,20] and contributes to disruptions in how increasingly complex information processing can take place. Multiple recent studies have begun to show that, particularly for youth growing up in highly impoverished environments where good nutrition is sporadically available at best, EdF is both increasingly apparent and often difficult to suppress.[20,21]

Finally, we should consider the effects of abuse and neglect on EF development in youth affected by homelessness. Homelessness in youth is often in response to an ongoing history of abusive and rejecting relationships with parents and caregivers. Recent research by Edmiston and colleagues and Pollak and colleagues has shown that child maltreatment influences, and ultimately produces lower levels of both gray and white matter development, as well as impairments in the ratio between the two, in the major structural regions that support EF.[39–41] Such changes are in line with research dating to the late 1980s by Greenough, which demonstrated the developmental impact of various stressors on the unfolding of multiple brain pathways.[42] Taken together, this research shows what has been suspected for years: trauma and abuse, and their correlates, have a substantially negative impact on opportunity and SES, and concurrently affect both the psychological and social worlds of impacted youth through disruption of the developing brain networks involved in behavioral and emotional regulation. This research highlights, in a remarkable way, the distinction that exists between our positive and negative experiences, and indicates how negative experiences substantially impact ongoing development across time. These results further push us to consider the complex biopsychosocial factors that underlie EF and its development across time, through a holistic view of the experience of trauma on young minds.

Taking these potential sources of impact together, we have hypothesized that homelessness during adolescence can negatively affect the emergence of EF, perhaps due to reduced opportunity for successful scaffolding and lack of resources that buffer and engage decision making and choice. Youth who experience homelessness may come to show a substantial diminishment in their EF. In line with this, our own work with urban African-American youth (ages 16–24) who are homeless indicates evidence of specific deficits in EF. Preliminary results on laboratory measures of EF (including the D-KEFS Sorting, Trailmaking, and Tower tasks, and the Iowa Gambling Task)[43] indicate EdF relative to broadly intact (low average range) intellectual and academic skill development.[44] In contrast, self-report of everyday EF, as assessed with the BRIEF, is much stronger; however, many youth overestimate their functional status and underreport difficulties.[45,46] The discrepancy between performance on hands-on measures and self-report appears to be rather significant in regard to understanding how, when confronted with a need to make a quick, strategic decision, poor choices can occur. This has further implications for understanding trajectories of emerging self-concept, competency, and belief in opportunity; all areas associated with and reflective of EF development and how it impacts movement towards independent adulthood.

The long-term impact of homelessness on EF development remains an area of particular concern. Adult homelessness has been strongly associated with both risk for violence and injury, including significant head injury, substance abuse and dependence, and diminished opportunity and eventual outcome.[47] And converging data suggest that increased periods of homelessness during adolescence are associated with a greater likelihood of continued homelessness during adulthood.[48] When considering an earlier history of negative developmental impact and increased risk for poor outcome, the long-term potential for making effective adult choices is significantly compromised, which hinders ultimate adaptation and functional outcome. As such, this domain of research stands as a societally important one for study, to reduce the potential that youth experiencing socioeconomic adversity have for a loss of choice and freedom.

If supported by further research, this will significantly impact our understanding of legal risk (e.g., culpability, judgment, and poor choices that get labeled as disruptive behavior), which is higher in homeless youth relative to housed peers. It is a complex interaction between these socio-environmental factors, involving genetic history (mediated by a combination of both biological and environmental risks) and opportunities (e.g., effective intervention and educational support). By understanding these intricate socio-environmental relationships and their influences on EF development, we may be able to determine more effective means of support and intervention for these vulnerable youth, and see a greater opportunity for developmental success. In theory, such research will lead to a reduction in negative outcomes such as substance abuse, poor sexual decision making, and crimes. As illustrated by the case of homeless youth, socio-environmental factors are critical to consider in the forensic context, from both contributory and preventative perspectives.

Case 3: Aggression and executive dysfunction – conduct disorder and substance use disorder

Youth who enter juvenile justice settings often present with a complex set of behavioral difficulties involving aggression, CD, and substance use. These overlapping risk behaviors present a challenge for the examining clinician, both in terms of understanding why a particular youth is presenting to the court and/or jail, and how to best dictate intervention, both in the immediate present and across time. To what extent are these behaviors due to environmental factors, and to what degree are they due to biological or genetic factors? And to what extent might an interactive model between these domains be more explanatory and helpful in identifying outcome? These considerations often play into the degree to which courts will consider the actions of youth to be open to treatment by mental health professionals. The extent to which youth can benefit from treatment often plays a role in granting some degree of sentencing leniency, at least to grant time for the youth to experience some treatment and observe if his or her behavior improves.

In such a context, multiple factors need to be considered. Consideration should be given to early childhood experiences and their effect. Having poor early developmental experiences can be one factor contributing to the complex of behaviors that often produce juvenile justice contact.[49,50] Family violence, parental substance use, perinatal substance exposure, poor parenting, neighborhood violence, and early traumatic events all can, either individually or in concert with other factors, lead to early behavioral problems, such as oppositionality, defiance, and other disruptive behaviors.[50] A subset of these children can progress to more serious violations of the rights of others and thereby begin to display CD.[49] This constellation of behaviors can then lead to contact with the legal system.

One of the ongoing challenges in working with at-risk youth involves differentiating those youth who present with CD and anti-social behaviors due to their context (i.e., living in a violent community or being around gangs) and those who have an underlying personality or temperamental risk for these behaviors, and which might be prodromal evidence of Antisocial Personality Disorder. Some investigators have moved toward using instruments like the Hare Psychopathy Checklist, Youth Version (PCL-YV) developed by Hare and colleagues.[51] Originally based on the concept of psychopathy as defined by Cleckley (1976), the PCL-Revised[52] was designed to assess adults in criminal justice settings.[53] The youth version is more problematic in that very little of the psychopathy construct has been understood within a developmental schema. Psychopathy, as a concept, also fails to account for the emerging executive, learning, and attentional systems that are important factors in understanding children's and adolescents' behaviors, as well as the pathways through which these systems can be disturbed by environmental and intrinsic factors. Currently, no widely available measure exists to assess whether CD behaviors in youth are due to personality or environmental factors.

The resulting situation is one in which the clinician must try to assess the degree to which personality and/or environment might play a role in the presentation of these behaviors. One approach to making this determination is to take a careful history from the subject as well as from collaterals. In the course of this assessment, the evaluating clinician should make note of instances where behavioral problems emerge and try to assess the degree to which these are context dependent or independent. Individuals with emerging personality disorders tend to show their behavioral issues independent of context, whereas those with a more likely environmental causation display behaviors in some type of dynamic relationship with the environment and its pattern of stressors.

Another schema that can be helpful in these evaluations involves the assessment of aggressive patterns, often a key component leading to CD and incarceration. While multiple nosological divisions of aggression could be made depending on the criteria and characteristics used, current research supports at least one key distinction between a form of aggression that is reactive, affective, defensive, or impulsive (RADI) and another form that is proactive, instrumental, or planned (PIP).[54,55] These two forms correspond to what we term "hot" and "cold" aggression, respectively, and are strongly associated with what has come to be conceptualized as aspects of "hot" and "cold" EF (see Chapter 1).[56-58] RADI or "hot" aggression is characterized by a rapid response to a perceived threat. The predominant emotions associated with it are anger and anxiety followed by a sense of guilt or remorse. Individuals with this aggressive pattern often describe themselves as unable to contain their anger and they feel regret after the act. They can often reflect, at times of calm, on the fact that their aggression may indeed be maladaptive and problematic.

Conversely, PIP or "cold" aggression can also be driven by anger, but is often associated with pleasure or disgust. Individuals with this pattern show little emotionality or guilt, and will often only exhibit emotions during the act of aggression itself. The PIP subtype is much rarer than the RADI subtype, and is often associated with psychopathy when it exists in a fixed or continuous form of behavior. Individuals often see their aggression as adaptive and helpful for their end goals despite consequences.

Research estimates show that the RADI subtype of aggression, as measured by components of the Achenbach Youth-Self Report (YSR), has a prevalence rate of almost 2% in a general high school population vs. over 9% among delinquent youth.[59] Similarly, PIP aggression was found in a little over 1% of a general high school population and 13% among delinquent youth. Finally, the condition where elements of both PIP and RADI are evident is present in a little over 1% of high school students and over 48% of delinquent youth.[60,61]

Despite these findings, several critics have challenged the two-factor model.[62] One group of authors has argued that researchers have confounded two dichotomies of information processing.[63,64] In automatic processing, responses to stimuli are learned repeatedly and so often that they become routine and, therefore, automatic. Controlled processing is thought to occur via EF that select a behavior appropriate to the stimulus. Bushman and Anderson argue that "hostile" aggression, or RADI aggression, is unreasoned and automatic, whereas "instrumental" or PIP aggression is reasoned and controlled, with most forms of aggression reflecting elements of both controlled and automatic processing.[62] It is possible that RADI and PIP exist as separate aggression pathways with both automatic and controlled elements. As such, the subtypes of aggression might be differentiated through their neural pathways and the relative weighting of automatic and controlled elements, with aggression as a final common output. These circuits could be the key point of differentiation between RADI and PIP as research continues to better define the basis of these pathways.

In the constellation of CD and aggression, a major additional factor that is often present is substance use. Comorbidity between CD and substance use disorders is quite high in large-scale studies of youth entering incarceration. Teplin and colleagues reported substance use in about 50% of 1829 Chicago youth presenting to juvenile hall (36% female, ages 10–18), with a majority using alcohol and cannabis.[65] These rates are consistent with findings from research done by Steiner and colleagues on 790 youth (18% female, ages 13–22) at the California Youth Authority.[66,67]

The presence of high rates of substance use can be seen as a bidirectional process in relationship to EdF. Exposure to substances can certainly exacerbate and affect EF (see Chapter 14).[68-70] This is particularly true for youth exposed to substances at early time periods when alcohol can be particularly toxic to brain development.[71,72] The converse side of this relationship is that EdF can increase the risk of drug and substance use.[73-75] Poor decision making results in greater risk-taking behavior, and substance use is part of this pathway. EdF can lead to a greater degree of drug experimentation and then consequently greater amounts of drug use.

The confluence of EdF, aggressive patterns, substance use, and CD all take place within a complex biopsychosocial context. The examining clinician, in response to the system for which she may be consulting, will likely be asked to make some type of determination about the degree to which these behavioral patterns are treatable. As a general rule, the treatment of substance use disorders should be the highest priority unless the aggressive pattern is such that it prevents any reasonable engagement with treatment.[49] If the aggression is at such a high level, then inpatient hospitalization, to ensure safety and gain control of the aggression, is likely warranted and may even be available through the justice system.

Substance abuse treatment is a good modality to start with, especially given the usual therapeutic approaches emphasize a patient-centered motivational structure, which helps the patient identify and define personal goals.[76] Harm reduction and abstinence approaches both likely have a role to play in a comprehensive substance abuse treatment model.[77] A consulting clinician must decide if acute detoxification is warranted. Indication for this would be that the subject has been actively using substances for long periods of time and has grown dependent on these substances. In these instances, a medical consultation with an experienced addiction medicine specialist may be warranted to help make a determination about the course of treatment. After acute detoxification, long-term outpatient treatment is indicated. Roughly 30–60 days after achievement of sobriety or a lower steady state of substance use, when the substance is metabolically cleared from the body, it may be beneficial to complete some type of neuropsychological assessment.[78] This is the point in time when substance-induced disorders often separate from independent psychological disturbances, and it brings an opportunity to better measure the youth's underlying EF and capacity for engagement. In presenting this data to the youth, it is beneficial to use a strengths-based perspective and help him understand how his cognitive functions, including EF, relate to the pattern of substance use, aggression, and conduct difficulties that have played out. From this point, appropriate referrals can be made depending on the diagnostic picture that emerges, and as the clinical evidence for one or more spectra of disorder are more visible.

Through the example of a youth with CD and substance use, the impact of aggression and EdF is illustrated. The mental health consultant's role in this instance is to initiate assertive steps towards intervention and assess the likelihood that intervention can arrest negative behavioral patterns and support more strategic, reflective, and responsible decision making. Research into the capacity for change in individuals with underlying susceptibility to aggression and conduct disturbances is mixed in its results; as we better understand the trajectories of EF development, we have opportunities for potential intervention success given early identification and engagement. It is that hopefulness we must convey as part of the consultation, as possible.

Summary and future directions

As noted at the beginning of this chapter, there has been much learned to date concerning the development of EF that has significant influence on how we serve as consultants to the educational, social welfare, and justice systems, and guide ongoing decision making and policy. Our emerging understanding of the brain and its developmental trajectories strongly influence how we appreciate the complexities of behavioral and cognitive development and what we communicate with others about risk and resilience. We know that there are a broad array of influences on how capability and capacity unfold; the developmental patterns that emerge after clear or subtle insults to the brain are varied. The neuropsychological and psychiatric consultant has the important task of responding to questions about how to understand these developmental idiosyncrasies and their implications. For it is this role held by developmentally oriented clinicians, as consultants to these enterprises, that is a truly important one for helping delineate the potential impact the variety of internal and external sources of influence may ultimately have on any particular child's path towards independence.

The three cases illustrate various areas in which the neuropsychologist or child psychiatrist may provide consultation. Case 1 presents an example of neuropsychological practice in a forensic setting. Neuropsychologists are frequently asked to determine the effects of illness, brain injury, or other trauma on current and future functioning. In these situations, the clinician must use her knowledge of neuroanatomy and the development of EF to inform her hypotheses, with a particular awareness that early insults affect the typical developmental trajectory. The effects of socioeconomic environmental factors on EF are presented in Case 2. Studies are noted that have shown that the environment can impact the development of cognitive functioning; however, few studies have examined the effects of homelessness on EF in children and adolescents. The findings from related studies suggest that factors associated with homelessness, such as educational instability, malnutrition, and lack of parental support, may impact the developmental trajectory of the PFC and other areas that contribute to EF. An improved understanding of these relations may help neuropsychologists identify and engage interventions that support developmental success. Finally, in Case 3, which describes the relation of EF to aggression and substance use, the consultant's role is discussed, to assess the effect of substance use, the need for treatment, and the likely effectiveness of treatment, as well as to facilitate treatment.

As can be seen across the three examples provided, the consultant role remains a difficult one, because the situations that affect and influence EF development are always complex and multifactorial. As we state above, extrapolating directly from the research comes with hazards, as variabilities seen with any individual child represent the array of a multiple set of contributions that can unfold developmentally across time, leading to her ultimate behavioral and regulatory presentation. We most often make determinations at one circumscribed period of time, and cannot always anticipate how growth into deficit or even such acquired stressors as homelessness or poor nutrition over a later period of time may serve to impact and alter brain growth and opportunity. As such, it remains crucial that the consultant share both the strengths and cautions that exist within the research and its interpretation more broadly, when providing guidance to the systems developed to address and care for the child at hand. It is also important to convey that there is opportunity underneath adversity for many of the youth we treat. The role of interpretation of deficits and strengths is one of conveying both what might be limiting in the big picture, but also what still remains possible, and helping the systems balance, as best possible, between these two poles.

References

1. Albert D, Steinberg L. Age differences in strategic planning as indexed by the tower of London. *Child Dev* 2011; **82**(5): 1501–17.

2. Casey BJ, Getz S, Galvan a. The adolescent brain. *Dev Res* 2008; **28**(1): 62–77.

3. Steinberg L. A behavioral scientist looks at the science of adolescent brain development. *Brain Cogn* 2010; **72**(1): 160–4.

4. Inside the teenage brain: *What's going on in there? How science may help to explain the mysteries of the teen years* [television

broadcast]. Frontline. Boston: Public Broadcasting Service; 2002 Jan 31.

5. Cohen S. States rethink charging kids as adults. *The Washington Post.* 2007 Dec 2 [cited 2011 Dec 22]; Available from http://www.washingtonpost.com/wp-dyn/content/article/2007/12/01/AR2007120100792.html

6. Begley S, Rogers A, Wingert P, Hayden T. Why the young kill. *Newsweek.* 1999 May 3: 52.

7. Wallis C. What makes teens tick. *Time Magazine.* 2004 Sep 26 [cited 2011 Dec 22]; Available from http://www.time.com/time/magazine/article/0,9171,994126,00.html#ixzz1hISUlzPF

8. Atkins v. *Virginia*, 536 US **304** (2002).

9. Roper v. *Simmons*, 543 US **551** (2005).

10. Steinberg L. Adolescent development and juvenile justice. *Ann Rev Clin Psychol* 2009; **5**: 459–85.

11. Giedd LN. Structural magnetic resonance imaging of the adolescent brain. *Ann NY Acad Sci* 2004; **1021**(1): 77–85.

12. Bernstein JH, Waber DP. Executive capacities from a developmental perspective. In Meltzer L, ed. *Executive Function in Education: From Theory to Practice.* New York, NY: Guilford Press; 2007, 39–54.

13. Stiles J, Jernigan TL. The basics of brain development. *Neuropsychol Rev* 2010; **20**(4): 327–48.

14. Klein-Tasman BP, Janke KM. Intellectual disabilities. In Hunter SJ, Donders J, eds. *Principles and Practice of Lifespan Developmental Neuropsychology.* Cambridge, UK; Cambridge University Press; 2010, 221–38.

15. Pennington BF. *Diagnosing Learning Disorders: A Neuropsychological Framework,* 2nd edn. New York, NY, USA: Guilford Press; 2009.

16. Lipina SJ, Colombo JA. *Poverty and Brain Development During Childhood: An Approach from Cognitive Psychology and Neuroscience.* Washington, DC, USA: American Psychological Association; 2009.

17. Farah MJ, Betancourt L, Shera DM, *et al.* Environmental stimulation, parental nurturance and cognitive development in humans. *Dev Sci* 2008; **11**(5): 793–801.

18. Heckman JJ. Skill formation and the economics of investing in disadvantaged children. *Science* 2006; **312**(5782): 1900–2.

19. Parke RD. Development in the family. *Ann Rev Psychol* 2004; **55**(1): 365–99.

20. Farah MJ, Noble KG, Hurt H. Poverty, privilege and brain development: Empirical findings and ethical implications. In Illes J, ed. *Neuroethics in the 21st Century.* New York: Oxford University Press; 2005.

21. Farah MJ, Noble KG, Hurt H. The developing adolescent brain in socioeconomic context. In Romer D, Walker EF, eds. *Adolescent Psychopathology and the Developing Brain: Integrating Brain and Prevention Science.* New York, NY, USA: Oxford University Press; 2007, 373–87.

22. Hyde J. From home to the street: Understanding young people's transitions into homelessness. *J Adolesc* 2005; **28**(2): 171–83.

23. Fowler PJ, Toro PA, Miles BW. Pathways to and from homelessness and associated psychosocial outcomes among adolescents leaving the foster care system. *Am J Publ Hlth* 2009; **99**(8): 1453–8.

24. Shelton KH, Taylor PJ, Bonner A, van den Bree M. Risk factors for homelessness: evidence from a population-based study. *Psychiatry Serv* 2009; **60**(4): 465–72.

25. Ferguson KM. Exploring family environment characteristics and multiple abuse experiences among homeless youth. *J Interpers Violence* 2009; **24**(11): 1875–91.

26. Paradise M, Cauce AM. Home street home: the interpersonal dimensions of adolescent homelessness. *Anal Soc Issues Publ Policy* 2002; **2**(1): 223–38.

27. Wright JD. Poverty, homelessness, health, nutrition, and children. In Kryder-Coe J, Salamon L, Molnar J, eds. *Homeless Children and Youth: A New American Dilemma.* New Brunswick, NJ: Trans-ACTION Books; 1991, 71–103.

28. Hackman DA, Farah MJ. Socioeconomic status and the developing brain. *Trends Cogn Sci* 2009; **13**(2): 65–73.

29. Fantuzzo J, Perlman S. The unique impact of out-of-home placement and the mediating effects of child maltreatment and homelessness on early school success. *Child Youth Serv Rev* 2007; **29**(7): 941–60.

30. Zima BT, Wells KB, Freeman HE. Emotional and behavioral problems and severe academic delays among sheltered homeless children in Los Angeles county. *Am J Publ Hlth* 1994; **84**(2): 260–4.

31. Buckner JC, Bassuk EL, Weinreb LF. Predictors of academic achievement among homeless and low-income housed children. *J Sch Psychol* 2001; **39**(1): 45–69.

32. Rubin DH, Erickson CJ, San Agustin M, Cleary SD, Allen JK, Cohen P. Cognitive and academic functioning of homeless children compared with housed children. *Pediatrics* 1996; **97**(3): 289–94.

33. Fosberg LB, Dennis DL. *Practical Lessons: The 1998 National Symposium on Homelessness Research*. Washington, DC: US Dept of Housing and Urban Development; 1999. Available from http://aspe.hhs.gov/pic/reports/aspe/6817.pdf#page=75

34. Milburn NG, Rotheram-Borus MJ, Rice E, Mallet S, Rosenthal D. Cross-national variations in behavioral profiles among homeless youth. *Am J Commun Psychol* 2006; **37**(1–2): 63–76.

35. Busen NH, Engebreston JC. Facilitating risk reduction among homeless and street-involved youth. *J Am Acad Nurse Pract* 2008; **20**(11): 567–75.

36. Rubin DH, Erickson CJ, San Agustin M, Cleary SD, Allen JK, Cohen P. Cognitive and academic functioning of homeless children compared with housed children. *Pediatrics* 1996; **97**(3): 289–94.

37. Teicher MH, Andersen SL, Polcari A, Anderson CM, Navalta CP, Kim DM. The neurobiological consequences of early stress and childhood maltreatment. *Neurosci Biobehav Rev* 2003; **27**(1–2): 33–44.

38. Mirsky AF. Perils and pitfalls on the path to normal potential: The role of impaired attention: homage to Herbert G. Birch. *J Clin Exp Neuropsychol* 1995; **17**(4): 481.

39. Edmiston EE, Wang F, Mazure CM, Mayes LC, Blumber HP. Corticostriatal-limbic gray matter morphology in adolescents with self-reported exposure to childhood maltreatment. *Arch Pediatr Adolesc Med* 2011: **165**(12): 1069–77.

40. Pollak SD, Cicchetti D, Klorman R, Brumaghim JT. Cognitive brain event-related potentials and emotion processing in maltreated children. *Child Dev* 1997; **68**(5): 773–87.

41. Pollak SD. Early adversity and mechanisms of plasticity: integrating affective neuroscience with developmental approaches to psychopathology. *Dev Psychopathol* 2005; **17**(3): 735–52.

42. Greenough WT, Black JE, Wallace CS. Experience and brain development. *Child Dev* 1987; **58**(3): 539–59.

43. Bechara A, Damasio AR, Damasio H, Anderson SW. Insensitivity to future consequences following damage to human prefrontal cortex. *Cognition* 1994; **50**(1–3): 7–15.

44. Edidin JP, Gustafson E, Karnik NS, Hunter SJ. Neurocognitive functioning in homeless youth. Poster to be presented at the International Neuropsychological Society 40th Annual Meeting; 2012 Feb 15–18; Montreal, Quebec, Canada.

45. Kruger J, Dunning D. Unskilled and unaware of it: How difficulties in recognizing one's own incompetence lead to inflated self-assessments. *J Pers Soc Psychol* 1999; **77**(6): 1121–34.

46. Pajare F. Self-efficacy beliefs and mathematical problem-solving of gifted students. *Contemp Educ Psychol* 1996; **21**(4): 325–44.

47. Hwang SW, Colantonio A, Chiu S, et al., The effect of traumatic brain injurt on the health of homeless people. *CMAJ* 2008; **179**(8): 779–84.

48. Chamberlain C, Johnson G. Pathways into adult homelessness. *J Sociol* 2011 Nov. doi:10.1177/1440783311422458.

49. Karnik NS, Steiner H. Aggression and its disorders. In Steiner H, ed. *Handbook of Developmental Psychiatry*. Singapore: World Scientific Publishing; 2011.

50. Steiner H, Karnik NS. Child and adolescent antisocial behavior. In Sadock B, Sadock V, eds. *Kaplan & Sadock's Comprehensive Textbook of Psychiatry*. Philadelphia: Lippincott, Williams & Wilkins; 2005.

51. Forth A, Kosson D, Hare RD. *The Hare Psychopathy Checklist: Youth Version (PCL-YV)*. Toronto, Ontario, Canada: Multi-Health Systems; 2003.

52. Hare RD. *Manual for the Revised Psychopathy Checklist* (2nd edn.). Toronto, ON, Canada: Multi-Health Systems; 2003.

53. Cleckley H. *The Mask of Sanity*, 5th edn. St. Louis, MO: Mosby; 1976.

54. Hinshaw SP, Lee SS. Conduct and oppositional defiant disorders. In Mash EJ, Barkley RA, eds. *Child Psychopathology*, 2nd edn. New York, NY: Guilford Press; 2003, 144–98.

55. Steiner H, Saxena K, Chang K. Psychopharmacologic strategies for the treatment of aggression in juveniles. *CNS Spectrums* 2003; **8**(4): 298–308.

56. Anderson PJ. Towards a developmental model of executive function. In Anderson V, Jacobs R, Anderson P, eds. *Executive Functions and the Frontal Lobes: A Lifespan Perspective*. Philadelphia, PA: Taylor & Francis; 2008, 3–21.

57. Crone EA. Executive functions in adolescence: Inferences from brain and behavior. *Dev Sci* 2009; **12**(6): 825–30.

58. Zelazo PD, Muller U. Executive function in typical and atypical development. In Goswami U, ed. *The Wiley-Blackwell Handbook of Childhood Cognitive Development*. 2nd edn. Oxford, UK: Blackwell Publishing Ltd.; 2011, 574–603.

59. Achenbach TM. *The Achenbach System of Empirically Based Assessment (ASEBA): Development, Findings, Theory, and Applications*. Burlington, VT: University of Vermont Research Center for Children, Youth and Families; 2009.

60. Soller MV, Karnik S, Steiner H. Psychopharmacologic treatment in juvenile offenders. *Child Adolesc Psychiatr Clin N Am* 2006; **15**(2): 477–99.

61. Steiner H, Saxena K, Medic S, Plattner B, Delizonna L: Proactive/reactive aggression and psychopathology in high school students. *Scientific Proceedings of the Annual Meeting of the American Psychiatric Association*, 2005.

62. Bushman BJ, Anderson CA. Is it time to pull the plug on hostile versus instrumental aggression dichotomy. *Psychol Rev* 2001; **108**(1): 273–9.

63. Norman D, Shallice T. Attention to action: willed and automatic control of behavior. In Davidson R, Schwartz G, Shapiro D, eds. *Consciousness and Self-regulation: Advances in Research and Theory*. Vol. 4. New York: Plenum Press; 1986.

64. Shiffrin RM, Schneider W. Controlled and automatic human information processing: II. Perceptual learning, autonomatic attending, and a general theory. *Psychol Rev* 1977; **84**(1): 127–90.

65. Teplin LA, Abram KM, McClleand GM, Dulcan MK, Mericle AA. Psychiatric disorders in youth in juvenile detention. *Arch Gen Psychiatry* 2002; **59**(12): 1133–43.

66. Karnik NS, Popma A, Blair J, Khanzode L, Miller SP, Steiner H. Personality correlates of physiological response to stress among incarcerated juveniles. *Zeit Kinder-Jugendpsychiatrie Psychother* 2008; **36**(3): 185–90.

67. Karnik NS, Soller M, Redlich A, *et al.* Prevalence of and gender differences in psychiatric disorders among juvenile delinquents incarcerated for nine months. *Psychiatry Serv* 2009; **60**(6): 838–41.

68. Hanson KL, Medina KL, Padula CB, Tapert SF, Brown SA. Impact of adolescent alcohol and drug use on neuropsychological functioning in young adulthood: 10-year outcomes. *J Child Adolesc Subst* 2011; **20**(2): 135–54.

69. Thoma RJ, Monnig MA, Lysne PA, *et al.*, Adolescent substance abuse: the effects of alcohol and marijuana on

neuropsychological performance. *Alcohol Clin Exp Res* 2011; **35**(1): 39–46.

70. Medina KL, Hanson KL, Schweinsburg AD, Cohen-Zion M, Nagel BJ, Tapert SF. Neuropsychological functioning in adolescent marijuana users: Subtle deficits detectable after a month of abstinence. *J Int Neuropsychol Soc* 2007; **13**(5): 807–20.

71. Fontes MA, Bolla KI, Cunha PJ, *et al.* Cannabis use before age 15 and subsequent executive functioning. *Br J Psychiatry* 2011; **198**(6): 442–7.

72. Gruber SA, Sagar KA, Dahlgren MK, Racine M, Lukas SE. Age of onset of marijuana use and executive function. *Psychol Addict Behav* 2011; **21**: 1–11.

73. Tarter RE, Kirisci L, Mezzich A, Cornelius JR, Pajer, Vanyukov M. Neurobehavioral disinhibition in childhood predicts early age at onset of substance use disorder. *Am J Psychiatry* 2003; **160**(6): 1078–85.

74. Nigg JT, Wong MM, Martel MM, *et al.* Poor response inhibition as a predictor of problem drinking and illicit drug use in adolescents at risk for alcoholism and other substance use disorders. *J Am Acad Child Psychol* 2006; **45**(4): 468–75.

75. Aytaclar S, Tarter RE, Kirisci L, Lu S. Association Between Hyperactivity and executive cognitive functioning in childhood and substance use in early adolescence. *J Am Acad Child Psychol* 1999; **38**(2): 172–8.

76. Lundahl BW, Kunz C, Brownell C, Tollefson D, Burke BL. A meta-analysis of motivational interviewing: twenty-five years of empirical studies. *Research on Social Work Practice.* 2010;**20**(2): 137–160. Available from: http://dx.doi.org/10.1177/1049731509347850.

77. Toumbourou JW, Stockwell T, Neighbors C, Marlatt GA, Sturge J, Rehm J. Interventions to reduce harm associated with adolescent substance use. *Lancet* 2007;**369**(9570): 1391–401. Review

78. Miller L. Neuropsychological assessment of substance abusers: *Rev Recommendations* 1985; **2**(1): 5–17.

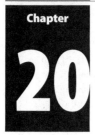

Chapter

20

Reflections on executive functioning

Elizabeth P. Sparrow and Scott J. Hunter

It can be argued that EF is the most important factor for successful adaptation to the human world. Although there are differing definitions and models for understanding EF (see Chapter 1), researchers and clinicians agree that intact EF skills are necessary for independently living as a responsible member of society who demonstrates appropriate and self-sustaining behavior. There remains debate regarding whether there is a unitary executive *function* (singular, comparable to a general factor), a non-unitary group of executive *functions* (plural), or a multifaceted cluster of separable but correlated executive functions;[1,2,3] however, all of the currently considered models agree that EF is complex, and multifactorial in its development and influence.

Executive functioning is complex and difficult to define

The challenge with any complex construct is creating a unitary definition or model that can account for all variations (see Chapter 1 for a review of historical and contemporary models). And, with regard to EF, the predominant definitions are filled with seeming contradictions and a focus on what may seem to be extremes of behavior. For example, a person with intact EF is described as flexible, able to adapt to changes in her environment; at the same time, she is persistent, and able to persevere (without becoming perseverative), and capable of self-monitoring and being strategic. This pattern of contrast within the goals of mental flexibility can be applied to skills such as consideration of a plan or goal, attention, concept, response set, even effort. Intact EF is also associated with being able to inhibit as well as initiate – again, seemingly opposite sides of the EF coin.

To illustrate this further, take the following example: imagine you are on the first day of a new job, and in your excitement, desirous of trying to emphasize an interest in everything about the field. While acknowledging your excitement, your department chair steps in and advises you to "pick one thing and stick with it," in order to maximize your professional opportunity and outcome. You follow this advice, and decide to focus all of your time and effort on creating a clinically informed, web-based model of the DSM-IV-TR that can be easily accessed and utilized. One year later you meet with the department chair again, to review your professional progress to date. You are feeling pleased that you followed his advice. Unfortunately, it becomes clear during the discussion that you failed to take into account that the DSM-IV-TR was currently being revised, and as a result, your incomplete model is already outdated. Given all the time you spent working on this project, your chair points out that you have not submitted any research manuscripts, and you have neglected to

Executive Function and Dysfunction, ed. Scott J. Hunter and Elizabeth P. Sparrow. Published by Cambridge University Press. © Cambridge University Press 2012.

teach any courses or advise any students. You counter by asking, "Hey, didn't you say to pick one thing and stick with it?" Your chair looks askance at your comment and just scowls at you.

As this hypothetical example illustrates, EF generally involves some degree of judgment, integration of situational contexts with previous knowledge and long-term goals, and juggling multiple demands. The downfall in judgment, strategy, and an appreciation of the "big picture" in the example given above is, in fact, a representation of how a disruption in EF can play out for any one person; it shows the contradictions inherent in both being focused and strategic, while failing to appreciate the full range of considerations and expectations that may be required on any given day, when being executive.

The terms "higher order" and "meta-" are often used when describing EF. The analogy of a CEO (chief executive officer) of a large corporation can be helpful for newcomers to the field when grasping the general ideas of EF; however, it may be more accurate to think of EF in terms of Luria's description of "the complex process of formation and *execution* of a program" (p. 219,[4] italics added for emphasis). Conceptually, EF is more about implementation than about knowledge, the appropriate application of information and behavior at the right time. Novel, nonroutine, and unstructured situations call for higher levels of EF. As tasks become automatic in their execution, in effect becoming "familiar habits," or are highly structured, EF demands decrease. Because EF can be so effortful and energy-consuming, it is only brought online as needed (which may be quite often during some tasks). EF is critical for purposeful, self-directed guidance of behavior, in order to reach a goal, as well as when forming a plan of action and identifying whether the goal has been met.

Executive functioning varies over development

The challenge to defining a complex construct grows greater when that construct also varies across time and setting. During typical development, there are many changes in EF (see Chapter 2). Given the shared timeline seen between these behavioral changes and the neuroanatomical changes that unfold (see Chapter 3), it is tempting to assume a causal link definitively exists between the two. However, this area of research is still young, and it is not yet clear how both the internal and external environments fully interact to influence the exact development of both EF as a behavior and the underlying neurofunctional processes that guide and direct its engagement. While we understand that there are genetically programmed contributions to the structural and functional expansions that take place neurodevelopmentally, we must also consider that any particular child's behavioral explorations and interactions with the external environment potentially lead to further facilitative (and potentially problematic) neurochemical and neuroanatomical changes that can influence EF. This complex interaction is not yet fully understood, nor effectively explicated, as a result.

Executive functioning is more than the frontal lobes

The field has progressed beyond the initial belief that a single cortical area, the PFC, is solely responsible for EF. It is now clear that many brain areas are involved in the network underlying EF, including various cortical, subcortical, and cerebellar regions interconnected by many white matter tracts. Yet, it remains still an open question as to what fully regulates and determines the broad expression of EF. While the "integrity of the whole brain is necessary for optimal performance on executive tasks"(p. 217),[1] we are still determining what fully defines that integrity.

Executive functioning is dissociable from IQ

Research into the behavioral aspects of EF is following the same path as has been seen with neuroanatomy and physiology; it is moving beyond the ideas that reference a single construct towards the delineation of separate, dissociable constructs. Yet debate remains. Most prominent in this debate are questions about the relationship between EF and IQ. A study of the IQ-EF relationship found that tests comprising the WM index accounted for most of the covariance between the two,[5] a conundrum as many conceptualize WM as part of EF. Although the study examined the contrast between EF (including WCST, Stroop Interference condition, COWAT, and Design Fluency) and non-EF measures (including Stroop color and Stroop word conditions, list-learning task, and RCFT-Copy), the majority of measures (particularly academic achievement) considered were also correlated with IQ; in other words, the correlations were not particularly unique to EF measures. This suggests that there remains a difficulty with fully parsing, in terms of both behavior and its definitions, what is separable as an indication of EF versus what is a component of being an intelligent individual. In general, sophisticated analyses have found that EF as a whole and IQ are not strongly correlated.[6,7,8] While there are some instances in which there are strong positive correlations between IQ and EF, such as certain EF tests correlating with IQ,[9,10] or EF correlating with IQ only in certain ranges of IQ,[11] there remain other indications of dissociability.

Stepping beyond these statistical analyses, there are a number of studies showing dissociation between EF and IQ in clinical populations. For example, one recent study reported average aspects of EF in the context of ID.[12] Examination of children and adolescents with ADHD has found EdF in the context of high IQ.[13] A general population study also found high percentages of children with significant IQ-EF discrepancies, in both directions.[8] Genetic studies have found evidence that EF and IQ are dissociable. A longitudinal study of children and their parents showed that although both IQ and aspects of EF are familial, EF was heritable even after controlling for IQ.[3] Twin studies have found additional support for the heritable nature of EF independent of IQ.[2,10]

Clinically, it is not uncommon to observe intact aspects of EF at the same time deficits are demonstrated (as discussed in Chapter 4 and in many chapters of Section II). A recent publication from an ongoing longitudinal twin study found support for unique genetic influences differentially impacting performance on different types of computerized EF tasks at 17 years old.[2]

Factors that impact executive functioning

There are a number of factors that influence levels of EF and EdF, including stable factors (such as demographics) and variable factors. Although the stable factors cannot be changed, awareness of them can improve interpretation of results. Variable factors represent an important area of development to be considered, particularly by clinicians who can target these factors in individual intervention plans, administrators who can use these factors to identify children who are at risk for EdF and proactively develop programs to reduce that risk, and researchers who can consider these factors as they systematically investigate methods of responding to EdF.

Stable factors associated with performance on EF tasks include *age, gender,* and *age by gender* interactions (see Chapters 2 and 4). *Ethnicity* has also been correlated with performance on some EF tasks. For example, a study of adolescent twins involving a computerized WCST found a significant effect for ethnicity ($p < 0.001$), with European Americans showing fewer perseverative errors than African Americans.[14] Another study of college students did not find that WCST performance varied by ethnicity, but did find significant effects for ethnicity on BADS subtests such as Zoo Map, with European Americans scoring higher than African Americans or Latino/a Americans.[15] Race was also a significant factor in an analysis of SES impacts on EF development.[16]

Another stable factor impacting EF is *genes*. Results from a recent twin study led to the conclusion that, "[EF skills are] ... among the most heritable psychological traits, possibly even more heritable than IQ." (p. 216).[2] A family study of parents and children also found high heritability estimates for EF.[3] These findings have encouraged consideration of EF as a possible endophenotype (i.e., a heritable, measurable construct that is closer to underlying biology and thus is more reliable than associated diseases, producing a larger genetic effect) for future research. This is not uniformly accepted, however, as heritability estimates are similar for actual disease conditions in some studies,[2] suggesting that it might be easier to use the actual disorder as the endophenotype rather than EF.

An interesting line of research is examining possible associations between *personality/ temperament* and EF.[17] Although the literature has many references to changes in personality after damage to the frontal lobes and subsequent EdF (including the well-known Phineas Gage[18]), few articles have considered relationships between existing personality features and level of EF (although see Rothbart and Posner's ongoing program of research examining the relationships between temperament and attention,[19,20] or work by J. Kagan[21] focusing on early expressions of anxiety as a temperamental feature and its impact across time on cognitive functioning). One of the recent publications in this area found EF performance was different for extraverts than for introverts, positing dopaminergic pathways as potential mediators of these correlations.[22] This domain is particularly relevant when considering the development of such lifelong difficulties as the disruptive behavior disorders, particularly sequelae predictive of Antisocial Personality Disorder (see Chapter 19).

Variable factors that impact EF include self-care, SES, and abuse, neglect, and trauma. Levels of these factors can exacerbate existing EdF, cause EdF, and even improve EF. It is critical to attend to these factors as they are changeable not only for children currently experiencing EdF but also for children who are at-risk for EdF. Exposure to *stress*, particularly when a child feels he has no control over the stress, negatively impacts EF.[23] A longitudinal study of childhood poverty found that chronic childhood stress was associated with decrements in WM assessed at 17 years old.[24] Current work by Hunter, Karnik, and Edidin, discussed in Chapter 19, focuses on the trajectories of EdF and resilience in EF that occur as a response to youth homelessness and accompanying psychopathology.

History of *trauma* (including *abuse and neglect*) also impacts EF. Children who were sexually or physically abused, or who witnessed domestic abuse ("familial" trauma) showed lower performance on WM, inhibition, auditory attention, and processing speed tasks than children exposed to "nonfamilial" trauma (i.e., car crash, natural disaster) or children without a trauma history.[25] Another study found that adolescents who retrospectively reported childhood physical abuse or neglect had increased rates of perseverative errors on the WCST.[26] The impact of *punitive discipline* on EF development has also been examined in a recent study; first graders in punitive schools (i.e., teachers disciplined students by beating with a stick, slapping the head, and pinching, an average of 40 punitive acts witnessed by students per day) had lower EF performance than first graders in non-punitive schools.[27] This is consistent with findings from a longitudinal study of parenting practices, namely that harsh parenting was associated with lower inhibitory control, and supportive parenting was associated with faster development of inhibitory control.[28] Similar conclusions were reached from a meta-analysis, that positive parental control (i.e., limit-setting, clear guidance and instructions) was positively associated with self-regulation and compliance in toddlers and negative parental control (i.e., coercion, criticism, hostility) was negatively associated with toddler self-regulation.[29]

Mood, both positive and negative, has also been shown to impact EF, although not necessarily in the direction one might predict.[30] Positive, happy mood has been associated with worse performance on WM tasks, impaired planning on Tower tasks, and increased inhibition cost on Stroop tasks. Positive mood seemed to facilitate creativity, however. Negative, sad mood was not consistently associated with EdF in the studies reviewed. Findings were mixed for effects of mood on verbal fluency and switching; positive mood seems to facilitate switching when switching to novel stimuli but impair switching when returning to familiar stimuli. Mitchell and Phillips hypothesize that this pattern of EdF in relation to positive mood may reflect a more heuristic, less rigorous processing style, in that positive mood is associated with reduced threat and low motivation to change a situation. *Social rejection* has also been demonstrated to negatively impact EF, particularly self-regulation, although this may be secondary to reduced motivation states as adding a cash incentive counteracted effects of the social rejection.[31]

Studies of *chronic pain* have found evidence of impaired attention, processing speed, speed of responding, mental flexibility, and verbal fluency.[32,33] A study of EF in people with rheumatoid arthritis found pain level was negatively correlated with performance on the Stroop ($p = 0.28$) and on WAIS-III Letter-Number Sequencing ($p = 0.002$); the significance of these findings was maintained even after controlling for age, education, and negative affect.[34] Positive affect was a moderating factor for this finding, with high positive affect and high pain associated with worse EF than low positive affect and high pain. It has even been suggested that EdF may play a role in the maintenance of chronic pain conditions.[33]

Sleep is another variable factor in EF, with sleep deprivation and disruption associated with decrements in EF.[35,36,37,38,39,40,41] Converging research strongly suggests that inadequate sleep, related to factors such as obstructive sleep apnea, snoring, and childhood obesity strongly impact both EF and behavioral regulation.[42,43,44] Another controllable factor in EF is *exercise and physical fitness*. A recent review concluded that aerobic fitness in childhood is associated with higher levels of cognitive functioning, including EF.[45] Children with higher aerobic fitness showed better performance on a selective attention task, with less impact from incongruent cues.[46] This finding has also been supported by longitudinal research that finds improvement in EF after children participate in an intense aerobic fitness program.[47] A study of sedentary, overweight children showed cognitive gains after participating in a 3-month afterschool physical fitness program.[48] These benefits do not seem to be limited to overweight children, as another study found cognitive improvement in children regardless of body-mass index after completion of a classroom-based exercise program.[49]

Another factor in EF that could potentially be changed is *SES*. A number of studies have consistently found associations between SES and EF across the lifespan;[50] these associations may be mediated by parent-child interactions,[51,52] parental education level,[53] amount of cognitive enrichment at home, or other factors. Educational factors that have been studied in relation to EF include length of schooling and quality of education. In studies that attempt to compare relative effects of *length of formal schooling* with effects of age on EF, it appears that there is some difference; children who have been in school longer do better on verbal fluency, WCST, WM, and mazes tasks than same-aged children in a lower grade.[54,55] This may reflect selection bias in terms of whether parents choose to enroll their children in school as soon as they are old enough, with a suspected bias toward delayed entry for children who are perhaps showing early signs of EdF. These fixed and variable factors impact EF, but the impact is not unidirectional.

Impact of executive deficits

EdF can impact nearly every aspect of everyday life. In addition to the impacts discussed in Chapter 4, EdF has been linked to outcome factors like level of education completed, financial security in adulthood, relationship status, substance use, criminal acts, medication adherence, health, and even moral development. A recent study found that, although "social and other noncognitive factors" taught in kindergarten (including paying attention in class, persisting on tasks, initiation, and behavioral self-control) are not necessarily linked with early childhood test scores, they are associated with markers of *adult "success,"* including college attendance, lifetime earnings, retirement savings, marriage rates, and homeownership at 27 years of age.[56] Other studies have reached similar conclusions, linking "noncognitive abilities" (e.g., motivation, risk-seeking, self-control, initiation, and persistence) to educational levels, teenage pregnancy, substance use, crime, and adult income (even after controlling for education).[57,58,59,60] What these studies call "noncognitive" factors certainly sound like EF. These types of findings from longitudinal studies encourage further investigation into early encouragement of EF, early identification of EdF, and early intervention for children with EdF, driven by the potential of significant long-term impact.

Less is known about the impact of EdF on *intrapersonal* factors, such as self-concept and self-reflection.[61] Clinical experience suggests that EdF can interfere with participation and compliance in psychotherapy. Several studies have reported on EdF as a suspected factor in medical noncompliance with treatment.[62,63] An emerging literature on EdF and *health* has linked individual differences in EF with successful implementation of diet[64,65,66,67,68,69] and exercise plans,[70,71] interrupting the substance use cycle,[72] smoking cessation,[73] binge-drinking,[74] and management of chronic illness.[75,76] Some have even posited that moral and ethical behavior relies on EF, describing the integration of contextual social knowledge, social semantic knowledge, and motivational/emotional states.[77,78]

It is possible for youth to *compensate* for EdF, particularly ones who are bright, but this can be at great cost. The cognitive resources consumed by an effort to compensate leave the individual less available for instruction and other problem-solving demands (including ones social and emotional). The cost incurred can also be seen in the development of secondary emotional issues; a child who is constantly told "you could do better if you tried," "stop being lazy and apply yourself," or, "you just need to get your act together and stop slacking off" is likely to internalize these negative statements[79] and show an enhanced vulnerability towards depression and anxiety.[80,81] This can also be associated with later self-confidence issues that further influence mood. These youth may be referred later in life for diagnosis and intervention as they struggle to meet life and educational demands (see comments on high school and college below).

Clinical implications of executive deficits

The neurodevelopmental and acquired disorders described in Section II of this volume share the common element of EdF, but there are many variations in both presentation and origin. The number of clinical conditions with EdF and the number of variations in presentation suggest the executive system is vulnerable, in terms of potential locations of insult and developmental periods which are sensitive. Within a diagnostic group or clinical condition, children may show different EF profiles. In general, existing psychological categorization systems are not based on cognitive profiles or neuroanatomical substrates, or even underlying deficits that lead to behavioral and emotional symptoms. Regardless, an understanding of EF and EdF can greatly improve understanding of why a child is struggling, and guide interventions including educational planning (see Chapters 17 and 18).

Executive dysfunction in high school and postsecondary education

When an adolescent or young adult's first evaluation occurs during high school, college, or some other advanced education program, it is possible that she is seeking the evaluation in response to exacerbation of EdF. Many times these individuals have attempted to compensate for their deficits, but with varied success. Academic under-achievement may be evident when comparing intellectual ability and academic knowledge with actual school performance. Eventually, the struggling individual reaches the point where the complexity and volume of work overwhelms his best efforts to compensate for EdF. Just as the transition to middle school stresses the already vulnerable functioning of a child with EdF (see Chapter 18), transitions to subsequent levels of education are stressful.[82] When an adolescent enters high school, he is often in a larger setting than he has experienced before. There are more distractions, such as extracurricular activities, driving, and dating. He also faces decreased structure and scaffolding from teachers and increased demands for planning and time management. High school usually represents a shift to long-term projects and exams that cover a wider range of information.

For individuals who continue to college, these stressors can intensify.[83] If living away from home, a college student must adjust to independent living without a parent who provides structure and support in areas like laundry, regular meals, and good sleep hygiene. College grades are often based on fewer data points, such as a single term paper, project, presentation, or final exam. Professors have less responsibility for an individual student's success, and may not be aware she is struggling until the end of a course. College students are expected to be fully independent adults; although advisors are assigned, they usually function as a source of information when the right questions are asked.

There is an emerging literature, particularly in the self-help genre, about surviving the adjustment to high school and beyond for people with ADHD,[84,85,86] ASD,[87,88,89,90] LD,[91,92,93,94,95,96] and executive deficits in general.[97,98] Although some of these books are diagnosis specific, the suggestions they provide may be helpful for many students with executive deficits. Yet, few of these self-help books share interventions that are well-tested and supported empirically. As a result, this area of intervention remains ripe for increased research and the development of empirically supported interventions to more effectively guide and enhance young adult EF development.

Executive dysfunction in correctional settings

Juvenile detainees show higher rates of psychiatric diagnoses than seen in the general population, particularly DBD and substance use disorders but also anxiety and affective disorders.[99] One study of 1440 juvenile detainees (10–18 years old) used a structured interview to assess DSM disorders in the past six months, and found 20% met criteria for an affective disorder, 22% for an anxiety disorder, and 44% for a DBD; 43% of the sample met criteria for at least two diagnoses.[100] The odds of having a psychiatric diagnosis were higher for juveniles sentenced to prison. A Swedish study found elevated rates of autism and ID among juvenile detainees.[101] A prospective study of arrests in a sample of boys with ADHD and a control group found the ADHD group had higher rates of offense and detention.[102] A review of lifetime arrest records for a sample of men with ADHD (no CD) showed significantly higher arrest rates, felony rates, convictions, and incarcerations relative to the non-ADHD sample.[103] While the existing literature does not address EdF explicitly, it seems reasonable to extrapolate that EdF might be a feature shared by many of these juvenile offenders.

Considering possible involvement of EdF in juvenile offenders is important not only for prevention of crime, but also for effective rehabilitation and release planning for those already in the juvenile justice system. A prospective study of children with ADHD found much higher rates of multiple arrests during a follow-up period relative to the control group.[102] A small study of 24 Canadian inmates found significant differences in WCST performance between recidivists and nonrecidivists.[104] Some studies have found associations between low levels of academic achievement and high rates of criminal offenses and recidivism.[105] Close examination of types of intervention suggests intervention can make a difference in recidivism rates;[106] for example, a study of juvenile offenders who received "wraparound planning" including involvement of families and mental health providers as well as other supports found reduced rates of recidivism, reduced odds of felony if arrested again, and less detention time served;[107] it is possible that some of the "supports" addressed unrecognized EdF. Taken as a whole, these limited findings suggest that understanding EdF in juvenile detainees and implementing specific interventions might lead to better outcomes; this certainly warrants further investigation.

Summary

EF is a complex construct with many facets, served by an intricate neurobiologic network that develops over the course of childhood, adolescence, and early adulthood. The behavioral manifestations of EF and EdF go through periods of rapid growth during this same time. Assessment of EF and EdF is a complex art and there is no gold standard test which can determine the presence of a deficit. Multiple clinical conditions involve EdF. Research to date indicates that interventions can be effective in preventing, reducing, and remediating EdF, including in the school setting. Forensic neuropsychologists are cautioned to think about the commonalities seen in group research as a starting point, and to also strongly consider individual difference factors that moderate the presentation of EdF for any particular individual. EdF impact many aspects of life, and many variables impact EF. Collaborative work among the professionals who help children and adolescents with EdF is key for making progress.[108] Overall, the most critical lesson to take from this volume is the importance of recognizing EdF (or the risk of EdF) and implementing intervention, so that opportunity and independence across time can be maximized and individually optimized, allowing for much greater success across time.

References

1. Jurado MB, Rosselli M. The elusive nature of executive functions: a review of our current understanding. *Neuropsychol Rev* 2007; **17**(3): 213–33. Epub 2007 Sep 5.

2. Friedman NP, Miyake A, Young SE, Defries JC, Corley RP, Hewitt JK. Individual differences in executive functions are almost entirely genetic in origin. *J Exp Psychol Gen* 2008; **137**(2): 201–25.

3. Jester JM, Nigg JT, Puttler LI, Long JC, Fitzgerald HE, Zucker RA. Intergenerational transmission of neuropsychological executive functioning. *Brain Cogn* 2009; **70**(1): 145–53. Epub 2009 Feb 24.

4. Luria AR. *The Working Brain*. Middlesex, England: Penguin Books, 1973.

5. Arffa S. The relationship of intelligence to executive function and non-executive function measures in a sample of average, above average, and gifted youth. *Arch Clin Neuropsychol* 2007; **22**(8): 969–78. Epub 2007 Oct 24.

6. Welsh MC, Pennington BF, Groisser DB. A normative-developmental study of executive function: a window on the prefrontal function in children. *Dev Neuropsychol* 1991; **7**: 131–49.

7. Ardila A, Pineda D, Rosselli M. Correlation between intelligence test scores and executive function measures. *Arch Clin Neuropsychol* 2000; **15**(1): 31–6.

8. Delis D, Lansing A, Houston WS, *et al.* Creativity lost: the importance of testing higher-level executive functions in school-age children and adolescents. *J Psychoeduc Assessm* 2007; **25** n1: 29–40.

9. Mahone EM, Hagelthorn KM, Cutting LE, *et al.* Effects of IQ on executive function measures in children with ADHD. *Child Neuropsychol* 2002; **8**(1): 52–65.

10. Friedman NP, Miyake A, Corley RP, Young SE, Defries JC, Hewitt JK. Not all executive functions are related to intelligence. *Psychol Sci* 2006; **17**(2): 172–9.

11. Foley J, Garcia J, Shaw L, Golden C. IQ predicts neuropsychologicalperformance in children. *Int J Neurosci* 2009; **119**(10): 1830–47.

12. Danielsson H, Henry L, Rönnberg J, Nilsson LG. Executive functions in individuals with intellectual disability. *Res Dev Disabil* 2010; **31**(6): 1299–304.

13. Brown TE, Reichel, Quinlan DM. Executive function impairments in high IQ children and adolescents with ADHD. *Open J Psychiatry* 2011; **1**(2): 56–65.

14. Anokhin AP, Golosheykin S, Grant JD, Heath AC. Developmental and genetic influences on prefrontal function in adolescents: a longitudinal twin study of WCST performance. *Neurosci Letters* 2010; **472**(2): 119–22.

15. Proctor A, Zhang J. Performance of three racial/ethnic groups on two tests of executive function: clinical implications for traumatic brain injury (TBI). *NeuroRehabilitation* 2008; **23**(6): 529–36.

16. Rhoades BL, Greenberg MT, Lanza ST, Blair C. Demographic and familial predictors of early executive function development: contribution of a person-centered perspective. *J Exp Child Psychol* 2011; **108**(3): 638–62.

17. Williams PG, Suchy Y, Rau HK. Individual differences in executive functioning: implications for stress regulation. *Ann Behav Med* 2009; **37**(2): 126–40.

18. Harlow JM. Recovery from the passage of an iron bar through the head. *Publ Massachusetts Med Soc* 1868; **2**: 327–47.

19. Posner MI, RothbartMK (2007). *Educating the Human Brain*. DC: APA.

20. Rothbart MK, Posner MI, Kieras J. Temperament, attention, and the development of self-regulation. In McCartney K., Phillips D. eds, *The Blackwell Handbook of Early Child Development*. London: Blackwell Press; 2006, 328–57.

21. Kagan J. *Galen's Prophecy: Temperament in Human Nature*. Cambridge, MA: Harvard University Press; 1994.

22. Campbell AM, Davalos DB, McCabe DP, Troup LJ. Executive functions and extraversion, *Personality Indiv Differences* 2011; **51**(6): 720–5.

23. Arnsten AF. The biology of being frazzled. *Science* 1998; **280**(5370): 1711–12.

24. Evans GW, Schamberg MA. Childhood poverty, chronic stress, and adult working memory. *Proc Natl Acad Sci USA* 2009; **106**(16): 6545–9.

25. DePrince AP, Weinzierl KM, Combs MD. Executive function performance and trauma exposure in a community sample of children. *Child Abuse Negl* 2009; **33**(6): 353–61.

26. Spann MN, Mayes LC, Kalmar JH, *et al.* Childhood abuse and neglect and cognitive flexibility in adolescents. *Child Neuropsychol* 2011. [Epub ahead of print]

27. Talwar V, Carlson SM, Lee K. Effects of a punitive environment on children's executive functioning: A natural experiment. *Soc Dev* 2011; **20**(4): 805–24.

28. Moilanen KL, Shaw DS, Dishion TJ, Gardner F, Wilson M. Predictors of longitudinal growth in inhibitory control in early childhood. *Soc Dev* 2009; **19**(2): 326–47.

29. Karreman A, van Tuijl C, van Aken MAG. and Deković M. Parenting and self-regulation in preschoolers: a meta-analysis. *Inf Child Dev* 2006; **15**: 561–79.

30. Mitchell RL, Phillips LH. The psychological, neurochemical and functional neuroanatomical mediators of the effects of positive and negative mood on executive functions. *Neuropsychologia* 2007; **45**(4): 617–29. Epub 2006 Sep 7.

31. Baumeister RF, DeWall CN, Ciarocco NJ, Twenge JM. Social exclusion impairs self-regulation. *J Pers Soc Psychol* 2005; **88**(4): 589–604.

32. Hart RP, Martelli MF, Zasler ND. Chronic pain and neuropsychological functioning. *Neuropsychol Rev* 2000; **10**(3): 131–49.

33. Solberg Nes L, Roach AR, Segerstrom SC. Executive functions, self-regulation, and chronic pain: a review. *Ann Behav Med* 2009; **37**(2): 173–83.

34. Abeare CA, Cohen JL, Axelrod BN, Leisen JC, Mosley-Williams A, Lumley MA. Pain, executive functioning, and affect in patients with rheumatoid arthritis. *Clin J Pain* 2010; **26**(8): 683–9.

35. Beebe DW. Cognitive, behavioral, and functional consequences of inadequate sleep in children and adolescents. *Pediatr Clin North Am* 2011; **58**(3): 649–65.

36. Beebe DW. A brief primer on sleep for pediatric and child clinical neuropsychologists. *Child Neuropsychol* 2011. [Epub ahead of print]

37. Bourke RS, Anderson V, Yang JS, *et al.* Neurobehavioral function is impaired in children with all severities of sleep disordered breathing. *Sleep Med* 2011; **12**(3): 222–9. Epub 2011 Feb 15.

38. Ståhle L, Ståhle EL, Granström E, Isaksson S, Annas P, Sepp H. Effects of sleep or food deprivation during civilian survival training on cognition, blood glucose and 3-OH-butyrate. *Wilderness Environ Med* 2011; **22**(3): 202–10.

39. Waters F, Bucks RS. Neuropsychological Effects of Sleep Loss: Implication for Neuropsychologists. *J Int Neuropsychol Soc* 2011; **4**: 1–16. [Epub ahead of print]

40. O'Brien LM. The neurocognitive effects of sleep disruption in children and adolescents. *Child Adolesc Psychiatr Clin N Am* 2009; **18**(4): 813–23.

41. Killgore WD, Grugle NL, Reichardt RM, Killgore DB, Balkin TJ. Executive functions and the ability to sustain vigilance during sleep loss. *Aviat Space Environ Med* 2009; **80**(2): 81–7.

42. Jiang F, VanDyke RD, Zhang J, Li F, Gozal D, Shen X. Effect of chronic sleep restriction on sleepiness and working memory in adolescents and young adults. *J Clin Exp Neuropsychol* 2011; **33**(8): 892–900.

43. Tauman R, Gozal D. Obstructive sleep apnea syndrome in children. *Expert Rev Respir Med* 2011; **5**(3): 425–40.

44. Spruyt K, Molfese DL, Gozal D. Sleep duration, sleep regularity, body weight, and metabolic homeostasis in school-aged children. *Pediatrics* 2011; **127**(2): e345–52.

45. Chaddock L, Pontifex MB, Hillman CH, Kramer AF. A review of the relation of aerobic fitness and physical activity to brain structure and function in children. *J Int Neuropsychol Soc* 2011; **17**(6): 975–85.

46. Chaddock L, Erickson KI, Prakash RS, *et al.* Basal ganglia volume is associated with aerobic fitness in preadolescent children. *Dev Neurosci* 2010; **32**(3): 249–56.

47. Tomporowski PD, Davis CL, Miller PH, Naglieri JA. Exercise and children's intelligence, cognition, and academic achievement. *Educ Psychol Rev* 2008; **20**(2): 111–31.

48. Davis CL, Tomporowski PD, McDowell JE, *et al.* Exercise improves executive function and achievement and alters brain activation in overweight children: a randomized, controlled trial. *Health Psychol* 2011; **30**(1): 91–8.

49. Hill LJ, Williams JH, Aucott L, Thomson J, Mon-Williams M. How does exercise benefit performance on cognitive tests in primary-school pupils? *Dev Med Child Neurol* 2011; **53**(7): 630–5.

50. Hackman DA, Farah MJ, Meaney MJ. Socioeconomic status and the brain: mechanistic insights from human and animal research. *Nat Rev Neurosci* 2010; **11**(9): 651–9.

51. Hughes C. Changes and challenges in 20 years of research into the development of executive functions. *Inf Child Dev* 2011; **20**(3): 251–71.

52. Carlson SM. Social origins of executive function development. In Lewis C, Carpendale JIM, eds., *Social Interaction and the Development of Executive Function. New Directions in Child and Adolescent Development* 2009; 123: 87–97.

53. Ardila A, Rosselli M, Matute E, Guajardo S The influence of the parents' educational level on the development of executive functions. *Dev Neuropsychol* 2005; **28**(1): 539–60.

54. McCrea SM, Mueller JH, Parrila RK. Quantitative analyses of schooling effects on executive function in young children. *Child Neuropsychol* 1999; **5**(4): 242–50.

55. Burrage MS, Ponitz CC, McCready EA, *et al.* Age- and schooling-related effects on executive functions in young children: a natural experiment. *Child Neuropsychol* 2008; **14**(6): 510–24.

56. Chetty R, Friedman JN, Hilger N, Saez E, Schanzenbach DW, Yagan D. How does your kindergarten classroom affect your earnings? Evidence from Project STAR. *NBER Working Paper* 16381, September 2010.

57. Borghans L, Duckworth AL, Heckman JJ, ter Weel B. The economics and psychology of personality traits. *J Hum Resources* 2008; **43**(4): 972–1059.

58. Bowles S, Gintis H, Osborne M. The determinants of earnings: A behavioral approach. *J Econ Lit* 2001; **39**(4): 11137–76.

59. Heckman JJ, Stixrud J, Urzua S. The effects of cognitive and noncognitive abilities on labor market outcomes and social behavior. *J Labor Econ* 2006; **24**(3): 411–82.

60. Cunha F, Heckman JJ. Investing in our young people. *NBER Working Paper* 16201, July 2010.

61. Lyons KE, Zelazo PD. Monitoring, metacognition, and executive function: elucidating the role of self-reflection in the development of self-regulation. *Adv Child Dev Behav* 2011; **40**: 379–412.

62. Zogg JB, Woods SP, Sauceda JA, Wiebe JS, Simoni JM. The role of prospective memory in medication adherence: a review of an emerging literature. *J Behav Med* 2011. [Epub ahead of print]

63. Stilley CS, Bender CM, Dunbar-Jacob J, Sereika S, Ryan CM. The impact of cognitive function on medication management: three studies. *Health Psychol* 2010; **29**(1): 50–5.

64. Nederkoorn C, Jansen E, Mulkens S, Jansen A. Impulsivity predicts treatment outcome in obese children. *Behav Res Ther* 2007; **45**(5): 1071–5.

65. Allan JL, Johnston M, Campbell N. Missed by an inch or a mile? Predicting the size of intention-behaviour gap from measures of executive control. *Psychol Hlth* 2011; **26**(6): 635–50. Epub 2011 May 24.

66. Hall PA. Executive control resources and frequency of fatty food consumption: Findings from an age-stratified community sample. *Health Psychol* 2011. [Epub ahead of print]

67. Davis C. Attention-deficit/hyperactivity disorder: associations with overeating and obesity. *Curr Psychiatry Rep* 2010; **12**(5): 389–95.

68. Pauli-Pott U, Albayrak O, Hebebrand J, Pott W. Association between inhibitory control capacity and body weight in overweight and obese children and adolescents: dependence on age and inhibitory control component. *Child Neuropsychol* 2010; **16**(6): 592–603.

69. Bruce AS, Black WR, Bruce JM, Daldalian M, Martin LE, Davis AM. Ability to delay gratification and BMI in preadolescence. *Obesity (Silver Spring)*. 2011; **19**(5): 1101–2.

70. Joseph RJ, Alonso-Alonso M, Bond DS, Pascual-Leone A, Blackburn GL. The neurocognitive connection between physical activity and eating behavior. *Obes Rev* 2011; **12**(10): 800–12.

71. Hall PA, Elias LJ, Fong GT, Harrison AH, Borowsky R, Sarty GE. A social neuroscience perspective on physical activity. *J Sport Exerc Psychol* 2008; **30**(4): 432–49.

72. Blume AW, Marlatt GA. The role of executive cognitive functions in changing substance use: what we know and what we need to know. *Ann Behav Med* 2009; **37**(2): 117–25.

73. Brega AG, Grigsby J, Kooken R, Hamman RF, Baxter J. The impact of executive cognitive functioning on rates of smoking cessation in the San Luis Valley Health and Aging Study. *Age Ageing* 2008; **37**(5): 521–5.

74. Mullan B, Wong C, Allom V, Pack SL. The role of executive function in bridging the intention-behavior gap for binge-drinking in university students. *Addict Behav* 2011; **36**(10): 1023–6.

75. Williams PG, Thayer JF. Executive functioning and health: introduction to the special series. *Ann Behav Med* 2009; **37**(2): 101–5.

76. Hall PA, Crossley M, D'Arcy C. Executive function and survival in the context of chronic illness. *Ann Behav Med* 2010; **39**(2): 119–27.

77. Moll J, Zahn R, de Oliveira-Souza R, Krueger F, Grafman J. Opinion: the neural basis of human moral cognition. *Nat Rev Neurosci* 2005; **6**(10): 799–809.

78. Barkley RA. *ADHD and the Nature of Self-Control*. New York: The Guilford Press; 1997.

79. Kelly K, Ramundo P. *You Mean I'm Not Lazy, Stupid or Crazy?! A Self-Help Book for Adults with Attention Deficit Disorder*. New York: Simon & Schuster; 1993.

80. Hammen C, Goodman-Brown T, Self-schemas and vulnerability to specific life stress in children at risk for depression. *Cog Tx and Res* 1990; **14**: 215–27.

81. Jacobs R, Reinecke M, Gollan J, Kane P. Empirical evidence of cognitive vulnerability for depression among children and adolescents: a cognitive science and developmental perspective. *Clin Psychol Rev* 2007; **28**: 759–82.

82. Rostain AL, Ramsay JR. College and high school students with attention-deficit/hyperactivity disorder: new directions in assessment and treatment. In *American College Health Association Professional Development Program – Use and Misuse of Stimulants: A Guide for School Health Professionals*. Englishtown, NJ, Princeton Media Associates; 2006, 7–16.

83. Brinckerhoff LC, Shaw SF, McGuire JM. Promoting access, accommodations, and independence for college students with learning disabilities. *J Learn Disabil* 1992; **25**(7): 417–29.

84. Maitland TEL, Quinn PO. *Ready for Take-Off: Preparing Your Teen With ADHD or LD for College*. Washington, DC, Magination Press; 2010.

85. Quinn PO, Maitland TEL. *On Your Own: A College Readiness Guide for Teens With ADHD/LD*. Washington, DC, Magination Press; 2011.

86. Quinn PO, Ratey N, Maitland TEL. *Coaching College Students with AD/HD:*

Issues and Answers. Silver Spring, Maryland: Advantage Books; 2000.

87. Wolf LE, Brown JT, Bork R. *Students with Asperger Syndrome: A Guide for College Personnel. Shawnee Mission*, Kansas: Autism Asperger Publishing Company; 2009.

88. Harpur J, Lawlor M, Fitzgerald M. *Succeeding in College with Asperger Syndrome: A Student Guide.* New York: Jessica Kingsley Publishers; 2004.

89. Freedman S. *Developing College Skills in Students With Autism and Asperger's Syndrome.* New York: Jessica Kingsley Publishers; 2010.

90. Palmer A. *Realizing the College Dream With Autism or Asperger Syndrome: A Parent's Guide to Student Success.* New York: Jessica Kingsley Publishers; 2006.

91. Chiang HM, Cheung YK, Hickson L, Xiang R, Tsai LY. Predictive factors of participation in postsecondary education for high school leavers with autism. *J Autism Dev Disord* 2011. [Epub ahead of print]

92. Murray C, Wren CT. Cognitive, academic, and attitudinal predictors of the grade point averages of college students with learning disabilities. *J Learn Disabil* 2003; **36**(5): 407–15.

93. Troiano PF, Liefeld J Ann, Trachtenberg JV. Academic support and college success for postsecondary students with learning disabilities. *J Coll Read Learn* 2010; **40**(2): 35–44

94. Ruban LM, McCoach DB, McGuire JM, Reis SM. The differential impact of academic self-regulatory methods on academic achievement among university students with and without learning disabilities. *J Learn Disabil* 2003; **36**(3): 270–86.

95. Allsopp DH, Minskoff EH, Bolt L. Individualized course-specific strategy instruction for college students with learning disabilities and ADHD: lessons learned from a model demonstration project. *Learn Disab Rese Pract* 2005; **20**(2): 103–18.

96. Skinner ME, Lindstrom BD. Bridging the gap between high school and college: strategies for the successful transition of students with learning disabilities. *Preventing School Failure* 2003; **47**(3): 132–7.

97. Dawson P, Guare R. *Smart but Scattered: The Revolutionary "Executive Skills" Approach to Helping Kids Reach Their Potential.* New York: The Guilford Press; 2009.

98. Cooper-Kahn J, Dietzel L. *Late, Lost, and Unprepared: A Parents' Guide to Helping Children with Executive Functioning.* Bethesda, MD: Woodbine House; 2008.

99. Teplin LA, Abram KM, McClelland GM, Dulcan MK, Mericle AA. Psychiatric disorders in youth in juvenile detention. *Arch Gen Psychiatry* 2002; **59**(12): 1133–43.

100. Washburn JJ, Teplin LA, Voss LS, Simon CD, Abram KM, McClelland GM. Psychiatric disorders among detained youths: a comparison of youths processed in juvenile court and adult criminal court. *Psychiatr Serv* 2008; **59**(9): 965–73.

101. Ståhlberg O, Anckarsäter H, Nilsson T. Mental health problems in youths committed to juvenile institutions: prevalences and treatment needs. *Eur Child Adolesc Psychiatry* 2010; **19**(12): 893–903. Epub 2010 Oct 15.

102. Satterfield JH, Hoppe CM, Schell AM. A prospective study of delinquency in 110 adolescent boys with attention deficit disorder and 88 normal adolescent boys. *Am J Psychiatry* 1982; **139**(6): 795–8.

103. Mannuzza S, Klein RG, Moulton JL 3rd. Lifetime criminality among boys with attention deficit hyperactivity disorder: a prospective follow-up study into adulthood using official arrest records. *Psychiatry Res* 2008; **160**(3): 237–46. Epub 2008 Aug 15.

104. Valliant PM, Freeston A, Pottier D, Kosmyna R. Personality and executive functioning as risk factors in recidivists. *Psychol Rep* 2003; **92**(1): 299–306.

105. Katsiyannis A, Ryan JB, Zhang D, Spann A. Juvenile delinquency and recidivism: the impact of academic achievement. *Read Writ Quart* 2008; *v* **24**(2): 177–96.

106. Redondo S, Sanchez-meca J, Garrido V. The influence of treatment programmes on the recidivism of juvenile and adult offenders: a European meta-analytic review. *Psycholo Crime Law* 1999; 5(3).

107. Pullmann MD, Kerbs J, Koroloff N, Veach-White E, Gaylor R, Sieler D. Juvenile offenders with mental health needs: reducing recidivism using wraparound. *Crime Delinq* 2006; 52: 375–97.

108. Banich MT. Executive function: the search for an integrated account. *Curr Directions Psychol Sci* 2009; 18(2): 89–94.

Appendix 1: Abbreviations used in the book

5-HT	Serotonin
5-HTT	Serotonin transporter
AAIDD	American Association on Intellectual and Developmental Disabilities
ABAS	Adaptive Behavior Assessment System
ABI	Acquired brain injury
ADEM	Acute disseminated encephalomyelitis
ACC	Anterior cingulate cortex
ACh	Acetylcholine
ADHD	Attention-Deficit/Hyperactivity Disorder
ADHD-C	ADHD, Combined type
ADHD-HI	ADHD, Predominantly Hyperactive-Impulsive type
ADHD-I	ADHD, Predominantly Inattentive type
ADOS	Autism Diagnostic Observation Schedule
AED	Antiepileptic drugs
AIDS	Acquired Immune Deficiency Syndrome
ALL	Acute lymphoblastic leukemia
AMAT-C	Amsterdam Memory and Attention Training for Children program
ANT	Amsterdam Neuropsychological Tasks
APFC	Anterior Prefrontal Cortex
APT	Attention Process Training
ARND	Alcohol-related neurodevelopmental disorder
ASD	Autism Spectrum Disorder(s)
ASEBA	Achenbach System of Empirically Based Assessment
AVM	Arteriovenous malformation
BADS	Behavioral Assessment of the Dysexecutive Syndrome
BASC	Behavior Assessment System for Children
BCECTS	Benign Childhood Epilepsy with Centrotemporal Spikes (a.k.a. Rolandic epilepsy)
BD	Bipolar Disorder
BFRS-R	Behavior Flexibility Rating Scale-Revised
BLLs	Blood lead levels
BOLD	Blood-oxygen-level dependence

BRIEF	Behavior Rating Inventory of Executive Function
CADS-IV	Conners' ADHD/DSM Scales
CANTAB	Cambridge Neuropsychological Test Automated Battery
CAI	Computer assisted instruction program
CAS	Das–Naglieri Cognitive Assessment System
CAT	Computerized attention training program
CBCL	Achenbach's Child Behavior Checklist
CBRS	Conners Comprehensive Behavior Rating Scales
CCC	Cognitive Complexity and Control theory
CCC-r	Cognitive Complexity and Control theory, Revised
CCRT	Computerized cognitive rehabilitation therapy
CCSS	Childhood Cancer Survivor Study
CCSS-NCQ	Childhood Cancer Survivor Study Neurocognitive Questionnaire
CCT	Children's Category Test
CCTT	Children's Color Trails Test
CD	Conduct Disorder
CDC	Centers for Disease Control and Prevention
CDI	Children's Depression Inventory
CELF	Clinical Evaluation of Language Fundamentals
CMS	Children's Memory Scale
CMU	Chronic marijuana use/users
CMV	Cytomegalovirus
CNS	Central nervous system
CO	Carbon monoxide
COWAT	Benton's Controlled Oral Word Association Test (a.k.a., Verbal Fluency)
CP	Cerebral Palsy
CPAT	Computerized Progressive Attention Training
CPRS	Conners' Parent Rating Scales
CPT	Continuous Performance Test/Task
CRP	Cognitive Remediation Program
CRS	Conners Rating Scales
CRT	Cranial/Craniospinal radiation therapy
CSF	Cerebrospinal fluid
CT	Computed tomography (a.k.a. CAT or computerized axial tomography)
CTOPP	Comprehensive Test of Phonological processing

CTRS	Conners' Teacher Rating Scale
CVLT	California Verbal Learning Test
CVLT-C	California Verbal Learning Test – Children's Version
DA	Dopamine
DBD	Disruptive Behavior Disorders
D-KEFS	Delis–Kaplan Executive Function System
DLPFC	Dorsolateral prefrontal cortex
DS	Down syndrome
DSM	*Diagnostic and Statistical Manual of Mental Disorders*
DSM-IV-TR	DSM, Fourth edition, Text revision
DSM-5	DSM, Fifth edition
DTI	Diffusion tensor imaging
EC	Conners Early Childhood
EdF	Executive dysfunction
EEG	Electroencephalography
ELBW	Extremely low birthweight
EF	Executive functioning
FA	Fractional anisotropy
FAS	Fetal Alcohol Syndrome
FASD	Fetal Alcohol Spectrum Disorder(s)
FLE	Frontal-lobe epilepsy
fMRI	Functional magnetic resonance imaging
FMRP	FraX Mental Retardation Protein
FPS	Family-centered problem-solving intervention
FraX	Fragile X Syndrome
GABHS	Group A β-hemolytic streptococcal infection
GAD	Generalized Anxiety Disorder
GCS	Glasgow Coma Scale
GDS	Gordon Diagnostic System
GED	Graduate Equivalency Diploma
HIE	Hypoxic–ischemic encephalopathy
HIV	Human immunodeficiency virus

ICPS	I Can Problem Solve curriculum
ID	Intellectual Disability
IQ	Intelligence Quotient
IVH	Intraventricular hemorrhage
K-CPT	Conners' Kiddie Continuous Performance Test
K-SADS	Kiddie-Schedule for Affective Disorders and Schizophrenia
LD	Learning Disorder/Disability
LTM	Long-term memory
MDD	Major Depressive Disorder
MEG	Magnetoencephalography
MFFT	Matching Familiar Figures Test
MR	Mental Retardation
MRI	Magnetic resonance imaging
MTA	Multimodal Treatment of Attention-Deficit/Hyperactivity Disorder study
NAA	*N*-acetyl-aspartate
NDD	Neurodevelopmental disabilities
NE	Norepinephrine
NEPSY	NEPSY: A Developmental Neuropsychological Assessment
NF-1	Neurofibromatosis, type 1
NIMH	National Institutes of Mental Health
OCD	Obsessive-Compulsive Disorder
OCP	Open Circle Program curriculum
ODD	Oppositional Defiant Disorder
OFC	Orbitofrontal prefrontal cortex
OTMT	Oral Trail Making Test
PANDAS	Pediatric Autoimmune Neuropsychiatric Disorder Associated with Streptococcal Infection
PATHS	Promoting Alternative Thinking Strategies curriculum
PBD	Pediatric Bipolar Disorder
PCBs	Polychlorinated biphenyls
PCE	Prenatal cocaine exposure
PDA	Personal digital assistant

PDD	Pervasive Developmental Disorder(s)
PDD-NOS	Pervasive Developmental Disorder, Not Otherwise Specified
PET	Positron emission tomography
PFC	Prefrontal cortex
PIP	Proactive, instrumental, or planned aggression
PKU	Phenylketonuria
PKC	Protein kinase C
PME	Prenatal marijuana exposure
PNE	Prenatal nicotine exposure
PTSD	Post-Traumatic Stress Disorder
PVL	Periventricular leukomalacia
RADI	Reactive, affective, defensive, or impulsive aggression
RAN/RAS	Rapid Automatized Naming and Rapid Alternating Stimulus
RD	Reading Disorder/Disability
RCFT	Rey Complex Figure Test
RFFT	Ruff Figural Fluency Test
ROCF	Rey–Osterreith Complex Figure
RT	Reaction/Response time
SAD	Separation Anxiety Disorder
SAS	Supervisory Attentional System
SB-IV	Stanford–Binet Intelligence Scale, 4th edn
SBH	Subcortical band heterotopia
SBM	Spina bifida with myelomeningocele
SCD	Sickle cell disease
SDB	Sleep disordered breathing
SES	Socio-economic status
SRSD	Self-Regulated Strategy Development model
SSRI	Selective serotonin reuptake inhibitor
STM	Short-term memory
Stroop	Stroop Color and Word Test
TAT	Thematic Apperception Test
TB	Tuberculosis
TBI	Traumatic brain injury
TDD	Temper Dysregulation Disorder with Dysphoria

TEA-Ch	Test of Everyday Attention for Children
TEC	Tasks of Executive Control
ToLC	Test of Language Competence
TLE	Temporal-lobe epilepsy
TMT	Trail-Making Test
TMT-A	Trail-Making Test, Part A
TMT-B	Trail-Making Test, Part B
TOLDX	Tower of London, Drexel University
TOPS	Teen Online Problem Solving Program
TOVA	Test of Variables of Attention
TPBA	Transdisciplinary Play-Based Assessment
TRF	Achenbach's Teacher's Report Form
TS	Tourette Syndrome (a.k.a. Tourette's Disorder)
VLBW	Very low birthweight
VLPFC	Ventrolateral prefrontal cortex
VMI	Beery–Buktenica Developmental Test of Visual–Motor Integration
VSAT	Visual Search and Attention test
WAIS	Wechsler Adult Intelligence Scale
WCST	Wisconsin Card Sorting Test
WIAT	Wechsler Individual Achievement Test
WISC	Wechsler Intelligence Scale for Children
WJ-Ach	Woodcock–Johnson Tests of Achievement
WJ-Cog	Woodcock–Johnson Tests of Cognitive Abilities
WM	Working memory
WMTB	Working Memory Test Battery for Children
WPPSI	Wechsler Preschool and Primary Scale of Intelligence
WRAML	Wide Range Assessment of Memory and Learning
WRAVMA	Wide Range Assessment of Visual Motor Ability
WS	Williams syndrome
YSR	Achenbach's Youth-Self Report

Appendix 2: Tests/tasks referenced in the book

Test Name	Reference
Achenbach System of Empirically Based Assessment (ASEBA; includes CBCL, TRF, & YSR)	• Achenbach TM, Rescorla L. *Manual for the ASEBA School-age Forms and Profiles.* Burlington, VT, University of Vermont, Research Center for Children, Youth, and Families, 2001.
Adaptive Behavior Assessment System, Second edition (ABAS-II)	• Harrison PL, Oakland T. *Adaptive Behavior Assessment System. Manual. 2nd edn.* San Antonio, TX: The Psychological Corporation, 2003.
Amsterdam Neuropsychological Tasks (ANT)	• deSonneville LMJ. Amsterdam neuropsychological tasks: A computer-aided assessment program. In den Brinker BPLM, Beck PJ, Brand AN, *et al.*, eds. *Cognitive Ergonomics, Clinical Assessment, and Computer-assisted Learning: Computers in Psychology.* Lisse, The Netherlands: Swets & Zeitlinger, 1999; 187–203.
A-not-B task	• Piaget, J. *The Construction of Reality in the Child.* New York: Basic Books, 1954. • Espy KA, Kaufmann PM, McDiarmid M, Glisky ML. Executive functioning in preschool children: A-not-B and other delayed response format task performance. *Brain Cogn* 1999; **41**(2): 178–99.
Antisaccade task	• Hallett, PE. Primary and secondary saccades to goals defined by instructions. *Vision Res* 1978;**18**(10): 1279–96.
Autism Diagnostic Observation Schedule (ADOS)	• Lord C, Rutter M, DiLavore PC, Risi S. *Autism Diagnostic Observation Schedule (ADOS).* Torrance, CA: Western Psychological Services, 2001.
Beery-Buktenica Developmental Test of Visual-Motor Integration (VMI)	• Beery KE. *The Beery–Buktenica Developmental Test of Visual–Motor Integration (VMI). 4th edn. rev.* Parsippany, NJ: Modern Curriculum Press, 1997.
Behavior Assessment System for Children, 2nd edition (BASC-2)	• Reynolds CR, Kamphaus RW. *Behavior Assessment System for Children. Examiner's Manual. 2nd edn.* Circle Pines, MN: AGS Publishing; 2004.
Behavior Flexibility Rating Scale-Revised (BFRS-R)	• Peters-Scheffer N, Didden R, Green VA, *et al.* The behavior flexibility rating scale, Revised: Factor analysis, internal consistency, inter-rater and intra-rater reliability, and convergent validity. *Res Dev Disabil* 2008; **29**(5): 398–407.
Behavior Rating Inventory of Executive Function (BRIEF, BRIEF-SR, BRIEF-P, BRIEF-A)	• Gioia GA, Isquith PK, Guy SC, Kenworthy L. *BRIEF: Behavior Rating Inventory of Executive Function.* Odessa, FL, Psychological Assessment Resources, 2000.

Test Name	Reference
	• Gioia GA, Espy KA, Isquith PK. *The Behavior Rating Inventory of Executive Function – Preschool (BRIEF-P)*. Odessa, FL, Psychological Assessment Resources, 2003. • Roth RM, Isquith PK, Gioia GA. *Behavior Rating Inventory of Executive Function – Adult (BRIEF-A)*. Lutz, FL: Psychological Assessment Resources, 2005.
Behavioral Assessment of the Dysexecutive Syndrome (BADS)	• Wilson BA, Alderman N, Burgess PW, Emslie H, Evans JJ. *Behavioral Assessment of the Dysexecutive Syndrome (BADS)*. Bury St. Edmunds, UK: Thames Valley Test Company, 1996. • Norris G, Tate, RL. The behavioural assessment of the dysexecutive syndrome (BADS): ecological, concurrent and construct validity. *Neuropsychol Rehabil* 2000; **10**(1): 33–45.
Behavioral Assessment of the Dysexecutive Syndrome (BADS-C)	• Emslie HC, Wilson FC, Burden V, Nimmo-Smith I, Wilson BA. *Behavioural Assessment of the Dysexecutive Syndrome in Children (BADS-C)*. Bury St. Edmunds, UK: Thames Valley Test Company, 2003. • Engel-Yeger B, Josman N, Rosenblum S. Behavioural assessment of the dysexecutive syndrome for children (BADS-C): An examination of construct validity. *Neuropsychol Rehabil* 2009; **19**(5): 662–76.
Brazelton Neonatal Behavioral Assessment Scale (BNBAS)	• Als H, Tronick E, Lester BM, Brazelton TB. The Brazelton neonatal behavioral assessment scale (BNBAS). *J Abnorm Child Psychol* 1977; **5**(3): 215–31.
Brown ADD Scales	• Brown TE. Brown *Attention Deficit Disorder Scales For Children And Adolescents. Examiner's Manual*. San Antonio, TX: The Psychological Corporation, 2001.
California Sorting Test	• Delis DC, Squire LR, Bihrle A, Massman P. Componential analysis of problem-solving ability: Performance of patients with frontal lobe damage and amnesic patients on a new sorting test. *Neuropsychologia* 1992; **30**(8): 683–97. *see also D-KEFS Tower*
California Verbal Learning Test: Second Edition (CVLT-2)	• Delis DC, Kramer JH, Kaplan E, Ober BA. *California Verbal Learning Test. 2nd edn*. San Antonio, TX: Psychological Corporation, 2000.
California Verbal Learning Test – Children's Version (CVLT-C)	• Delis DC, Kramer JH, Kaplan E, Ober BA. *The California Verbal Learning Test. Children's Version (CVLT-C)*. San Antonio, TX: Psychological Corporation, 1994.
Cambridge Neuropsychological Tests Automated Battery (CANTAB)	• Sahakian BJ, Owen AM. Computerised assessment in neuropsychiatry using CANTAB. *J Roy Soc of Med* 1992; **85**:399–402.

Test Name	Reference
	• Luciana M, Nelson CA. Assessment of neuropsychological function through use of the cambridge neuropsychological testing automated battery: Performance in 4- to 12-year-old children. *Dev Neuropsychol* 2002; **22**(3): 595–624.
Category test	• Reitan RM, Wolfson D. *The Halstead–Reitan Neuropsychological Test Battery: Theory And Clinical Interpretation.* Tucson, AZ, Neuropsychology Press, 1993. • DeFilippis NA, McCampbell E. *The Booklet Category Test.* Odessa, FL: Psychological Assessment Resources, Inc., 1979. • Choca J, Laatsch L, Garside D, Arnemann C. CAT; *The Computer Category Test. Examiner's Manual.* North Tonawanda, NY: Multi-Health Systems, Inc., 1994.
Child Behavior Checklist (CBCL)	*see Achenbach System of Empirically Based Assessment*
Children's Category Test (CCT)	• Boll T. *Children's Category Test. Manual.* San Antonio, TX: Psychological Corporation, 1993.
Children's Color Trails Test (CCTT)	• Llorente AM, Williams J, Satz P, D'Elia L. *Children's Color Trails Test (CCTT).* Los Angeles: Western Psychological Services, 1998. *see also Trail Making Test*
Children's Depression Inventory (CDI)	• Kovacs, M. *Manual For The Children's Depression Inventory.* North Tonawanda, NY: Multi-Health Systems, 2001. • Kovacs M. *Children's Depression Inventory (CDI). Technical Manual Update.* North Tonawanda, NY: Multi-Health Systems, 2003.
Children's Memory Scale (CMS)	• Cohen M. *Children's Memory Scale (CMS).* San Antonio, TX: The Psychological Corporation, 1997.
Clinical Evaluation of Language Fundamentals (CELF)	• Semel E, Wiig E. *Clinical Evaluation Of Language Functions. (CELF).* Ohio, Charles Merrill, 1980. • Semel E, Wiig E, Secord W. *Clinical Evaluation Of Language Fundamentals. Revised. (CELF-R).* New York: The Psychological Corporation, 1987. • Semel E, Wiig E, Secord W. *Clinical Evaluation Of Language Fundamentals. 3rd edn. (CELF-3).* San Antonio, TX: The Psychological Corporation, 1995. • Semel E, Wiig E, Secord WA. *Clinical Evaluation of Language Fundamentals. 4th Edn. (CELF-4).* San Antonio, TX: The Psychological Corporation, 2003.
Clock-drawing	• Goodglass H, Kaplan E. *The Assessment of Aphasia and Related Disorders.* Philadelphia: Lea & Febiger, 1983. Cohen MJ, Ricci CA, Kibby MY, Edmonds JE. Developmental progression of clock face drawing in children. *Child Neuropsychol* 2000; **6**(1): 64–76.

Test Name	Reference
Cognitive Assessment System (CAS)	• Naglieri JA, Das JP. *Cognitive Assessment System*. Itasca, IL: Riverside Publishing, 1997.
Color Trails Test	• Maj M, D'Elia L, Satz P, Janssen R, Zaudig M, Uchiyama C, *et al*. World Health Organization, Division of Mental Health/Global Programme on AIDS. Evaluation of two new neuropsychological tests designed to minimize cultural bias in the assessment of HIV-1 seropositive persons: A WHO study. *Arch Clin Neuropsychol* 1993; **8**(2): 123–35. • D'Elia LF, Satz P, Uchiyama CL, White T. *Color Trails Test. Professional Manual*. Odessa, FL: Psychological Assessment Resources, 1996. *see also Trail Making Test*
Comprehensive Test of Phonological Processing (CTOPP)	• Wagner RK, Torgesen JK, Rashotte CA. CTOPP: *Comprehensive Test of Phonological Processing. Examiner's Manual*. Pro-Ed: Austin, TX, 1999.
Conflicting Motor Response	• Christensen AL. *Luria's Neuropsychological Investigation*. Copenhagen: Munksgaard, 1979. *see also portions of NEPSY-2 Manual Motor Sequences*
Conners 3rd Edition (Conners 3)	• Conners CK. *Conners 3rd edn. (Conners 3) Manual*. North Tonawanda, NY: Multi-Health Systems, Inc., 2008.
Conners Comprehensive Behavior Rating Scales (Conners CBRS)	• Conners, CK. *Conners Comprehensive Behavior Rating Scales (Conners CBRS) Manual*. North Tonawanda, NY: Multi-Health Systems, Inc., 2008.
Conners CPT-II	• Conners CK, MHS Staff. *Conners' Continuous Performance Test. Version 5 for Windows, 2nd edn. (Conners CPT-II v5)*. North Tonawanda, NY: Multi-Health Systems, Inc., 2000.
Conners K-CPT	• Conners CK, MHS Staff. *Conners' Kiddie Continuous Performance Test (K-CPT)*. North Tonawanda, NY: Multi-Health Systems, Inc., 2001.
Conners Early Childhood Rating Scales (Conners EC)	• Conners CK. *Conners Early Childhood (Conners EC) Manual*. North Tonawanda, NY: Multi-Health Systems, Inc., 2009.
Conners Parent Rating Scales – Revised (CPRS-R)	*see Conners Rating Scales – Revised*
Conners Rating Scales – Revised (CRS-R; includes CADS-IV, CPRS-R, CTRS-R)	• Conners C. *Conners' Rating Scales. Technical manual. Rev (CRS-R)*. North Tonawanda, NY: Multi-Health Systems, Inc., 1997.
Conners Teacher Rating Scales – Revised (CTRS-R)	*see Conners Rating Scales – Revised*
Conners' ADHD/DSM-IV Scales (CADS-IV)	*see Conners Rating Scales – Revised*
Continuous Performance Tests (CPTs)	*see Conners CPT-II, Conners K-CPT, Gordon Diagnostic System, Tests of Variables of Attention*

Test Name	Reference
Controlled Oral Word Association Test (COWAT; a.k.a. "FAS" or "first letter fluency")	• Benton AL, Hamsher, K. *Multilingual Aphasia Examination 2nd edn*. Iowa City, IA: AJA Associates, 1976. • Ruff, RM, Light, RH, Parker, SB, Levin, HS. Benton controlled oral word association test: reliability and updated norms. *Arch Clin Neuropsychol* 1996; **11**(4): 329–38. *see also portions of D-KEFS VerbalFluency, NEPSY-II Word Generation*
Delis-Kaplan Executive Function System (D-KEFS)	• Delis D, Kaplan E, Kramer J. *Delis–Kaplan Executive Function System. Examiner's Manual*. San Antonio, TX: Psychological Corporation, 2001.
Design Fluency	• Jones-Gotman M, Milner B. Design fluency: the invention of nonsense drawings after focal cortical lesions. *Neuropsychologia* 1977; **15**:653–74. *see also D-KEFS Design Fluency, NEPSY Design Fluency, RFFT*
Dichotic listening task	• Bryden, MP. An overview of the dichotic listening procedure and its relation to cerebral organization. In Hugdahk, ed. *Handbook of Dichotic Listening: Theory, Method, And Research*. London: John Wiley, 1988; 1–43.
Digit Symbol Substitution Test	*see Wechsler scales, Coding*
Go/No-Go task	• Luria AR. *Higher Cortical Functions in Man*. New York: Basic Books, 1980. *see also TEC*
Gordon Diagnostic System (GDS)	• Gordon M. *The Gordon Diagnostic System*. DeWitt, NY: Gordon Systems, 1983.
Grooved Pegboard Test	• Reitan RM, Davison LA. *Clinical Neuropsychology: Current Status and Applications. Appendix*. Washington, DC: VH Winston and Sons, 1974. • Knights RM, Norwood J. *Revised Smoothed Normative Data On The Neuropsychological Test Battery For Children*. Ottawa, Canada, Knights RM, Norwood J; 1980. • Trites R. *Grooved Pegboard Test. Instruction/Owner's Manual*. Lafayette, IN: Lafayette Instruments, 1989.
Hayling task	• Burgess PW, Shallice T. Response suppression, initiation and strategy use following frontal lobe lesions. *Neuropsychologia* 1996; **34**(4): 263–73.
Matching Familiar Figures Test (MFFT)	• Kagen J. *Matching Familiar Figures Test*. Cambridge, MA, Harvard University, 1965. • Arizmendi T, Paulsen K, Domino G. The matching familiar figures test: a primary, secondary, and tertiary evaluation. *J Clin Psychol* 1981; **37**(4): 812–18.
Mesulam's Tests of Directed Attention	• Mesulam M-M. A cortical network for directed attention and unilateral neglect. *Ann of Neurol* 1981; **10**:309–25.

Test Name	Reference
n-back task	• Owen AM, McMillan KM, Laird AR, Bullmore E. N-back working memory paradigm: A meta-analysis of normative functional neuroimaging studies. *Hum Brain Mapp* 2005; **25**(1): 46–59. *see also TEC, TEA-Ch Code Transmission*
NEPSY	• Korkman M, Kirk U, Kemp, S. *NEPSY: A Developmental Neuropsychological Assessment. Manual.* San Antonio, TX, Psychological Corporation, 1998. Korkman M, Kirk U, Kemp, S. *Nepsy-II. Clinical and Interpretive Manual. 2nd edn. (NEPSY-II).* San Antonio, TX: Harcourt Assessment, 2007.
Object Alternation Task	• Freedman M, Black S, Ebert P, Binns M. Orbitofrontal function, object alternation and perseveration. *Cereb Cortex* 1998; **8**(1): 18–27.
Oral Trail Making Test (OTMT)	• Ricker JH, Axelrod, BN. Analysis of an oral paradigm for the trail making test. *Assessment.* 1994; **1**(1): 51–5. • Ricker JH, Axelrod BN, Houtler BD. Clinical validation of the oral trail making test. *Neuropsychiatry Neuropsychol Behav Neurol* 1996; **9**:50–3. • Mrazik M, Millis S, Drane DL. The oral trail making test: effects of age and concurrent validity. *Arch Clin Neuropsychol* 2010; **25**(3): 236–43.
Penn Conditional Exclusion Test	• Kurtz MM, Ragland JD, Moberg PJ, Gur RC. The penn conditional exclusion test: a new measure of executive-function with alternate forms of repeat administration. *Arch Clin Neuropsychol* 2004; **19**(2): 191–201.
Porteus Maze Test	• Porteus SD. *The Maze Test and Clinical Psychology.* Palo Alto, CA: Pacific Books, 1959. • Porteus S D. *Porteus Maze Test. Fifty Years' Application.* New York: Psychological Corporation, 1965.
Posner task	• Posner MI, Walker JA, Friedrich FJ, Rafal RD. Effects of parietal injury on covert orienting of attention. *J Neurosci* 1984; **4**(7): 1863–74.
Purdue Pegboard	• Purdue Research Foundation. *Purdue Pegboard Test.* Lafayette, IN, Lafayette Instruments. Tiffin J. *Purdue Pegboard. Examiner's Manual.* Rosemont, IL: London House, 1968. • Gardner RA, Broman M. The purdue pegboard: Normative data on 1334 school children. *J Clin Child Psychol* 1979; **8**(3): 156–62.
Rapid Automatized Naming and Rapid Alternating Stimulus (RAN/RAS)	• Denckla MB, Rudel RG. Rapid automatized naming (R.A.N): Dyslexia differentiated from other learning disabilities. *Neuropsychologia* 1976; **14**:471–9.

Test Name	Reference
	• Wolf M, Denckla MB. *RAN/RAS: Rapid Automatized Naming and Rapid Alternating Stimulus Tests*. Austin, TX: Pro-Ed, 2005. • Norton ES, Wolf M. Rapid automatized naming (RAN) and reading fluency: implications for understanding and treatment of reading disabilities. *Annu Rev Psychol* (First published online as a *Review in Advance* on August 11, 2011);63 (Volume publication date January 2012): 427–52. *see also CTOPP Rapid Naming, NEPSY-II Speeded Naming*
Raven's Progressive Matrices	• Raven JC. *Guide to the Standard Progressive Matrices*. London, HK Lewis, 1960. • Raven JC, Court JH, Raven J. *Manual for Raven's Progressive Matrices*. London: HK Lewis, 1976.
Repetitive patterns or Recurrent series writing	• Luria AR. *Higher Cortical Functions in Man. Rev and Expanded. 2nd edn.* New York: Consultants Bureau, 1980; 223–4, 424. • Lezak MD, Howieson DB, Loring DW, Hannay HJ, Fischer J. *Neuropsychological Assessment. 4th ed.* New York: Oxford University Press, 2004; 632.
Rey Complex Figure Test (RCFT); Rey-Osterrieth Complex Figure (ROCF)	• Osterrieth PA. Le test de copie d'une figure complexe. *Archives de Psychologie* 1944; **30**:206–356. • Meyers JE, Meyers, KR. *Rey Complex Figure Test and Recognition Trial.* Odessa, FL: Psychological Assessment Resources, 1995. • Bernstein JH, Waber D. *DSS-ROCF: The Developmental Scoring System for the Rey-Osterrieth Complex Figure.* Lutz, FL: Psychological Assessment Resources, Inc., 1996. • Knight JA, Kaplan E. *The Handbook of Rey–Osterrieth Complex Figure Usage: Clinical and Research Applications.* New York, NY: John Wiley & Sons, Inc., 2003.
Ruff Figural Fluency Test (RFFT)	• Ruff RM, Allen CC, Farrow CE, Nieman H, Wylie T. Figural fluency: Differential impairment in patients with left versus right frontal lesions. *Arch Clin Neuropsychol.* 1994; **9**(1): 41–55. *see also Design Fluency*
Schedule for Affective Disorders and Schizophrenia for School-Age Children (Kiddie-SADS, K-SADS)	• Kaufman J, Birmaher B, Brent D, *et al.* Schedule for affective disorders and schizophrenia for school-age children – present and lifetime version (K-SADS-PL): initial reliability and validity data. *J Am Acad Child Adolesc Psychiatry* 1997; **36**:980–8.
Seashore Rhythm Task	• Reitan RM, Wolfson D. *The Halstead-Reitan Neuropsychological Test Battery: Theory and Clinical Interpretation.* Tucson, AZ: Neuropsychology Press, 1993. • Reitan RM, Wolfson D. (1989). The seashore rhythm test and brain functions. *Clin Neuropsychol.* 1989; **3**:70–8.

Test Name	Reference
Sorting tasks	*See California Sorting Task, Delis-Kaplan Executive Function System Sorting, Wisconsin Card Sorting Task*
Span tasks (digits, words, spatial)	*See Wechsler Intelligence Scales*
Sternberg Memory Test	• Sternberg S. Memory scanning: Mental process revealed by reaction-time experiments. *Am Sci* 1969; **57**(4):421–57.
Stop-signal task	• Schachar R, Logan G. Impulsivity and inhibitory control in normal development and childhood psychopathology. *Dev Psychol* 1990; **26**:710–20.
Stroop Color-Word Test	• Stroop JR. Studies of interference in serial verbal reactions. *J Exp Psychol.* 1935;18(6): 643–62. • Golden CJ. *Stroop Color and Word Test: A Manual for Clinical and Experimental Uses.* Wood Dale, IL: Stoelting, 1978. • Golden CJ, Freshwater SM, Golden Z. *Stroop Color and Word Test, Children's Version.* Wood Dale, IL: Stoelting, 2003. *see also D-KEFS Color-Word Interference*
Tasks of Executive Control (TEC)	• Isquith PK, Roth RM, Gioia GA. *Tasks of Executive Control (TEC).* Odessa, FL: PAR Inc., 2010. *see also go/no-go task, n-back task*
Teacher's Report Form (TRF)	*see Achenbach System of Empirically Based Assessment*
Test of Everyday Attention for Children (TEA-Ch)	• Manly T, Robertson IH, Anderson V, Nimmo-Smith I. *The Test of Everyday Attention for Children (TEA-Ch).* Bury St. Edmunds, UK: Thames Valley Test Company, 1999. • Manly T, Anderson V, Nimmo-Smith I, Turner A, Watson P, Robertson IH. The differential assessment of children's attention: the test of everyday attention for children (TEA-Ch), normative sample and ADHD performance. *J Child Psychol Psychiatry* 2001; **42**(8): 1065–81.
Test of Language Competence (ToLC)	• Wiig E, Secord W. *Test of Language Competence.* San Antonio, TX: Psychological Corporation, 1989.
Test of Variables of Attention (TOVA)	• Greenberg LM, Waldman ID. Developmental normative data on the test of variables of attention (T.O.V.A.). *J Child Psychol Psychiatry* 1993; **34**(6): 1019–30.
Thematic Apperception Test (TAT)	• Murray HA. *Thematic Apperception. Test Manual.* Cambridge, MA: Harvard University Press, 1943.
Tinkertoy task	• Lezak DM. The problem of assessing executive functions. *Int J Psychol* 1982; **17**:281–97.
Tower of Hanoi	• Anderson JR, Douglass S. Tower of Hanoi: evidence for the cost of goal retrieval. *J Exp Psychol Learn Mem Cogn* 2001; **27**(6): 1331–46.

Test Name	Reference
	• Bull R, Espy KA, Senn TE. A comparison of performance on the towers of London and Hanoi in young children. *J Child Psychol Psychiatry* 2004; **45**(4): 743–54.
Tower of London	• Shallice T. Specific impairments of planning. *Phil Trans Roy Soc Lond. Series B Biol Sci.* 1982; **298**(1089): 199–209. • Baker K, Segalowitz SJ, Ferlisi MC. The effect of differing scoring methods for the tower of London task on developmental patterns of performance. *Clin Neuropsychol* 2001; **15**(3): 309–13. • Bull R, Espy KA, Senn TE. A comparison of performance on the towers of London and Hanoi in young children. *J Child Psychol Psychiatry* 2004; **45**(4): 743–54. • Culbertson WC, Zillmer EA. *Tower of London: Drexel University (TOLDX). 2nd edn.* North Tonawanda, NY: Multi-Health Systems, 2005.
Tower tasks	*See D-KEFS Tower, NEPSY Tower, Tower of Hanoi, Tower of London.*
Trail Making Test (TMT)	• *Army Individual Test Battery. Manual of Directions and Scoring.* Washington, DC: War Department, Adjutant General's Office, 1944. • Reitan RM, Davidson LA, eds. *Clinical Neuropsychology: Current Status And Applications.* New York: JohnWiley & Sons, 1974; 53–89. • Rourke BP, Finlayson MAJ. Neuropsychological significance of variations in patterns of academic performance: verbal and visual–spatial abilities. *J Abnorm Child Psychol* 1978; **6**(1). *see also CMS Sequences, Children's Color Trails, Color Trails, D-KEFS Trail Making Test, OTMT*
Transdisciplinary Play-Based Assessment, Second Edition (TPBA2)	• Linder TW. *Transdisciplinary Play-Based Assessment (TPBA). 2nd edn.* Baltimore, MD: Paul H. Brookes Publishing Co., 2008.
Verbal Fluency tasks (first letter, phonemic, semantic)	*see COWAT, D-KEFS Verbal Fluency, NEPSY-II Word Generation*
Visual Search and Attention Test (VSAT)	• Trenerry MR, Crosson B, DeBoe J, Leber WR. *Visual Search and Attention Test.* Odessa, FL: Psychological Assessment Resources, 1990.
Wechsler Adult Intelligence Scale (WAIS)	• Wechsler D. *The Measurement of Adult Intelligence.* Baltimore, MD: Williams & Wilkins, 1939. • Wechsler, D. *Wechsler Bellevue Intelligence Scale.* New York, NY: The Psychological Corporation, 1939. • Wechsler D. *Wechsler Adult Intelligence Scale. Rev. (WAIS-R).* San Antonio, TX: Psychological Corporation, 1981.

Test Name	Reference
	• Wechsler D. *Wechsler Adult Intelligence Scale. 3rd edn. (WAIS-III)*. San Antonio, TX: Psychological Corporation, 1997. • Wechsler D. *Wechsler Adult Intelligence Scale. 4th edn. (WAIS-IV)*. San Antonio, TX: Harcourt Assessment, Inc., 2008. • Wechsler D. *Wechsler Adult Intelligence Scale. Technical and Interpretive Manual. 4th edn. (WAIS-IV)*. San Antonio, TX: Harcourt Assessment, Inc., 2008.
Wechsler Individual Achievement Test (WIAT)	• Wechsler DL. *Wechsler Individual Achievement Test (WIAT)*. San Antonio, TX: Psychological Corp, 1992. • Wechsler DL. *Wechsler Individual Achievement Test. 2nd edn. (WIAT-II)*. San Antonio, TX: Psychological Corp, 2002. • Wechsler D. *Wechsler Individual Achievement Test. 3rd Ed. (WIAT-III)*. San Antonio, TX: The Psychological Corporation, 2009.
Wechsler Intelligence Scale for Children (WISC)	• Wechsler D. *Wechsler Intelligence Scale for Children (WISC)*. New York: The Psychological Corporation, 1949. • Wechsler D. *Wechsler Intelligence Scale For Children. Rev. (WISC-R)*. San Antonio, TX: The Psychological Corporation, 1974. • Wechsler D. *Wechsler Intelligence Scale for Children. 3rd Ed. (WISC-III)*. San Antonio, TX: The Psychological Corporation, 1991. • Wechsler D. *Wechsler Intelligence Scale for Children. 4th edn. (WISC-IV)*. San Antonio, TX: The Psychological Corporation, 2003. • Wechsler D. *Wechsler Intelligence Scale for Children. Technical and Interpretive Manual. 4th edn. (WISC-IV)*. San Antonio, TX, The Psychological Corporation, 2003. • Wechsler D. *Wechsler Intelligence Scale for Children, 4th Ed. Integrated (WISC-IV-Int): Technical And Interpretative Manual*. San Antonio, TX: Harcourt Assessment, Inc., 2004.
Wechsler Preschool and Primary Scale of Intelligence (WPPSI)	• Wechsler D. *Wechsler Preschool and Primary Scale of Intelligence (WPPSI)*. San Antonio, TX: The Psychological Corporation, 1967. • Wechsler D. *Wechsler Preschool and Primary Scale of Intelligence, Rev. (WPPSI-R)*. San Antonio, TX: • The Psychological Corporation, 1989. • Wechsler D. *Wechsler Preschool and Primary Scale of Intelligence, 3rd edn. (WPPSI-III)*. San Antonio, TX: The Psychological Corporation, 2002.
Wide Range Assessment of Memory and Learning (WRAML)	• Sheslow D, Adams W. *Wide Range Assessment of Memory and Learning*. Wilmington, DE: Jastak Associates, 1990.

Test Name	Reference
Wide Range Assessment of Visual Motor Abilities (WRAVMA)	• Adams W, Sheslow D. *Wide Range Assessment of Visual Motor Abilities (WRAVMA)*. Wilmington, DE: Wide Range, Inc., 1995.
Wisconsin Card Sorting Task (WCST)	• Berg EA. A simple objective technique for measuring flexibility in thinking. *J Gen Psychol* 1948; **39**:15–22. • Grant DA, Berg EA. *Wisconsin Card Sorting Test*. Odessa, FL: Psychological Assessment Resources, 1993. • Heaton RK, Chelune GJ, Talley JL, Kay GG, Curtiss G. *Wisconsin Card Sorting Test. Manual. Rev. and Expanded*. Odessa, FL: Psychological Assessment Resources, 1993. • Heaton RK, PAR Staff. *Wisconsin Card Sorting Test. Computer Version 4, Research edn. (WCST: CV4)*. Odessa, FL: Psychological Assessment Resources, 2003.
Woodcock-Johnson Tests of Achievement (WJ-Ach)	• Woodcock RW, Johnson MB. *Woodcock–Johnson Psycho-Educational Battery*. Chicago, IL: Riverside Publishing, 1977. • Woodcock RW, Johnson MB. *Woodcock–Johnson Tests of Achievement. Rev.* Allen, TX: DLM; 1989. • Mather N, Woodcock RW. *Woodcock–Johnson Tests of Achievement, 3rd edn., Examiner's Manual*. Itasca, IL: Riverside Publishing, 2001.
Woodcock-Johnson Tests of Cognitive Ability (WJ-Cog)	• Woodcock RW, Johnson MB. *Woodcock–Johnson Psycho-Educational Battery*. Chicago, IL: Riverside Publishing, 1977. • Woodcock RW, Johnson MB. *Woodcock-Johnson Psycho-Educational Battery, Rev. (WJ-R)*. Chicago, IL: Riverside Publishing, 1989. • Woodcock RW, McGrew KS, Mather N. *Woodcock-Johnson Tests of Cognitive Ability, 3rd edn.* Itasca, IL: Riverside Publishing, 2001.
Working Memory Test Battery for Children (WMTB)	• Pickering SJ, Gathercole SE. *Working Memory Test Battery for Children*. London: Psychological Corporation, 2001.

Index

Note: page numbers in *italics* refer to figures and tables